Teaching Atlas of Interventional Radiology

Non-Vascular Interventional Procedures

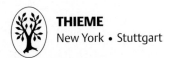

THIEME
New York • Stuttgart

Teaching Atlas of Interventional Radiology

Non-Vascular Interventional Procedures

Saadoon Kadir, M.D.
Interventional Radiologist
North County Radiology
Interventional Radiologist
Cardinal Glennon Children's Hospital
St. Louis, Missouri
Clinical Professor of Radiology
Saint Louis University
  School of Medicine
St. Louis, Missouri

Thieme Medical Publishers, Inc.
333 Seventh Ave.
New York, NY 10001

Vice President, Production and Electronic Publishing: Anne T. Vinnicombe
Production Editor: Print Matters, Inc.
Sales Director: Ross Lumpkin
Associate Marketing Director: Verena Diem
Chief Financial Officer: Peter van Woerden
President: Brian D. Scanlan
Compositor: Compset
Printer: Edwards Brothers

Library of Congress Cataloging-in-Publication Data

Teaching atlas of interventional radiology : non-vascular interventional procedures /
   [edited by] Saadoon Kadir.
       p. ; cm.
   Includes bibliographical references and index.
   ISBN 1-58890-056-8 (US)—ISBN 3-13-107972-X (GTV)
   1. Interventional radiology—Atlases. I. Kadir, Saadoon.
   [DNLM: 1. Radiology, Interventional—Atlases. WN 17 T2527 2005]
   RD33.55.T43 2005
   617′05—dc22

                                   2005050645

Printed in the United States
5 4 3 2 1
TMP ISBN 1-58890-056-8

GTV ISBN 3 13 10792 X

CONTENTS

PREFACE

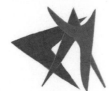

"For every disease there is a cure. . . ."
—*Hadith*

This second volume of the *Teaching Atlas of Interventional Radiology* discusses non-vascular diseases. The format of the previous volume, *Diagnostic and Therapeutic Angiography*, has been retained to provide practical information and solutions to problems arising in everyday practice. This format is being adapted increasingly because of its usefulness for teaching purposes. The cases selected for this volume represent situations that can be expected in a busy interventional practice. There is emphasis on the clinical aspects of the diseases and treatment options as well as technical aspects of the therapeutic procedures. It is increasingly necessary, that the interventional radiologists also assume the role of a *clinician*.

This volume of the *Teaching Atlas of Interventional Radiology* is intended for physicians in training and those in clinical practice. As with the previous book, it is not intended to provide comprehensive coverage of the field but covers a range of diseases seen in a busy clinical practice.

I wish to express my sincere appreciation to the section editors and the authors for sharing their experiences, for their patience and help in bringing this project to completion. The completion of this book would have been difficult without the support from my family, in particular, from my best friend and wife, Salma.

Saadoon Kadir, M.D.

CONTRIBUTORS

Editor

Saadoon Kadir, M.D.
Interventional Radiologist
North County Radiology
Interventional Radiologist
Cardinal Glennon Children's Hospital
St. Louis, Missouri
Clinical Professor of Radiology
Saint Louis University
    School of Medicine
St. Louis, Missouri

Section Editors

Saadoon Kadir, M.D.
Interventional Radiologist
North County Radiology
Interventional Radiologist
Cardinal Glennon Children's Hospital
St. Louis, Missouri
Clinical Professor of Radiology
Saint Louis University
    School of Medicine
St. Louis, Missouri

Carl F. Beckmann, M.D.
Department of Diagnostic Radiology
Lahey Clinic Medical Center
Burlington, Massachusetts

John D. Bennett, M.D., C.M., F.R.C.P.C.
Department of Diagnostic Radiology
St. Joseph's Hospital
University of Western Ontario
London, Ontario, Canada

Moulay A. Meziane, M.D.
Department of Radiology
The Cleveland Clinic Foundation
Cleveland, Ohio

Contributors

Okan Akhan, M.D.
Professor of Radiology
Department of Radiology
Hacettepe University
    School of Medicine
Ankara, Turkey

Sulaiman Al-Basam, M.D., F.R.C.P.C.
Department of Diagnostic Radiology
St. Joseph's Hospital
London, Ontario, Canada

Kamran Ali, M.D.
Clinical Assistant Professor
Department of Diagnostic Radiology
University of Kansas
    School of Medicine
Wichita, Kansas

Murray Asch, M.D., F.R.C.P.C.
Department of Medical Imaging
Division of Vascular and Interventional
    Radiology
University of Toronto
Toronto, Ontario, Canada

Hilary M. Babcock, M.D.
Instructor
Department of Medicine
Division of Infectious Diseases
Washington University
    School of Medicine
St. Louis, Missouri

Carl F. Beckmann, M.D.
Department of Diagnostic Radiology
Lahey Clinic Medical Center
Burlington, Massachusetts

John D. Bennett, M.D.C.M., F.R.C.P.C.
Department of Diagnostic Radiology
St. Joseph's Hospital
University of Western Ontario
London, Ontario, Canada

Joachim Berkefeld, M.D.
Institute for Neuroradiology
Johann Wolfgang Goethe-Universität
Frankfurt am Main, Germany

Bruce R. Carr, M.D.
Professor
Department of Obstetrics and Gynecology
University of Texas Southwestern
   Medical Center
Dallas, Texas

I. W. Choo, M.D.
Department of Radiology
College of Medicine, Sung Kyun Kwan
   University
Samsung Medical Center
Seoul, Korea

Anne Cotten, M.D.
Department of Skeletal Radiology
Hopital Roger Salengro-C.H.R.U. de Lille
Lille-Cedex, France

Kevin W. Dickey, M.D., F.S.C.V.I.R.
Department of Radiology
Dartmouth University
   School of Medicine
Dartmouth Hitchcock
   Medical Center
Lebanon, New Hampshire

Ana Echenique, M.D.
Department of Radiology
University of Miami School of Medicine
South Florida Medical Imaging
Miami, Florida

Masafumi Fukagawa, M.D., Ph.D., F.J.S.I.M.
Associate Professor and Director
Division of Nephrology and Dialysis Center
Kobe University School of Medicine
Kobe, Japan

Ziad W. Ghamra, M.D.
Department of Pulmonary and
   Critical Care Medicine
The Cleveland Clinic Foundation
Cleveland, Ohio

Robert N. Gibson, M.D., F.R.A.N.Z.C.R., D.D.U.
Professor, Department of Radiology
University of Melbourne School of Medicine
Royal Melbourne Hospital and Western
   Hospital Clinical School
Parkville, Victoria, Australia

Amanjit Gill, M.D.
Assistant Professor
Radiology Department
University of Texas Medical Branch
Galveston, Texas

Ruffin J. Graham, M.D.
Department of Radiology
Section of Thoracic Imaging
The Cleveland Clinic Foundation
Cleveland, Ohio

Rolf Günther, M.D.
Professor
Department of Diagnostic Radiology
Technical University
Aachen, Germany

Hani M. Jneid, M.D.
Division of Cardiology
University of Louisville School of Medicine
Louisville, Kentucky

Corey J. Jost, M.D.
Department of Vascular
   and General Surgery
The Wichita Clinic Murdock
Wichita, Kansas

John Kachura, M.D., F.R.C.P.C.
Assistant Professor
Department of Medical Imaging
Faculty of Medicine
University of Toronto
Toronto General Hospital
Toronto, Ontario, Canada

Vishvanath C. Karande, M.D.
Center for Human Reproduction
Hoffman Estates, Illinois

Nigar Kirmani, M.D.
Associate Professor
Department of Medicine
Division of Infectious Diseases
Washington University School
   of Medicine
St. Louis, Missouri

Roman I. Kozak, M.D., F.R.C.P.C.
Assistant Professor
Department of Diagnostic Radiology
St. Joseph's Hospital
University of Western Ontario
London, Ontario, Canada

Stewart Kribs, M.D., F.R.C.P.C.
Department of Diagnostic Radiology
London Health Sciences Center
University of Western Ontario
London, Ontario, Canada

Robert E. Lambiase, M.D.
Associate Professor
Department of Diagnostic Imaging
Brown University Medical School
Rhode Island Hospital
Providence, Rhode Island

Fah Sean Leong, M.D.
Department of Diagnostic Radiology
Lahey Clinic Medical Center
Burlington, Massachusetts

Tito Livraghi, M.D.
Department of Radiology
Azienda Ospedaliera "Ospedale Civile"
  di Vimercate
Milan, Italy

Marc Lüchtenberg, M.D.
Clinic of Ophthalmology
Johann Wolfgang Goethe-Universität
Frankfurt am Main, Germany

Lindsay Machan, M.D.
Associate Professor
Department of Radiology
University of British
  Columbia Hospital
Vancouver, British Columbia, Canada

Martin G. Mack, M.D.
Department of Radiology
University Hospital
Johann Wolfgang Goethe-Universität
Frankfurt am Main, Germany

Mohammed Maroof, M.D.
Associate Professor
Department of Anesthesiology
University of North Carolina
Memorial Hospital
Chapel Hill, North Carolina

John P. McGahan, M.D.
Professor
Department of Radiology
University of California
Davis Medical Center
Sacramento, California

Atul C. Mehta, M.D., F.C.C.P.
Professor
Head, Section of Bronchology
Department of Pulmonary and
  Critical Care Medicine
The Cleveland Clinic Foundation
Cleveland, Ohio

Moulay A. Meziane, M.D.
Department of Radiology
The Cleveland Clinic Foundation
Cleveland, Ohio

Christopher P. Molgaard, M.D.
Department of Diagnostic Radiology
Lahey Clinic Medical Center
Burlington, Massachusetts

Douglas J. Moote, M.D., F.R.C.P.C.
Clinical Assistant Professor
Diagnostic Radiology
Yale University School of Medicine
Jefferson X-Ray Group
Hartford, Connecticut

William B. Morrison, M.D.
Associate Professor
Department of Radiology
Director of Musculoskeletal Imaging
Thomas Jefferson University Hospital
Philadelphia, Pennsylvania

Sudish C. Murthy, M.D., Ph.D.
Department of Thoracic and
  Cardiothoracic Surgery
The Cleveland Clinic Foundation
Cleveland, Ohio

Charles O'Malley, M.D.
Department of Diagnostic Radiology
The Cleveland Clinic Foundation
Cleveland, Ohio

Edgar Turner Overton, M.D.
Instructor
Department of Medicine
Division of Infectious Diseases
Washington University School of Medicine
St. Louis, Missouri

David J.M. Peck, M.D., F.R.C.P.C.
Assistant Prosessor
Department of Diagnostic Radiology
London Health Sciences Centre
University of Western Ontario
London, Ontario, Canada

Noel Peng, M.D.
National Fertility Center of Texas
Dallas, Texas

Richard N. Rankin, M.B., Ch.B., F.R.C.P.C.
Professor
Department of Diagnostic Radiology
London Health Sciences Centre
University of Western Ontario
London, Ontario, Canada

Walter M. Romano, M.D., F.R.C.P.C.
Associate Professor
Department of Diagnostic Radiology
St. Joseph's Hospital
University of Western Ontario
London, Ontario, Canada

Bipin D. Sarodia, M.D.
Cardinal Health Alliance
Muncie, Indiana

Matthias H. Schmidt, M.Sc., M.D., F.R.C.P.C.
Department of Diagnostic Imaging
IWK Health Centre
Halifax, Nova Scotia, Canada

Mark E. Schweitzer, M.D.
Professor
Departments of Radiology and
  Orthopedic Surgery
New York University School of Medicine
Hospital for Joint Diseases/Orthopedic
  Institute
New York, New York

Josef Tacke, M.D.
Department of Diagnostic Radiology
Technical University
Aachen, Germany

Suzuka Taki, M.D.
Department of Radiology
Kanazawa Medical University
Ishikawa Japan

Tapani Tikkakoski, M.D., Ph.D.
Associate Professor
Department of Radiology
Oulu University
Keski-Pohjanmaa Central Hospital
Kokkola, Finland

Khaled K. Toumeh, M.D.
Clinical Assistant Professor
Department of Diagnostic Radiology
University of Kansas School
  of Medicine
Wichita, Kansas

Katsuo Usuda, M.D., F.C.C.P.
Department of Pulmonary and
  Critical Care Medicine
The Cleveland Clinic Foundation
Cleveland, Ohio

Thomas J. Vogl, M.D.
Department of Radiology
University Hospital
Johann Wolfgang Goethe-Universität
Frankfurt am Main, Germany

Christoph Wald, M.D., Ph.D.
Assistant Professor of Radiology
Tufts University School of Medicine
Department of Diagnostic Radiology
Lahey Clinic Medical Center
Burlington, Massachusetts

Dominik Weishaupt, M.D.
Institute of Diagnostic Radiology
University Hospital
Zurich, Switzerland

Gerhard R. Wittich, M.D.
Gulf Imaging Associates
Bayshore Medical Center
Pasadena, Texas

Shozo Yano, M.D., Ph.D.
Division of Nephrology and
  Dialysis Center
Kobe University
  School of Medicine
Kobe, Japan

SECTION I
Neck and Thorax

CHAPTER 1 Nasolacrimal Duct Strictures

Joachim Berkefeld and Marc Lüchtenberg

Clinical Presentation

A 29-year-old woman presented with epiphora of her left eye necessitating dabbing of the tears more than 10 times a day. Epiphora, painful swelling in the left lacrimal sac region, and purulent discharge from the canaliculi had started 7 months earlier after an upper respiratory tract infection. Acute dacryocystitis was diagnosed and she was treated with antibiotic and decongestant eye drops as well as irrigation. The symptoms of acute inflammation resolved but epiphora persisted, not responding to the conservative treatment.

Radiological Studies

The lower lacrimal punctum and canaliculus were intubated with the plastic sheath of a 24 gauge catheter needle. Distension dacryocystography with digital subtraction imaging using constant contrast injection revealed complete obstruction of the distal nasolacrimal duct and a visible stump of the duct below the widened lacrimal sac. The contours of the sac and the ductal lumen were smooth, without filling defects or deformities. There were no canalicular or lacrimal sac stenoses. The dacryocystograms showed no contrast passage into the inferior nasal meatus but there was reflux through the canaliculi (**Fig. 1-1**).

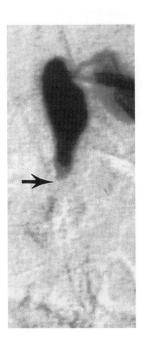

Figure 1-1 Distension dacryocystogram shows complete obstruction of the distal left nasolacrimal duct (arrow) and dilation of the lacrimal sac.

3

Diagnosis

Obstruction of nasolacrimal duct above the level of Hasner's valve

Treatment Options

The acute dacryocystitis was treated successfully by antibiotics, decongestants, and irrigation. However, this conservative therapy was not successful for the epiphora. Persistent symptoms together with the dacryocystographic finding of complete nasolacrimal duct obstruction established the indication for recanalization of the ductal system. Treatment options included an open or endoscopic surgical procedure or balloon dilatation. Open or endoscopic surgical dacryocystorhinostomy has high technical success and post-procedure patency rates but requires general anesthesia. The surgical procedure is associated with a risk of eyelid deformity secondary to scarring. Our experience with balloon dacryocystoplasty suggested that recanalization of focal occlusions of the distal nasolacrimal duct were technically feasible with a reasonable long-term outcome. Therefore, the less invasive balloon dilatation was chosen as the first treatment option.

Treatment

Surface anesthesia (Proxymetacain eye drops) was applied to the left eyelid and also injected through the intubated canaliculus. The nasal mucosa was anesthetized with lidocaine spray. The upper punctum was dilated with a conical dilator and the plastic sheath of a 22 gauge catheter needle (Surflo, Terumo) was inserted into the opening. A 0.014 in. steerable guide wire with hydrophilic coating and a flexible, shapeable tip (Transend X, Target-Boston-Scientific, Freemont, CA) was inserted (alternatively, a stiffer 0.014 in. extra-support cardiac wire Choice, Boston-Scientific, Watertown, MA) could be used). The wire was angled upward together with the cannula and pushed forward into the stump of the nasolacrimal duct. The cannula was advanced over the wire as far as possible. Under

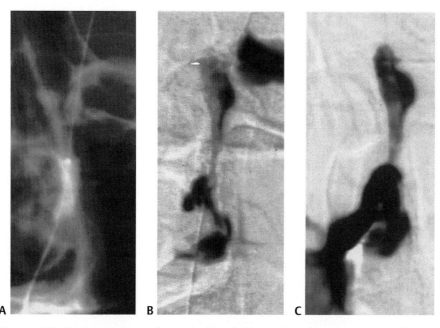

Figure 1-2 (**A**) Image shows the angioplasty balloon inflated in the obstructed duct segment. (**B**) Postdilatation dacryocystogram shows a recanalized nasolacrimal duct. (**C**) After removal of the guide wire, the duct lumen is widely patent and there is free flow of contrast material into the inferior nasal meatus.

the guidance of the cannula, the hydrophilic wire easily passed the initial portion of the occluded duct. Despite a moderate amount of resistance at Hasner's valve, the guide wire could be advanced into the inferior nasal meatus. The curved tip was then manipulated out through the nasal cavity using lateral fluoroscopy. A 3 mm × 2 cm small-vessel angioplasty balloon catheter (Crosssail, Guidant, Temescula, CA) was inserted via the nasal cavity and inflated up to 8 atm. Repeated dacryocystograms after balloon dilatation showed recanalization of the occluded duct segment and normal contrast flow into the inferior nasal meatus (**Fig 1-2**). Clinically, there was complete resolution of the epiphora immediately after the dacryocystoplasty. No recurrence has been observed during the follow-up period of 6 months.

Discussion

Epiphora, persistent tearing of the eye, is due to an imbalance between the production and drainage of the lacrimal fluid. It is a frequent symptom in patients seen in an ophthalmology practice. Lacrimal duct obstruction is a major cause of epiphora. Obstruction develops frequently as sequelae to acute or chronic dacryocystitis. Other causes include posttraumatic (after facial fractures), maxillary sinus surgery, and congenital stenoses.

Acute inflammatory changes (swelling, skin discoloration, and purulent discharge) frequently resolve with conservative therapy (antibiotics, decongestants, and irrigation). Emergency surgical drainage of an empyema is necessary only occasionally. Chronic dacryocystitis is associated with thickening of mucosal folds in the lacrimal sac or the nasolacrimal duct. Obstructions develop mainly in areas of physiological narrowing, namely, at the junction of the lacrimal sac and nasolacrimal duct (valve of Krause) or at the outlet of the nasolacrimal duct (valve of Hasner). Retention of viscous mucus or calculus formation (dacryocystolithiasis) may further impede drainage of lacrimal fluid.

A dacryocystogram is necessary to assess the degree and the location of ductal obstruction in patients who have failed conservative treatment of epiphora. Our experience and data from the literature indicate that fluoroscopically guided balloon dacryocystoplasty is a viable alternative to operative treatment, especially in cases fulfilling the criteria listed in **Table 1-1**. A technical success rate of 90% and long-term improvement in 70 to 80% can be expected, if these criteria are used for patient selection. Current data suggest that balloon dacryocystoplasty is an alternative to open or endonasal surgery in 30 to 50% of the patients presenting with epiphora.

As an alternative to the technique described (i.e., the use of steerable micro guide wires for recanalization), some authors have described the use of 0.021 in. hydrophilic-coated guide wires or special ball-tip wires. Both of these seem to be more traumatic to the ductal structures.

Table 1-1   Indications and Contraindications for Dacryocystoplasty

Indications

Partial obstruction of the nasolacrimal duct or the lower portion of the
    lacrimal sac
Complete obstruction of the distal nasolacrimal duct with a visible stump
Adult age of the patient
Absence of active inflammation
Absence of findings indicating posttraumatic obstruction
Absence of filling defects on dacryocystography that would indicate the presence
    of dacryocystolithiasis
Absence of high-grade or diffuse obstruction in the canaliculi or lacrimal sac

Contraindications

Active dacryocystitis
Posttraumatic stenoses (occurring after facial bone fractures)

Complete obstruction of the entire nasolacrimal duct can also be recanalized if the lesion allows passage of a guide wire. However, long-term follow-up of such cases showed recurrence of clinical symptoms in excess of 50%. The use of metallic or plastic nasolacrimal duct stents can improve technical success rates, but the long-term outcome is limited because of stent obstruction due to incrustation or overgrowth of granulation tissue.

Calculi have been removed in an occasional case by forceful irrigation after dilatation of the lumen. Dilatation of canalicular stenoses is also technically feasible, but the long-term results are unknown. Therefore, widespread use of these techniques is presently not recommended.

Endoscopically guided mechanical or laser-assisted dacryocystoplasty may be complementary to or an alternative to the radiological technique and has the advantage of directly visualizing dacryoliths or lesions of the ductal wall. Technical and clinical success rates appear to be similar to those of the radiological technique. The main advantage of the interventional radiological approach is that the level of invasiveness is relatively low. The procedure is well tolerated by most of the patients and can be performed on an outpatient basis using surface anesthesia.

PEARLS AND PITFALLS_____

- Epiphora due to obstruction of the lacrimal draining system is frequently caused by sequelae of acute or chronic dacryocystitis.
- Balloon dacryocystoplasty is a minimally invasive alternative to operative dacryocystorhinostomy in patients who have failed conservative management.
- High technical and clinical success rates can be expected in circumscribed stenoses or distal occlusions of the nasolacrimal duct.
- Interventional treatment is contraindicated in the presence of active dacryocystitis or bony narrowings. The application of the interventional radiological approach for occlusions of the entire nasolacrimal duct, canalicular stenoses, and dacryolithiasis is of questionable benefit.

Further Reading

Berkefeld J, Kirchner J, Müller HM, et al. Balloon dacryocystoplasty: indications and contraindications. Radiology 1997;205:791–796

Ilgit ET, Yüksel D, Ünal M, et al. Transluminal balloon dilation of the lacrimal draining system for the treatment of epiphora. AJR Am J Roentgenol 1995;165:1517–1524

Janssen AG, Mansour K, Krabbe GJ, et al. Dacryocystoplasty: treatment of epiphora by means of balloon dilation of the obstructed nasolacrimal duct system. Radiology 1994;193:453–456

Lee JM, Song HY, Han YM, et al. Balloon dacryocystoplasty: results in the treatment of complete and partial obstructions of the nasolacrimal system. Radiology 1994;192:503–508

Meyer-Rüsenberg HW, Emmerich KH, Lüchtenberg M, et al. Endoscopic laser dacryocystoplasty: methodology and outcome after 3 months [in German]. Ophthalmologe 1999;96:332–334

Song HY, Jin YH, Kim JH, et al. Nonsurgical placement of a nasolacrimal polyurethane stent: long-term effectiveness. Radiology 1996;200:759–763

Sprekelsen MB, Barberan MT. Endoscopic dacryocystorhinostomy: surgical technique and results. Laryngoscope 1996;106:187–189

Wilhelm KE, Hofer U, Textor HJ, et al. Dacryoliths: nonsurgical fluoroscopically guided treatment during dacryocystoplasty. Radiology 1999;212:365–370

Wilhelm KE, Hofer U, Textor HJ, et al. Nonsurgical fluoroscopically guided dacryocystoplasty of common canalicular obstructions. Cardiovasc Intervent Radiol 2000;23:1–8

CHAPTER 2 Percutaneous Parathyroid Ablation
Shozo Yano and Masafumi Fukagawa

Clinical Presentation

A 51-year-old man who had been on maintenance hemodialysis for 17 years was referred for the evaluation of hyperparathyroidism. Despite medical treatment that included phosphate binders and oral active vitamin D sterols, serum levels of intact parathyroid hormone (PTH) remained between 600 and 800 pg/mL with evidence for high turnover bone disease (i.e., elevated serum alkaline phosphatase and skeletal changes on bone radiographs). Intravenous vitamin D therapy (calcitriol 1 μg, three times per week at the end of each hemodialysis treatment) not only failed to suppress PTH secretion but led to marked hypercalcemia and hyperphosphatemia (calcium corrected for albumin 11.0 mg/dL, phosphate 6.0 mg/dL).

Radiological Studies

Ultrasonography demonstrated marked enlargement of the left lower parathyroid gland (**Fig. 2-1A**). A round, encapsulated mass that demonstrated increased vascularity was present within the gland (**Fig. 2-1B**), suggesting the presence of a nodule. The left upper and right lower parathyroid glands (not shown) were also mildly enlarged.

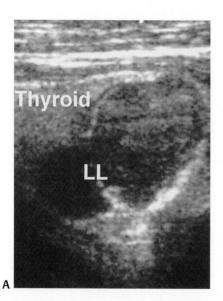
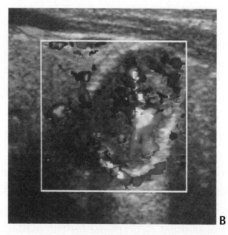

A B

Figure 2-1 (**A**) Sagittal sonogram shows an enlarged left lower parathyroid gland (LL). The volume of the gland was estimated to be 1.5 cm³. An encapsulated nodule with slightly higher echogenicity is demonstrated within the gland. (**B**) Power Doppler in the sagittal plane shows increased vascularity, especially in the encapsulated lesion.

Diagnosis

Parathyroid hyperplasia (nodular) with secondary hyperparathyroidism due to chronic renal failure

Treatment

Using ultrasound guidance, a 21 gauge needle designed for percutaneous injection therapy was inserted into the center of the enlarged left lower parathyroid gland. About 1 mL of 90% ethanol with 1% lidocaine added was slowly injected into the gland. The needle, which is designed for percutaneous injection therapy (Hakko Shoji, Tokyo, Japan), has an occluded tip and three side holes. A follow-up examination 1 month after treatment demonstrated a marked decrease in the size of the gland and its blood supply (**Figs. 2-2A,B**). Serum PTH level fell from 634 to 253 pg/mL and serum calcium decreased to 10.2 mg/dL after the ethanol injection.

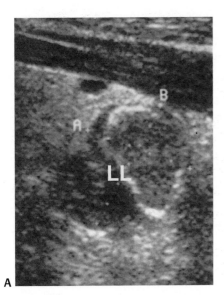
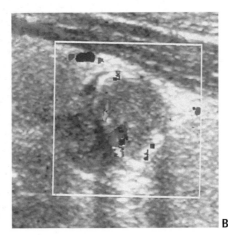

A   B

Figure 2-2 (**A**) Sonogram obtained 1 month after percutaneous ethanol injection therapy (PEIT) shows reduction in the volume of the gland (0.9 cm^3). (**B**) Power Doppler image obtained 1 month after PEIT shows markedly diminished blood flow to the gland.

Discussion

High turnover bone disease is one of the most important complications of chronic hemodialysis. This abnormality is caused by high levels of PTH secreted from enlarged parathyroid glands. Such patients are routinely treated by oral active vitamin D sterols, phosphate binders, and, in severe cases, intravenous vitamin D therapy.

Patients refractory to intravenous vitamin D therapy usually have marked parathyroid hyperplasia. Recent data suggest that these glands are composed of nodular hyperplasia with a lower density of vitamin D and calcium-sensing receptors, thus the resistance to medical therapy. It is therefore important to recognize the presence of nodular hyperplasia for the management of severe secondary hyperparathyroidism.

In the clinical setting, the most convenient parameter for the determination of a hyperplastic parathyroid gland is its size, which is easily assessed by ultrasonography. A gland volume of 0.5 cm^3 or diameter of 1 cm is highly suspicious for nodular hyperplasia. In addition, the presence of a nodule is occasionally suspected by the shape of the gland and by the presence of increased vascularity, even in smaller glands.

Selective percutaneous ethanol injection therapy (PEIT) is a technique for managing patients with severe secondary hyperparathyroidism due to nodular hyperplasia who are refractory to medical therapy. With this therapy, glands with nodular hyperplasia are "selectively" destroyed by ethanol injected under ultrasonographic guidance. The other glands with diffuse hyperplasia can then be controlled by medical therapy. This technique is safe and has found widespread use, especially in Japan. Patients with three or more glands with nodular hyperplasia may not be candidates for PEIT. Such patients may be better managed by parathyroidectomy. If PTH levels do not decrease after successful PEIT, the presence of ectopic parathyroid gland(s) should be searched by Technetium 99m methoxyisobutylisonitrile (MIBI) scintigraphy, computed tomography, or magnetic resonance imaging.

Major complications of PEIT of the parathyroid gland are pain and recurrent nerve palsy. These occur as a result of ethanol leaking from the injected gland and along the PEIT needle tract. To avoid this risk and prevent leakage of ethanol from the gland, the needle tip position must be confirmed to be within the gland before injecting the ethanol. The amount of ethanol used for the initial injection should be <90% of the estimated volume of the parathyroid gland ($\frac{\pi}{6} \times a \times b \times c$, where a, b, and c represent the diameters of the gland, in three dimensions). Additional ethanol injection should be done by using minimal amounts at the site where residual blood supply is demonstrated. With such precautions, a skilled operator can perform PEIT with a low risk of complications.

Another intervention for hyperplastic parathyroid glands in uremic patients is direct vitamin D injection therapy. With this form of therapy, a very high concentration of calcitriol or maxacalcitol is achieved in the parathyroid glands. Reports indicate that this therapy can not only suppress PTH secretion but can also restore the gland's responsiveness to medical therapy, suggesting the possible upregulation of the calcitriol receptor. Furthermore, regression of parathyroid hyperplasia has been demonstrated by this therapy. In addition to vitamin D analogues, injection of other agents, such as adenovirus and calcimimetics, has been tried in animal models.

PEARLS AND PITFALLS

- Size, shape, and blood supply of the parathyroid gland are the most useful parameters for assessment of parathyroid hyperplasia in uremic patients.
- Patients with nodular hyperplasia (involving at least one gland) are refractory to medical therapy. With PEIT, glands with nodular hyperplasia are destroyed by ethanol injection and those with diffuse hyperplasia are managed by medical therapy.
- Complications from leakage of ethanol into surrounding tissues can be avoided by optimizing the volume and site of injection.
- Persistence of high PTH levels despite effective destruction of nodular hyperplasia suggests the presence of ectopic glands beyond the reach of ultrasonography.

Further Reading

Fukagawa M. Cell biology of parathyroid hyperplasia in uremia. Am J Med Sci 1999;317:377–382

Fukagawa M, Kazama JJ, Shigematsu T. Management of the patients with advanced secondary hyperparathyroidism: the Japanese approach. Nephrol Dial Transplant 2002;17:1553–1557

Fukagawa M, Kitaoka M, Inazawa T, et al. Imaging of the parathyroid in chronic renal failure: diagnostic and therapeutic aspects Curr Opin Nephrol Hypertens 1997;6:349–355

Fukagawa M, Kitaoka M, Tominaga Y, et al. Japanese Society for Parathyroid Intervention: guideline for percutaneous ethanol injection therapy of the parathyroid glands in chronic dialysis patients. Nephrol Dial Transplant 2003;18(Suppl 3):iii31–iii33

Fukagawa M, Kitaoka M, Yi H, et al. Serial evaluation of parathyroid size by ultrasonography is another useful marker for the long-term prognosis of calcitriol pulse therapy in chronic dialysis patient. Nephron 1994;68:221–228

Kakuta T, Fukagawa M, Fujisaki T, et al. Prognosis of parathyroid function after successful percutaneous ethanol injection therapy (PEIT) guided by color Doppler flow mapping in chronic dialysis patients. Am J Kidney Dis 1999;33:1091–1099

Kitaoka M. Ultrasonographic diagnosis of parathyroid glands and percutaneous ethanol injection therapy. Nephrol Dial Transplant 2003;18(Suppl 3):ii27–ii30

Kitaoka M, Fukagawa M, Kurokawa K. Direct injection of calcitriol into parathyroid hyperplasia in chronic dialysis patients with severe parathyroid hyperfunction. Nephrol 1995;1:563–568

Kitaoka M, Fukagawa M, Ogata E, et al. Reduction of functioning parathyroid cell mass by ethanol injection in chronic dialysis patients. Kidney Int 1994;46:1110–1117

Shiizaki K, Hatamura I, Negi S, et al. Percutaneous maxacalcitol injection therapy regress hyperplasia of parathyroid and induces apoptosis in uremia. Kidney Int 2003;64:992–1003

CHAPTER 3 Thyroid Biopsy

Suzuka Taki

Clinical Presentation

A 57-year-old woman presented with a right neck nodule. Physical examination revealed right cervical adenopathy. There was no history of thyroid disease, previous malignancy, or neck irradiation.

Radiological Studies

An ultrasound examination of the neck was obtained and showed a 1.5 cm diameter lymph node. An echogenic band was seen in the enlarged node, which suggested benign lymphadenopathy (**Fig. 3-1**). Incidental to this finding, a 6 mm diameter hypoechoic nodule with calcification was detected in the right lobe of the thyroid gland. The margins of this nodule were poorly defined (**Fig. 3-2**). These findings were strongly suggestive of a carcinoma.

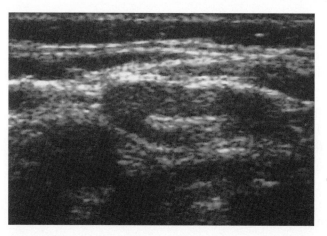

Figure 3-1 Sonogram shows an enlarged cervical node containing a high echo band, which suggests benign lymphadenopathy.

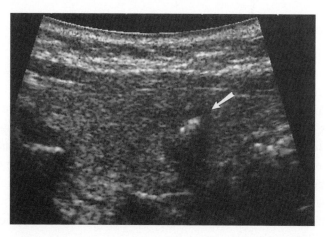

Figure 3-2 Sagittal sonogram of the right thyroid lobe shows a 6 mm nodule with calcification (arrow). The margins are not well defined.

Diagnosis

Papillary microcarcinoma of the thyroid

Treatment

An ultrasound-guided core biopsy was performed using a cutting needle. Both the thyroid nodule and the lymph node were biopsied. Histology confirmed the diagnosis of a papillary microcarcinoma of the thyroid. The lymph node showed benign inflammation. The patient underwent a subtotal thyroidectomy and modified lymph node dissection.

Discussion

Papillary carcinoma is the most common thyroid malignancy. It is a well-differentiated tumor that disseminates via the lymphatics. Women (all ages) are affected two to three times more frequently than men. It occurs more frequently in patients who have received radiation.

The World Health Organization Histological Classification published in 1988 defines papillary microcarcinoma (PMC) as a "papillary carcinoma 1.0 cm or less in diameter." The prognosis of PMC is extremely good and the postsurgical cause-specific 10-year survival rate is between 96 and 99.8%. The 18- to 20-year tumor recurrence rate is only 6 to 7%.

Most PMCs are discovered incidentally during routine or postoperative follow-up cervical sonography. Although the presence of calcification, irregular margins and absence of a halo are useful signs for diagnosing papillary carcinoma, some benign lesions (e.g., degenerated adenomas) can have a similar appearance. On the other hand, some thyroid carcinomas may have a regular margin and no calcification. In the absence of reliable clinical or radiological signs for distinguishing between benign and malignant nodules, ultrasound-guided fine needle aspiration biopsy (FNAB) and large needle core biopsy (LNCB) have assumed an important role in the management of thyroid nodules.

Sonographic guidance offers the advantage of precisely targeting small lesions and reducing complications. FNAB has long been a standard technique for the diagnosis of thyroid nodules. However, it provides only a cytological diagnosis. With improvements in biopsy needles, the LNCB technique has become safer, more accurate, and easier to perform.

Technique for Thyroid Biopsy

Ultrasound-guided LNCB of the thyroid is based on the principle of the fine needle biopsy technique. The patient is placed in a spine position with the neck extended. After the skin is prepped and sterile draped, 3 to 4 mL subcutaneous lidocaine 1% is applied for anesthesia. A 2 mm skin incision is made with an 18 gauge injection needle tip or a scalpel blade. The biopsy needle is then inserted under continuous ultrasound monitoring. The needle tip is brought to the selected prefiring location and the biopsy gun is fired. As soon as the biopsy needle is withdrawn, manual pressure is applied to the biopsy site to prevent bleeding. The specimen is carefully removed from the biopsy needle (avoiding damage) and placed upon sterile dry paper. The biopsy specimen and paper are then placed in 10% formalin. Two to three tissue samples are obtained from each lesion. After the biopsy, a pressure dressing is applied. The patient is observed for 30 to 60 minutes while maintaining a supine position.

For LNCB, we use a spring-activated, short-throw (1.1 cm excursion), 18 gauge trucut type needle (Acecut, TSK Laboratory International Inc., Vancouver, BC, Canada). A sample from this type of needle can contain approximately three to five normal thyroid follicles in its width. For the ultrasound guidance, a high frequency (7.5–10.0 MHz), small-size sector or curved-array transducer with a needle guide attachment is used (**Fig. 3-3**). These transducers enable us to choose the easiest and safest biopsy route. A sector or curved-array transducer provides a wide view and depth (i.e., of the direction of the needle) from the small contact area.

It is essential to use a needle-guide device. If the freehand technique is used, there is a risk that the postfiring needle tip position is not seen as it passes through the imaging plane. A trajectory angle of ~40 degrees against the skin surface is suitable for thyroid biopsy. If possible, an angle-adjustable needle-guide device should be used. When determining the approach route and prefiring needle tip position, care should be taken to avoid the carotid artery. In addition, the needle tip should not pass through the gland. If the needle passes through the thyroid gland, the recurrent nerve, esophagus, trachea, or vertebral artery could be injured.

LNCB allows accurate histological diagnosis, which also enables us to identify benign conditions. The patient presented had lymph node enlargement >1 cm. One of the factors affecting the prognosis of PMC is the presence of clinically apparent lymph node metastasis. LNCB biopsy of the lymph node at the same sitting helps to decide whether an extended operation is necessary.

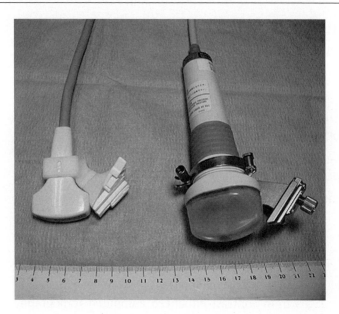

Figure 3-3 Transducers used for thyroid biopsy with biopsy guides attached.

PEARLS AND PITFALLS

- Ultrasound-guided needle biopsy is the procedure of choice for establishing the diagnosis of thyroid papillary microcarcinoma.
- The prognosis of thyroid papillary microcarcinoma is extremely good with a postsurgical 10-year survival of between 96 and 99.8%.
- Large needle core biopsy is preferred because it provides a histological diagnosis that is more reliable than the cytological diagnosis provided by fine needle aspiration biopsy.

Further Reading

Franklin NT, Tublin ME. Thyroid sonography: current applications and future directions. AJR Am J Roentgenol 1999;173:437–443

Screaton NJ, Berman LH, Grant JW. US-guided core-needle biopsy of the thyroid gland. Radiology 2003;226:827–832

Taki S, Kakuda K, Kakuma K, et al. Thyroid nodules: evaluation with US-guided core biopsy with an automated biopsy gun. Radiology 1997;202:874–877

CHAPTER 4 Mediastinal Biopsy

Ruffin J. Graham and Moulay A. Meziane

Clinical Presentation

A 32-year-old man with acquired immunodeficiency syndrome (AIDS) presented with a 2-day history of fever, chills, dyspnea upon exertion, and general malaise. Four months prior to onset of the present illness, he had been treated for *Pneumocystis carinii* pneumonia. At the current admission to the hospital, his CD4 count measured 36 cells/mL.

Radiological Studies

The posteroanterior (PA) chest radiograph demonstrates a widening of the superior mediastinum (**Fig. 4-1A**). The right paratracheal stripe has an irregular, lobulated contour suggestive of lymphadenopathy. The lungs appear clear. Images from contrast-enhanced computed tomography (CT) (**Figs. 4-1B,C**) confirm the presence of homogeneous, infiltrating soft tissue masses or lymphadenopathy in the superior mediastinum, right paratracheal and subcarinal regions, and right hilum. Small bilateral pleural effusions are also present.

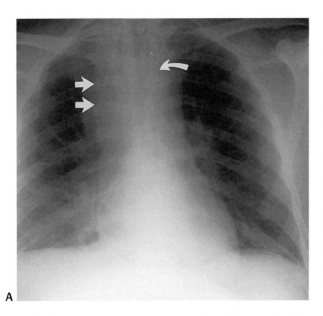

A

Figure 4-1 (**A**) Posteroanterior radiograph of the chest demonstrates right paratracheal soft tissue mass (straight arrows). The trachea (curved arrow) is displaced to the left. (**B**) Contrast-enhanced computed tomographic (CT) image at the level of the manubrium demonstrates soft tissue masses in the right paratracheal region (thick arrow). The left brachiocephalic vein (thin arrow) is densely enhanced by the contrast bolus. A pleural effusion is seen (arrowheads). (**C**) Contrast-enhanced CT image at the subcarinal level demonstrates additional soft tissue masses in the right hilum (thin straight arrow) and subcarinal region (curved arrow). Bilateral pleural effusions are layering posteriorly (arrowheads). These CT findings suggest mediastinal lymphadenopathy.

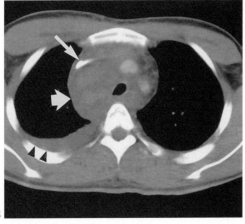

B

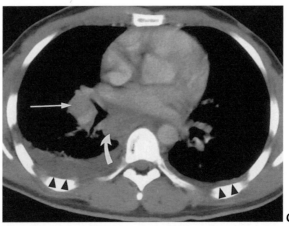

C

Differential Diagnosis

Given the clinical history and radiographic findings, the major differential diagnostic considerations are a neoplastic process and opportunistic infection. Neoplastic causes of mediastinal lymphadenopathy in the AIDS population include Kaposi's sarcoma and non-Hodgkin's lymphoma. The principal infectious causes include tuberculosis (*Mycobacterium tuberculosis*) and *Mycobacterium avium-intracellulare* (MAI) infection. The differences in the treatment regimens for these diagnoses render tissue diagnosis (i.e., biopsy) essential.

The imaging studies suggest that the diagnostic workup could be accomplished by fiberoptic bronchoscopy, percutaneous fine needle aspiration biopsy (FNAB), or mediastinoscopy. Bronchoscopy with transbronchial fine needle aspiration was performed initially but failed to yield malignant cells. Microbiological studies were also negative. Because of the patient's depleted, immunosuppressed condition, a CT-guided FNAB of the mediastinal lymph nodes was attempted before mediastinoscopy. With the patient in the prone position on the CT table, a right paravertebral approach was selected for biopsy (**Fig. 4-2**). Aspirated samples again disclosed no malignant cells, but acid-fast bacilli were identified. Further analysis with DNA probe provided the diagnosis of MAI infection.

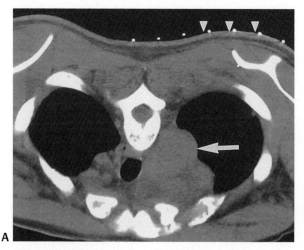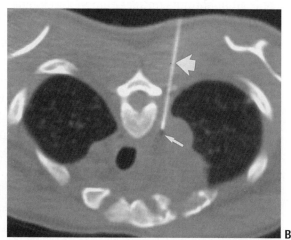

Figure 4-2 (**A**) With the patient in the prone position, a right paravertebral approach is planned for percutaneous biopsy of the right paratracheal lymphadenopathy (arrow). Radiopaque marking strip (arrowheads) is placed on the patient's back. (**B**) A 19 gauge needle has been inserted into the right paratracheal mass (thick arrow). Streaky low attenuation (small arrow) or "tip artifact" confirms presence of needle tip in the mass. The use of lung windows during the procedure assists in maintaining an extrapleural course for the needle.

Diagnosis

Mycobacterium avium-intracellulare infection

Discussion

MAI is an atypical mycobacterium of the nonphotochromogen group. The organism is typically found in soil and water and colonizes the respiratory or gastrointestinal (GI) tract by inhalation or ingestion of aerosolized bacteria. Direct human to human transmission has not been demonstrated (Goodman, 1991). The major risk factor for disseminated infection is the level of immune dysfunction, best reflected by the CD4 cell count (Horsburgh, 1991). MAI infection indicates advanced immunosuppression, occurring when the CD4 count falls below 60 cells/mL. Epidemiological studies suggest that

MAI infection will develop in 15 to 24% of patients with AIDS. It is the AIDS-defining disease in 4% of patients (Horsburgh, 1991).

Radiographic and imaging studies are often important in establishing the diagnosis of MAI infection in AIDS patients because of the frequently non-specific clinical symptoms (fever, weight loss, abdominal pain). The chest radiograph is abnormal in up to 80% of AIDS patients with MAI infection. The most common radiographic pattern is one of interstitial lung disease—diffuse, bilateral reticulonodular infiltrates. Miliary disease and cavitary nodules or infiltrates are rare. Mediastinal lymphadenopathy has been reported radiographically in 6 to 20% of patients with AIDS and MAI infection. CT is a more sensitive method of detecting mediastinal lymphadenopathy and may also be helpful in narrowing the diagnostic likelihood of MAI infection. In one study reviewing 96 chest CT scans in patients with AIDS, Sider et al identified 33 cases with mediastinal lymphadenopathy, nine of which were secondary to MAI infection. The other major causes were AIDS-related lymphoma (10 cases) and tuberculosis (5 cases) (Sider et al, 1993).

Regardless of the patient population, mediastinal masses most often represent benign or malignant neoplasms, lymphadenopathy (neoplastic, inflammatory, etc.), cysts, cardiovascular lesions, or esophageal abnormalities. The exact incidence of each of these abnormalities is difficult to determine because published surgical series tend to be biased toward lesions requiring biopsy or resection. The patient's age is an important consideration in developing a working differential diagnosis. In adults, 60 to 70% of primary mediastinal masses are benign. Masses of thymic origin, neurogenic tumors, lymphomas, and germ cell neoplasms are most common. In children, malignant tumors predominate, particularly lymphomas and neuroblastomas (Hoffman et al, 1993).

Once the presence of a mediastinal mass has been confirmed radiographically, precise anatomical location of the mass (i.e., anterior, middle, or posterior mediastinum) becomes essential in further narrowing the differential diagnosis. For example, lymphadenopathy is by far the most common cause of a middle mediastinal mass, and ~80% of posterior mediastinal masses are neurogenic tumors. Cross-sectional imaging techniques may be helpful in further characterizing the mass. Indeed, the CT or magnetic resonance imaging (MRI) appearance of some mediastinal masses may be so characteristic that the need for more invasive imaging or biopsy may be obviated or even contraindicated. Aneurysms and hiatal hernias are common examples.

In most cases, institution of medical or surgical therapy for a mediastinal soft tissue mass requires a specific diagnosis based on cytological or histological features. Coincident with the development of improved cytological techniques, FNAB has emerged as a well-tolerated, reliable technique for sampling mediastinal soft tissue masses.

There are two major considerations in planning for FNAB of a mediastinal mass. First, the radiologist must determine if the lesion is accessible by the percutaneous route. Access to mediastinal masses is limited by the bony thorax, by adjacent vascular structures, and occasionally by the small size of some masses. These same factors favor the use of small needles (19 gauge or smaller) and limit the use of core biopsy techniques. In dealing with each of these challenges, CT has been invaluable in extending the uses of FNAB (Westcott, 1988). CT is the most useful method of localizing mediastinal masses and for planning the most direct and safest route of access to the lesion. Most lesions are approached by a parasternal or paravertebral approach, preferably avoiding the pulmonary parenchyma to limit the chance for iatrogenic pneumothorax. Although fluoroscopy or ultrasound may be used to guide some percutaneous biopsies, CT guidance is the preferred method for small (≤2 cm) mediastinal masses and masses that are immediately adjacent to major cardiovascular structures (Westcott, 1988).

After determining that a mediastinal mass is accessible to percutaneous biopsy, the second major consideration for the radiologist is to exclude contraindications to the procedure based on the imaging findings or the patient's clinical history. If the imaging findings are insufficient to exclude a vascular nature to the mass, then FNAB should not be attempted. Clinical factors that serve as reliable contraindications to percutaneous FNAB include severely compromised pulmonary function, coagulopathy, pulmonary hypertension, and inability of the patient to cooperate for the procedure (Hoffman et al, 1993; Westcott, 1988).

Most published reports about the diagnostic accuracy of percutaneous mediastinal biopsy are limited to experience with FNAB. The diagnostic accuracy for mediastinal soft tissue masses is 85 to 90% (Adler et al, 1983; Weisbrod et al, 1984; Herman et al, 1991; Böcking et al, 1995; Zafar and Moinuddin, 1995). The yield is particularly high for metastatic carcinoma, germ cell tumors, and benign cysts (Herman et al, 1991). Percutaneous FNAB has not achieved the same high levels of diagnostic accuracy for lymphoma that it has for carcinoma (Adler et al, 1983; Westcott, 1988; Weisbrod et al, 1991). The more undifferentiated the cell type constituting the lymphoma, the easier it is to make a diagnosis by cytology. Similarly, non-Hodgkin's lymphomas are more easily diagnosed by small needle (19 gauge or smaller) sampling than are Hodgkin's lymphomas (Westcott, 1988). In cases of well-differentiated or Hodgkin's lymphomas, larger needles or core biopsy techniques may be necessary for examining tissue architecture or identifying Reed-Sternberg cells. Even then, it may not be possible to make a definitive diagnosis. Thymomas, while less problematic than lymphomas, may also require sampling by large needles for accurate diagnosis, particularly those with a predominance of lymphocytic components (Herman et al, 1991). **Table 4-1** shows a summary of technical parameters surrounding percutaneous biopsy of the mediastinum.

There are few data on the accuracy of FNAB in determining the cause of nonneoplastic lymphadenopathy. In one report of 22 patients with mediastinal lymphadenopathy secondary to tuberculosis, a true positive diagnostic rate for percutaneous FNAB was 66% and the false-negative rate was 34% (Khan et al, 1994). The rates for fiberoptic bronchoscopy and mediastinoscopy were 20% and 75%, respectively.

Complications

Published reports indicate that percutaneous FNAB of mediastinal masses is a safe and well-tolerated procedure (Adler et al, 1983; Weisbrod et al, 1984; Herman et al, 1991; Böcking et al, 1995; Zafar and Moinuddin, 1995). Pneumothorax is the most common complication, occurring in ~10 to 20% of cases. Whenever possible, the pulmonary parenchyma should be avoided when planning a route of access. When that is not possible, preexisting lung disease—particularly emphysema—appears to be the most significant risk factor for developing a pneumothorax (Westcott, 1988). The use of small needles and limiting the number of passes may also decrease the incidence of pneumothorax. Less frequent complications include hemoptysis and minor mediastinal hemorrhage. There have been two reports of bloody pericardial effusion with pericardial tamponade (Weisbrod et al, 1984; Man et al, 1998). Both developed almost immediately following small needle biopsy of lymphoma in the anterior mediastinum and were treated by pericardiocentesis. Neither case resulted in death.

When compared with fiberoptic bronchoscopy or mediastinoscopy, the use of percutaneous FNAB in the diagnostic workup of mediastinal masses will vary based on local practice patterns and operator experience. Needle aspiration of the mediastinum can be performed transbronchially, but this approach is usually limited to middle mediastinal masses or masses adjacent to large airways. It is usually more costly than FNAB. Mediastinal FNAB is faster, safer, less expensive, and better tolerated than surgery or mediastinoscopy. General anesthesia and hospitalization are not required. FNAB also provides more flexible access to all parts of the mediastinum in comparison with mediastinoscopy. The latter may still be necessary for the staging of lung carcinomas without evidence of mediastinal disease or in the patient with a mediastinal mass who has undergone a nondiagnostic FNAB (Westcott, 1988).

Table 4-1 Summary of Parameters Guiding Percutaneous Mediastinal Biopsy

Parameter	Clinical Standard
INDICATIONS	
	Cell typing of suspected malignant soft tissue masses
	Confirming diagnosis of probable benign lesions
	Staging neoplasms
	Obtaining bacteriologic material for suspected infectious processes
CONTRAINDICATIONS	
Absolute	Inability to exclude vascular nature of the mass based on imaging features
Relative	Severe pulmonary dysfunction
	Coagulopathy
	Hypertension
	Inability of patient to cooperate for procedure
IMAGING GUIDANCE	
	Computed tomography has broadest applications
	Fluoroscopy or ultrasound may occasionally be used
ROUTE OF ACCESS	
Parasternal	For anterior mediastinal masses
Paravertebral	For posterior mediastinal masses
Parasternal or paravertebral	For middle mediastinal masses
NEEDLE CHARACTERISTICS	
Fine needle aspiration biopsy (19 gauge or smaller)	For most lesions
Core-biopsy sampling	May be necessary in suspected cases of lymphoma or thymoma
COMPLICATIONS	
	Pneumothorax (10–20% of cases)
	Minor hemorrhage
	Catastrophic hemorrhage (rare)
DIAGNOSTIC YIELD	
	Metastatic disease (90–95%)
	Germ cell tumors (90–95%)
	Thymoma (70–75%)
	Lymphoma (50–60%)
	Infectious causes (not well documented)

We believe that the greatest limitations of percutaneous FNAB of mediastinal masses are sampling errors and inadequate cytological interpretation. Increasing experience and resulting improvement in the expertise on the part of physicians performing and interpreting the biopsies present the surest means to achieving reproducible results and a high degree of technical excellence (Weisbrod et al, 1984).

PEARLS AND PITFALLS_____

- CT-guided fine needle aspiration biopsy of mediastinal masses can be used for obtaining tissue samples for differentiating between tumor and infection in immunocompromised patients.
- Diagnostic accuracy for mediastinal soft tissue masses is between 85 and 90%. The yield is higher for metastatic carcinoma and germ cell tumors and lower for lymphoma and lymphadenopathy secondary to tuberculosis.
- Most lesions are approached by a parasternal or paravertebral approach, avoiding the pulmonary parenchyma to limit the possibility of a pneumothorax.

- Access to mediastinal masses may be limited by the bony thorax, adjacent vascular structures, and small size of some masses.
- Contraindications to percutaneous fine needle aspiration biopsy include severely compromised pulmonary function, coagulopathy, pulmonary hypertension, and inability of the patient to cooperate for the procedure.

Further Reading

Adler OB, Rosenberger A, Peleg H. Fine-needle aspiration biopsy of mediastinal masses: evaluation of 136 experiences. AJR Am J Roentgenol 1983;140:893–896

Böcking A, Klose KC, Kyll HJ, et al. Cytologic versus histologic evaluation of needle biopsy of the lung, hilum and mediastinum. Acta Cytol 1995;39:463–471

Goodman PC. Mycobacterial disease in AIDS. J Thorac Imaging 1991;6:22–27

Herman SJ, Holub RV, Weisbrod GL, et al. Anterior mediastinal masses: utility of transthoracic needle biopsy. Radiology 1991;180:167–170

Hoffman OA, Gillespie DJ, Aughenbaugh GL, et al. Primary mediastinal neoplasms (other than thymoma). Mayo Clin Proc 1993;68:880–891

Horsburgh CR. Mycobacterium avium complex infection in the acquired immunodeficiency syndrome. N Engl J Med 1991;324:1332–1338

Khan J, Akhtar M, von Sinner WN, et al. CT-guided fine needle aspiration biopsy in the diagnosis of mediastinal tuberculosis. Chest 1994;106:1329–1332

Man A, Schwarz Y, Greif J. Case report: cardiac tamponade following fine needle aspiration (FNA) of a mediastinal mass. Clin Radiol 1998;53:151–152

Sider L, Gabriel H, Curry DR, et al. Pattern recognition of the pulmonary manifestations of AIDS on CT scans. Radiographics 1993;13:771–784

Weisbrod GL, Lyons DJ, Tao LC, et al. Percutaneous fine-needle aspiration biopsy of mediastinal lesions. AJR Am J Roentgenol 1984;143:525–529

Westcott JL. Percutaneous transthoracic needle biopsy. Radiology 1988;169:593–601

Zafar N, Moinuddin S. Mediastinal needle biopsy. Cancer 1995;76:1065–1068

CHAPTER 5 Mediastinal Abscess

Ruffin J. Graham and Moulay A. Meziane

Clinical Presentation

Six weeks after cardiac transplantation, this patient presented with severe chest pain and fever of 38.7°C. Two weeks earlier, gram-negative septicemia was diagnosed for which he had been placed on antibiotics.

Radiological Studies

Contrast-enhanced computed tomography (CT) revealed a well-circumscribed right paracardiac mass with a central region of lower density (**Fig. 5-1**). The CT appearance of this lesion was suggestive of an abscess. Because of his immunosuppressed condition, the transplant service requested percutaneous drainage as an initial therapeutic measure.

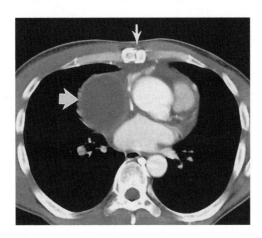

Figure 5-1 Contrast-enhanced CT demonstrates a right paracardiac fluid collection (thick arrow). Note the median sternotomy defect (small arrow).

Diagnosis

Postsurgical mediastinal abscess

Treatment

With the patient in the supine position, a repeat scan was obtained after placement of radiopaque markers on the anterior chest wall for determination of the access route (**Fig. 5-2**). A right parasternal approach was selected for drainage. For this approach, it was important to identify the internal mammary vessels to avoid injury during the drainage procedure. An 18 gauge needle was inserted into the abscess during expiration to minimize transgression of the pleural space. Foul-smelling, purulent fluid was easily aspirated and a sample was sent for microbiological examination. A guide wire was then advanced into the abscess cavity through the needle and the track was dilated to 11F. A 10F locking pigtail catheter was inserted into the abscess and sewn in position (**Fig. 5-3**). Bacteriologic studies failed to identify a specific organism. However, the patient defervesced following drainage catheter placement. One week later, he underwent successful elective surgical irrigation and debridement of the mediastinum.

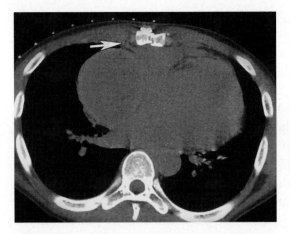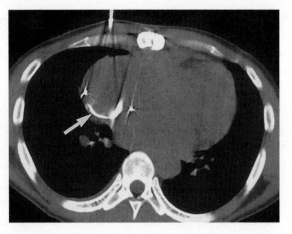

Figure 5-2 A radiopaque marker has been placed on the anterior chest wall for a right parasternal approach for drainage of the abscess. Arrow points to the internal mammary vessels.

Figure 5-3 After aspiration of a sample of the purulent fluid for microbiological examination, a 10F pigtail catheter (arrow) has been inserted for drainage of the abscess.

Discussion

Mediastinal abscesses are rare. Typically, these develop as sequelae to acute mediastinitis, which occurs most commonly as a postoperative infection following median sternotomy for open-heart surgery. Approximately 4% of post-sternotomy patients experience superficial wound infections after cardiac operations, and in 1 to 2%, the infection extends into the mediastinum (Davis and Sabiston, 1997). Acute mediastinitis may also result from esophageal or tracheobronchial perforation, penetrating trauma, and direct spread of infection into the mediastinum from contiguous anatomical spaces (e.g., the neck, pleura, retroperitoneum, etc.) (Breatnach et al, 1986). Regardless of the cause, mediastinal abscess is a serious complication that can often be fatal (Gobien et al, 1984).

Early diagnosis of acute mediastinitis and mediastinal abscess is critical to successful management. Clinical symptoms include chest pain, fever, chills, tachycardia, and leucocytosis. If undiagnosed, it may progress to shock. In the post-sternotomy patient, local erythema about the sternum and sternal instability (i.e., a "click") may be present, but these findings are unreliable for assessing the presence of mediastinal infection (Goodman et al, 1983). Plain radiographs of the chest and sternum are also of limited value in diagnosing mediastinitis. For example, a thin lucency in the sternum is commonly present in the post-sternotomy patient and does not indicate sternal dehiscence.

CT has assumed a central role in the diagnostic workup of patients with suspected acute mediastinitis and abscess formation. In the patient with esophageal perforation, the contrast esophagogram remains the essential radiographic study for suggesting the site of perforation. However, CT is helpful in identifying the presence of an extra-esophageal fluid collection or abscess. The accuracy and specificity of CT in demonstrating signs of mediastinitis or the presence of an abscess in post-sternotomy patients have been more problematic. In this setting, CT appears to have three major advantages (Kay et al, 1983). First, a normal CT scan in the post-sternotomy patient reliably excludes the possibility of acute mediastinitis. Second, CT is helpful in localizing wound infections as superficial (presternal) or deep (retrosternal). When CT demonstrates intact retrosternal soft tissue planes, wound infections require only superficial drainage. Third, CT provides an accurate, noninvasive method for diagnosing the presence or absence of a mediastinal fluid collection or abscess thereby reducing the delay for initiating appropriate therapy. However, it should be cautioned that some CT abnormality is evident in the anterior mediastinum of the great majority of patients who have undergone median sternotomy (Goodman et al, 1983). Minor abnormalities include a slight induration of mediastinal fat planes, pericardial thickening, and scattered minute air collections. Small defects in sternal closure are also common. Conversely, complete loss of integrity of anterior mediastinal fat planes or the presence of indistinct masses or encapsulated fluid implies acute mediastinitis (Goodman et al, 1983). When the imaging findings are equivocal, the clinical condition of the patient assumes primary importance in determining whether percutaneous drainage or reoperation is necessary for a mediastinal fluid collection.

Once the diagnosis has been made, drainage of the abscess is mandatory. Acute post-sternotomy mediastinitis/abscess has a reported mortality of up to 70%, and traditional therapy has included reoperation, mediastinal irrigation and drainage, and secondary wound closure. In a few selected cases, it may be possible to perform percutaneous abscess drainage, either as a curative step or to provide palliation prior to elective surgical debridement. CT of the thorax is virtually required to determine whether percutaneous abscess drainage is feasible. The procedure itself may be performed under CT guidance or with a combination of CT guidance and fluoroscopic observation.

In reviewing the CT of a patient with a suspected mediastinal abscess, there are three major considerations that determine whether a patient can safely undergo percutaneous abscess drainage (Gobien et al, 1984). First, a needle (and subsequent catheter) trajectory must be feasible that avoids any injury to cardiovascular or tracheobronchial structures. Second, a course extrinsic to the pleura must be selected. Third, it is desirable to establish gravity-dependent drainage once the catheter has been placed. However, the patient's clinical condition (e.g., an intubated patient) may limit options regarding his position during or after percutaneous abscess drainage.

Gobien et al described their results in aspirating and draining suspected mediastinal abscesses in 12 patients (Gobien et al, 1984). Nine of these patients were found to have mediastinal abscesses on CT-guided aspiration. In six, percutaneous abscess drainage was attempted immediately after the diagnostic aspiration, using a combination of CT and fluoroscopic guidance. In five patients, the abscess resolved after percutaneous drainage and the remaining patient experienced clinical improvement and later underwent elective surgical debridement. In these six patients, the drainage catheters remained in place for an average of 35 days (range 5–91).

Technique for Percutaneous Abscess Drainage

The technique of percutaneous abscess drainage has been well described, although the available literature discussing specific application to the mediastinum is limited (Gobien et al, 1984; Mueller and von Sonnenberg, 1990). In the mediastinum, CT guidance is preferred because visualization of vital cardiovascular structures is optimized and is not limited by the bony thorax. The patient may be placed in the prone, supine, or decubitus position to optimize the route of access. An 18 to 20 gauge needle is placed in the fluid collection and a sample is aspirated to determine if the fluid is infected. A Gram stain should be obtained if there is any doubt. Sterile fluid collections or hematomas are better left to resolve without percutaneous drainage. Once the infected nature of the fluid has been confirmed, a drainage catheter can be placed over a guide wire using the Seldinger technique. Prior to catheter insertion, the track is successively dilated. A 10 or 12F drainage catheter suffices for most mediastinal collections. The trocar method of catheter placement should not be attempted in the mediastinum. The drainage catheter may be left in place until resolution of the abscess or until elective surgical drainage can be attempted more safely. A repeat CT is the best imaging method for evaluating resolution of the abscess.

- Mediastinal abscesses develop as sequelae to acute mediastinitis and are most frequently seen after median sternotomy for open-heart surgery.
- Although most patients undergo operative management, percutaneous catheter drainage is applicable to some patients either as a curative procedure or in preparation for surgical drainage and debridement.
- CT is essential for planning and is preferred for guiding the procedure. An initial diagnostic aspiration is performed with an 18 or 20 gauge needle. If the aspirate is infected, a 10 or 12F drainage catheter is placed using the Seldinger technique.

Further Reading

Breatnach E, Nath PH, Delany DJ. The role of computed tomography in acute and subacute mediastinitis. Clin Radiol 1986;37:139–145

Davis RD, Sabiston DC. The mediastinum. In: Sabiston DC, ed. Textbook of Surgery: The Biological Basis of Modern Surgical Practice. 15th ed. Philadelphia, PA: WB Saunders; 1997:1906–1942

Gobien RP, Stanley JH, Gobien BS, et al. Percutaneous catheter aspiration and drainage of suspected mediastinal abscesses. Radiology 1984;151:69–71

Goodman LR, Kay HR, Teplick SK, et al. Complications of median sternotomy: computed tomographic evaluation. AJR Am J Roentgenol 1983;141:225–230

Kay HR, Goodman LR, Teplick SK, et al. Use of computed tomography to assess mediastinal complications after median sternotomy. Ann Thorac Surg 1983;36:706–714

Mueller PR, von Sonnenberg E. Interventional radiology in the chest and abdomen. N Engl J Med 1990;322:1364–1373

CHAPTER 6 Pleural Biopsy

Sudish C. Murthy, Hani M. Jneid, and Ziad W. Ghamra

Clinical Presentation

A 35-year-old woman presented to her local hospital with a 2-week history of dyspnea, dry cough, and dull chest pain. She had failed a 5-day course of oral azithromycin for presumed tracheobronchitis. There was no history of fever, night sweats, weight loss, trauma, exposure to sick contacts, or recent foreign travel. She was a lifelong nonsmoker and had no known toxic environmental or occupational exposures. Her father had worked at a steel mill and had reportedly had significant asbestos exposure. Her past medical history was notable for Crohn's disease that was in remission. Workup revealed a large, right-sided pleural effusion for which a chest tube was placed. Pleural fluid analysis demonstrated a chylothorax (pH 7.26, RBC 79,000, WBC 4400, LDH 398, protein 2.6 mg/dL, triglyceride 715 mg/dL, chylomicron positive). Cytology was negative for malignancy. Chemical pleurodesis with doxycycline was attempted. One month after her initial admission, she was transferred for further evaluation.

On examination, the patient was afebrile, cachectic, and bedridden and had a serum albumin <2 mg/dL. Renal function and urinalysis were normal. Chest tube drainage was >1000 mL/day and a repeat pleural fluid cytology was also negative for malignancy.

Radiological Studies

Magnetic resonance imaging (MRI) of the chest revealed a right posteromedial pleural mass, which was suspicious for a malignancy (**Fig. 6-1**). The lesion appeared to invade the posterior mediastinum and the posteromedial aspect of the right hemidiaphragm. Transdiaphragmatic involvement was suspected.

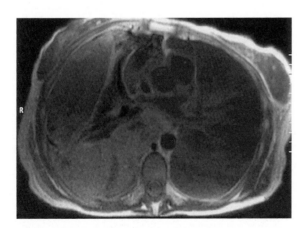

Figure 6-1 Magnetic resonance scan demonstrates a right posterior pleural mass with extension into the mediastinum and retroperitoneum.

24

Diagnosis

Spontaneous chylothorax secondary to suspected malignancy (lymphoma vs mesothelioma)

Treatment

The patient underwent mediastinoscopy, pleuroscopy, and biopsy of the chest mass. Frozen sections revealed N2 positive, epithelioid-type mesothelioma. Four grams of talcum were insufflated into the hemithorax to effect pleurodesis. Postoperatively, the patient was maintained on total parenteral nutrition but continued to have high output through the chest tube (>500 mL/day). She refused radiation therapy. One week after the talc pleurodesis, the chest tube was removed. Reaccumulation of fluid with shortness of breath necessitated placement of an indwelling pleural catheter 2 days later (PleurXTM, Denver Biomedical, Denver, CO) under local anesthesia. The patient was subsequently discharged home on a fat-free diet and was begun on experimental chemotherapy the following week.

Discussion

Diagnosis and treatment of pleural space disease represent a common referral for the thoracic surgeon. When an effusion is present, thoracentesis is the first diagnostic maneuver. Diagnostic yield for thoracentesis approaches 75% and complication rate is <5%. Pleuroscopy is reserved for diagnostic failures of thoracentesis or if therapeutic intervention is indicated. Diagnostic yield of pleuroscopy approaches 100% and pathological studies are not simply limited to cytology. The large pleural biopsies obtained during pleuroscopy can facilitate lymphoma subtyping and cytokeratin staining (to differentiate adenocarcinoma from mesothelioma). Thus pleuroscopy with biopsy was essential in this chapter.

The thoracic duct courses along the right side of the aorta in the lower chest. The duct coalesces to form the cisterna chyli and emerges through the aortic hiatus. The duct decussates to the left side of the midline at T4 and ascends toward the confluence of the left internal jugular and subclavian veins. Iatrogenic injury to the duct, and consequent chylothorax, can occur during esophageal or pulmonary surgery. Spontaneous chylothorax, however, is an uncommon entity. Underlying mediastinal malignancy is frequently discovered, and lymphoma is identified in over 70% of cases. Mesothelioma is a rarely reported cause of spontaneous chylothorax.

The association of malignant mesothelioma with occupational asbestos exposure was first recognized in 1960, though exposure can only be elicited in 70 to 80% of cases. Family members of people with a history of asbestos exposure have a higher incidence of malignant mesothelioma than the general population. Radiographic findings include unilateral cicatricial thickening of the pleura that can be confused with fibrothorax or pleural carcinomatosis (**Fig. 6-2**). Pleural effusion is variably present.

Multimodality therapeutic approaches for malignant mesothelioma incorporating surgery, chemotherapy, and radiation therapy have been described. Because of transdiaphragmatic extension, this patient's tumor was classified as stage IV and few therapeutic options are available. The management of chylothorax secondary to malignancy presents a formidable challenge. Standard therapy entails pleurodesis, pleural drainage, and total parenteral nutrition. Because this patient failed the standard approach, a pleurocutaneous shunt was eventually placed, which allowed for long-term control of the pleural space and alleviation of symptoms. Radiation therapy to the tumor and thoracic duct may also be considered in refractory cases.

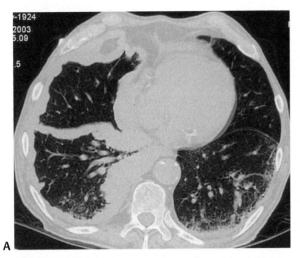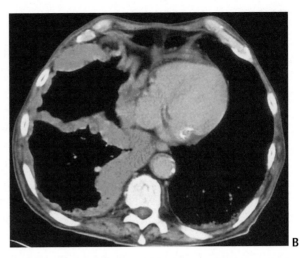

Figure 6-2 (A,B) Computed tomography of the chest (**A**, lung and **B**, mediastinal window setting) from a different patient shows the classic appearance of advanced pleural mesothelioma.

Technique for Pleural Biopsy

An alternative method is the imaging-guided percutaneous notched stylet cutting needle biopsy. Computed tomography or ultrasound is used for guidance and a tissue core is obtained with an 18 or 14 gauge spring-loaded needle. This method also permits safe biopsy of the pleura with a thickness of <5 mm. Patient positioning for biopsy is determined by the location of the area to be biopsied. After an appropriate skin prep and application of local anesthesia, the needle can be advanced into a pleural nodule in a more or less perpendicular fashion. In cases with pleural thickening without a nodule, the needle is advanced along the plane of the pleura so as to permit biopsy of a longer section.

The procedure can be performed on an outpatient basis; the patient is discharged after 4 hours if there are no complications (i.e., pneumothorax) on the postbiopsy chest radiograph. Satisfactory material can be obtained in the presence of nonnecrotic lesions and provides a sensitivity of ~88%. The complication rate is low, around 3%.

PEARLS AND PITFALLS

- The choice of technique (operative versus percutaneous) to diagnose pleural-based disease is dependent upon the suspected etiology. For instance, pleural carcinomatosis and tuberculous empyema can usually be identified by percutaneous biopsy. However, a lymphoma diagnosis and subsequent typing generally require a tissue sample larger than what can be obtained from percutaneous biopsy.
- Differentiating adenocarcinoma from mesothelioma can be difficult and often requires a larger tissue sample.
- Because intercostal neurovascular bundles travel toward the center of the intercostal space posteriorly, attempts at percutaneous access to the pleural space should be made more laterally to avoid injury. This decreases the chance of post-procedure hemothorax.
- The intercostal neurovascular bundle can be difficult to identify even when ultrasound-guided techniques are used.

Further Reading

Adams RF, Gleeson FV. Percutaneous image-guided cutting-needle biopsy of the pleura in the presence of a suspected malignant effusion. Radiology 2001;219:510–514

Chahinian AP, Pajak TF, Holland JF, et al. Diffuse malignant mesothelioma: prospective evaluation of 69 patients. Ann Intern Med 1982;96:746–755

Chen WJ, Mottet NK. Malignant mesothelioma with minimal asbestos exposure. Hum Pathol 1978; 9:253–258

Epler GR, Fitzgerald MX, Gaensler EA, et al. Asbestos-related disease from household exposure. Respiration (Herrlisheim) 1980;39:229–240

Rusch VW. A proposed new international TNM staging system for malignant pleural mesothelioma. From the International Mesothelioma Interest Group. Chest 1995;108:1122–1128

Screaton NJ, Flower CD. Percutaneous needle biopsy of the pleura. Radiol Clin North Am 2000; 38:293–301

Valentine VG, Raffin TA. The management of chylothorax. Chest 1992;102:586–591

Wagner E. Das tuberkelahnliche Lymphädenom. Arch Heilk 1870;11:495–525

Wagner JC, Sleggs CA, Marchand P. Diffuse pleural mesothelioma and asbestos exposure in the North Western Cape Province. Br J Ind Med 1960;17:260–271

Yates DH, Corrin B, Stidolph PN, et al. Malignant mesothelioma in southeast England: clinicopathological experience of 272 cases. Thorax 1997;52:507–512

CHAPTER 7 Pleurodesis

Sudish C. Murthy

Clinical Presentation

A 46-year-old woman was referred for the management of shortness of breath. Her past medical history was remarkable for metastatic atypical ovarian cancer with signet ring and neuroendocrine features that had failed platinum-based chemotherapy. She denied fevers, cough, night sweats, or recent weight loss. On physical examination, she was afebrile and mildly tachypneic. Breath sounds were markedly diminished bilaterally and the abdomen was distended but nontender.

Radiological Studies

The frontal chest radiograph demonstrated bilateral pleural effusions (right > left) (**Fig. 7-1**). The decubitus image demonstrated no fluid locculation (**Fig. 7-2**). Chest computed tomography (CT) (not shown) suggested some pleural thickening.

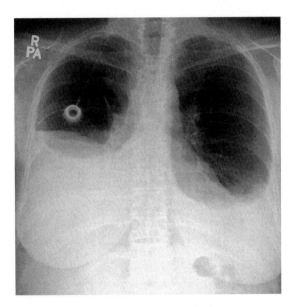

Figure 7-1 Upright chest radiograph demonstrates a large right- and a smaller left-sided pleural effusion.

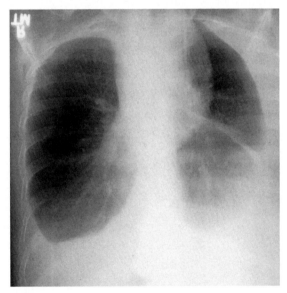

Figure 7-2 Lateral decubitus radiograph demonstrates a free-flowing right-sided effusion. Loculation of the fluid is present on the left.

Diagnosis

Malignant pleural effusion

Treatment

The patient was taken to the operating room for a right-sided pleuroscopy and talcum pleurodesis. Cytology examination of the fluid confirmed a malignant pleural effusion (MPE). The postoperative course was significant for transient fever to 39°C and hypoxia that persisted for 5 days. She was

28

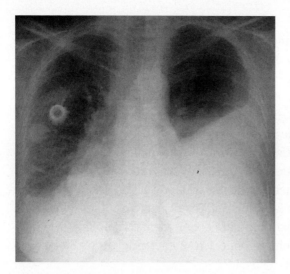 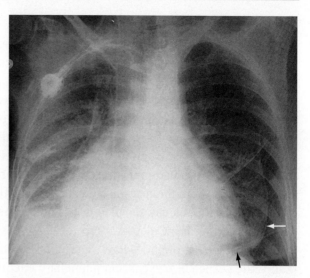

Figure 7-3 Following right-sided talcum pleurodesis, there is an increase in the left pleural effusion.

Figure 7-4 Chest radiograph following placement of the left pleural catheter. The lung remains unexpanded (arrows) demonstrating the entrapped lung syndrome.

treated with intravenous steroids and was discharged home on the seventh postoperative day. After the right-sided pleurodesis, there was an increase in the left-sided pleural effusion (**Fig. 7-3**). This was managed by the percutaneous placement of a drainage catheter. The chest radiograph obtained following catheter placement demonstrated entrapped lung syndrome (**Fig. 7-4**).

Discussion

Pleural effusion is the most common manifestation of pleural disease. Movement of fluid into and out of the pleural space represents a complex balance between hydrostatic and osmotic forces. Any process that alters this balance may result in a pleural effusion. Pleural effusions are routinely classified as transudative or exudative. Medical therapy is standard for transudative effusions, which are most often associated with pulmonary embolus, heart failure, and renal insufficiency. Exudative effusions have higher protein concentrations (>3 g/dL) and often require therapeutic intervention. Exudative effusions accompany pleural malignancy, pleural space infection (empyema), and pulmonary inflammation (parapneumonic effusion).

Because of the recurrent nature of MPE, a one-time drainage is seldom sufficient. Consequently, MPE represents the most common indication for pleurodesis. Talc poudrage performed through a pleuroscope is over 90% effective in controlling MPE. Talcum powder is 30 to 50% more efficacious than either tetracycline or bleomycin to effect pleural symphysis. Over 50% of patients are febrile after talc insufflation. Complications, though rare, include granulomatous inflammation, reexpansion pulmonary edema, adult respiratory distress syndrome (ARDS), and cerebral microemboli. This chapter illustrates the pulmonary dysfunction that can accompany the procedure. Treatment for this patient's "talc reaction" included high-dose intravenous steroids and expectant management.

In some patients with pleural carcinomatosis, the visceral pleura can become involved and severely restricts lung expansion. This leads to entrapped lung syndrome and these patients are not amenable to pleurodesis. However, most of these patients experience some relief of dyspnea with the drainage of the effusion, although a post-procedure chest radiograph may show incomplete reexpansion of the lung (**Figs. 7-3** and **7-4**). This phenomenon was demonstrated after drainage of this patient's left-sided effusion. Patients can be treated with a chronic indwelling pleurocutaneous catheter, which is managed at home and accessed once or twice weekly.

Technique for Percutaneous Pleurodesis

Pleurodesis can also be performed percutaneously using a 10 or 12 French, multiple-hole, pigtail-type catheter. This is used in patients who are unable to undergo general anesthesia or tolerate a large diameter chest tube. With the patient in the upright (sitting) position, sonography is used to assess the effusion and location of the costophrenic sulcus. After determination of the access site (around the tenth intercostal space, via a posterolateral approach), the skin is prepped and a fenestrated drape is placed. Following the application of local anesthesia, a 10 or 12 French multipurpose drainage catheter is inserted into the pleural space using either the trocar or the Seldinger technique. The catheter tip is positioned in the most dependent portion (i.e., the posterolateral costophrenic sulcus). This may necessitate fluoroscopic guidance. The catheter is then placed on suction. Once the output decreases to ±100 mL/day, the pleurodesis procedure is performed. Drainage of >1500 mL of effusion during one sitting is avoided as it can result in reexpansion pulmonary edema. Therefore, for large-volume effusions, a preprocedure thoracentesis should be done 1 to 2 days prior to pleurodesis to reduce the chance of reexpansion pulmonary edema.

The pleurodesis procedure is performed with the patient in the supine position, under conscious sedation. A slurry is prepared by mixing 5 g of talc in ~100 mL saline. The slurry is injected in 3 to 4 aliquots ~5 to 7 minutes apart. Rotation of the patient (altering position for each subsequent injection) allows greater dispersal of the talc mixture. Upon completion of the injections, the catheter is clamped and returned to suction after 6 to 8 hours. A completion chest radiograph is obtained to determine and document the presence of residual fluid. In most treated cases, the suctioned fluid volume drops and remains <100 mL per 24 hours, permitting removal of the catheter.

PEARLS AND PITFALLS_____

- Operative and percutaneous techniques for pleurodesis are useful tools in the management of patients with recalcitrant malignant pleural effusions. There are no randomized studies to compare these two techniques.
- Drainage of >1500 mL of effusion during one sitting can result in reexpansion pulmonary edema. Therefore, for large-volume effusions, a preprocedure thoracentesis should be done 1 to 2 days prior to pleurodesis to reduce the chance of reexpansion sequelae.
- 1 to 5 g of talcum are sufficient to promote pleural symphysis, and use of more than 10 g has been associated with talcum-related complications.
- Entrapped lung syndrome is a contraindication for pleurodesis. Insufflation of talcum into the hemithorax in these cases can lead to talcum-related complications without any therapeutic benefit.
- Loculated effusions should raise suspicion of entrapped lung and should be tapped prior to attempting pleurodesis. For entrapped lung syndrome, other percutaneous strategies exist.

Further Reading

Andrews CO, Gora ML. Pleural effusions: pathophysiology and management. Ann Pharmacother 1994;28:894–903

Bloom AI, Wilson MW, Kerlan RK Jr, et al. Talc pleurodesis through small-bore percutaneous tubes. Cardiovasc Intervent Radiol 1999;22:433–436

Clementsen P, Evald T, Grode G, et al. Treatment of malignant pleural effusion: pleurodesis using a small percutaneous catheter: a prospective randomized study. Respir Med 1998;92:593–596

Idell S. Evaluation of perplexing pleural effusions. Contemp Intern Med 1994;6:31–39

Scherer LA, Battistella FD, Owings JT, et al. Video-assisted thoracic surgery in the treatment of posttraumatic empyema. Arch Surg 1998;133:637–642

Walker-Renard PB, Vaughan LM, Sahn SA. Chemical pleurodesis for malignant pleural effusions. Ann Intern Med 1994;120:56–64

Yim APC, Liu H-P. Complications and failures of video-assisted thoracic surgery: experience from two centers in Asia. Ann Thorac Surg 1996;61:538–541

CHAPTER 8 Management of Central Airway Obstruction with Stents

Bipin D. Sarodia, Katsuo Usuda, and Atul C. Mehta

Clinical Presentation

A 44-year-old nonsmoker white female with no significant past medical history presented with complaints of dry cough and shortness of breath (New York Heart Association NYHA class III) that was worse when lying flat. The symptoms were progressive over 4 years, during which she was treated, without improvement, for suspected asthma with bronchodilator inhalers and prednisone. She also had pain in small joints and the knees and hearing difficulty. Her physical examination was unremarkable except for mild tachypnea with inspiratory stridor and a saddle nose deformity. Routine laboratory tests were normal except for mild anemia. Spirometry revealed a forced vital capacity (FVC) of 1.79 L (62% predicted), forced expiratory volume in one second (FEV$_1$) was 0.56 L (23% predicted), and the FEV$_1$:FVC was 31%, with no response to bronchodilator. Bronchoscopy revealed dynamic collapse of the tracheobronchial tree, including the cartilaginous portion during expiration, causing ~50% obstruction of the distal trachea and both main stem bronchi. There was no endobronchial mass lesion.

Radiological Studies

Chest radiographs and computed tomography (CT) of the chest were unremarkable except for narrowing of the upper trachea (5 mm anteroposterior diameter) and a small right lower lobe infiltrate. Ventilation-perfusion lung scan and CT of the paranasal sinuses were normal.

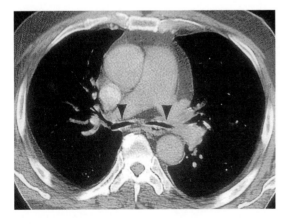

Figure 8-1 Chest computed tomographic scan from a patient with relapsing polychondritis shows severe narrowing of both main stem bronchi (arrowheads). The diameter measured 7 mm.

Diagnosis

Dynamic tracheobronchial obstruction secondary to relapsing polychondritis

Treatment

The patient had been treated with bronchodilator inhalers and multiple courses of prednisone followed by methotrexate over a 4-year period, without any obvious benefit. Continuous positive airway pressure therapy allowed her to sleep in the supine position, yet did not relieve her daytime symptoms of cough and dyspnea. Because of persistent symptoms, she underwent placement of self-expandable stents: a 2 cm × 10 mm diameter stent in the left main stem bronchus, and three 4 cm × 12 mm diameter stents in the trachea extending from 2 cm below the vocal cords to the carina. A stent was not placed in the right main stem bronchus to avoid blockage of the right upper lobe bronchus. **Figs. 8-2** to **8-4** show the stent deployment procedure and results.

At 3-month follow-up, there was marked improvement in the dyspnea, but she had persistent cough and mild right-sided wheezing. Chest radiographs showed the stents in their original positions and minimal bibasilar atelectasis. Bronchoscopy revealed persistent dynamic collapse of the right main stem bronchus causing 50% obstruction. This was relieved by the placement of a 2 cm × 10 mm diameter stent. The right upper lobe bronchus was partly covered by the stent, but its ventilation was maintained through the wire mesh of the bare metal stent. Spirometry performed at 3 months and 1 year after the initial stent placement revealed significant improvement in the airflow without significant response to a bronchodilator (**Table 8-1**).

At 30 months follow-up after the first stent placement, she has been symptom free except for a mild cough, and has not required an emergency room visit or hospitalization. She is able to accomplish all her activities of daily living and is a full-time employee performing an office job. Bronchoscopy revealed the airways to be patent with near total epithelialization of the stents.

Table 8-1   Spirometry Before and After Stent Placement

Spirometry	Baseline	At 3 Months	At 1 Year
FVC	1.79 (62%)	2.13 (74%)	2.00 (70%)
FEV$_1$	0.56 (23%)	1.02 (41%)	1.36 (55%)
Ratio	31%	48%	68%

Numbers in parentheses indicate % predicted values.

FEV$_1$, forced expiratory volume in 1 second; FVC, forced vital capacity.

Discussion

Overview of Central Airway Obstruction

There are three categories of central airway obstruction (CAO), which may be caused by benign or malignant disease processes: (1) intraluminal obstruction, (2) extrinsic compression, and (3) chondromalacia. In addition, a combination of factors may exist. **Table 8-2** lists the different etiologies of CAO. Symptoms include wheezing, stridor, dyspnea, postobstructive pneumonia, hypoxia, and respiratory insufficiency.

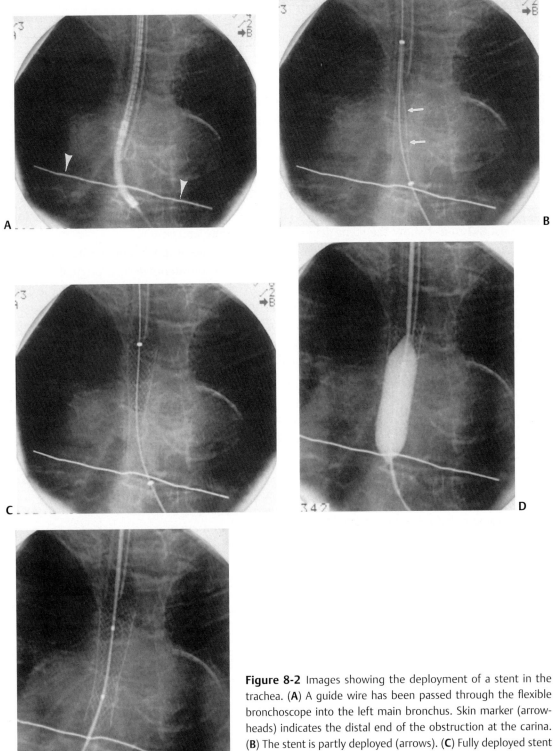

Figure 8-2 Images showing the deployment of a stent in the trachea. (**A**) A guide wire has been passed through the flexible bronchoscope into the left main bronchus. Skin marker (arrowheads) indicates the distal end of the obstruction at the carina. (**B**) The stent is partly deployed (arrows). (**C**) Fully deployed stent with its distal end just above the carina. (**D**) Angioplasty balloon dilating the narrowed segment to fully expand the stent. (**E**) The fully expanded stent.

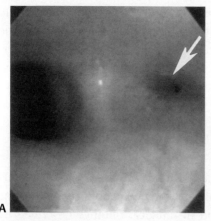
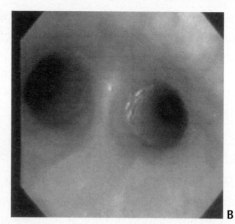

Figure 8-3 (**A**) Bronchoscopic view before and (**B**) after stent placement. Prior to stenting, there is near-total collapse of the right main stem bronchus (arrow). Following stent placement, it is wide open. A stent was previously placed in the left main stem bronchus. (See Color Plate 8–3A,B.)

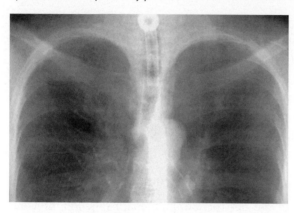

Figure 8-4 Chest radiograph obtained following stent placement in a different patient with relapsing polychondritis shows metallic stents in the trachea, left main stem bronchus, and bronchus intermedius. The tracheostomy tube is passing through the upper part of the tracheal stent.

Table 8-2   Etiology of Central Airway Obstruction

Malignant Disorders		Benign Disorders
Primary bronchogenic carcinoma	Granulation	Miscellaneous
Mucoepidermoid carcinoma	Endobronchial tuberculosis	Tracheopathia osteoplastica
Bronchial carcinoid	Wegener's granulomatosis	Amyloidosis
Contiguous tumor spread	Fungal infection	Relapsing polychondritis
Thyroid carcinoma	Sarcoidosis	Tracheobronchomalacia
Esophageal carcinoma	Iatrogenic obstruction	Postinfection
Head and neck carcinoma	Postintubation	Posttrauma
Thymoma	Posttracheostomy	Congenital
Thymic carcinoma	Post–sleeve resection	Foreign body
Germ cell tumor	Posttransplantation	Congenital
Malignant lymphoma	Benign tumor	Vascular anomaly
Metastases	Papilloma	Membranous web
Breast cancer	Hamartoma	Cartilage deformity
Colon cancer	Fibroma	
Renal cell carcinoma	Papillomatosis	
Sarcoma		

The diagnosis is frequently suspected by the findings on the chest radiographs. Imaging workup of these patients includes CT and magnetic resonance imaging (MRI). Additional studies may include virtual bronchoscopy (providing a road map for bronchoscopy), endobronchial ultrasound (for determining the degree of tracheobronchial wall invasion as well as treatment planning), and transbronchial needle aspiration (for establishing the etiology) (Choi et al, 2002; Grenier et al, 2002; Herth et al, 2002; Boiselle et al, 2002, 2003; Britt, 2004).

Relapsing Polychondritis

This is a rare, benign, multisystem disorder presumed to be of autoimmune etiology. It is characterized by recurrent, progressive inflammation and degeneration of cartilage and connective tissue. The diagnosis is based upon a constellation of clinical features and histological findings described by McAdam et al (1976) and Damiani and Levine (1979). These include polychondritis (auricular, nasal, laryngeal, tracheobronchial; nonerosive, seronegative inflammatory polyarthritis; ocular inflammation (uveitis); and cochlear and vestibular damage.

Airway manifestations are present in ~50% of patients. These lead to obstruction of the tracheobronchial tree and are most serious, predicting a poor prognosis. The narrowed coronal diameter of the trachea may be visible on the chest radiographs. CT may demonstrate diffuse, smooth thickening of the tracheobronchial wall causing narrowing and deformity of the airway lumen (see **Fig. 8-1**). No single medical or surgical treatment is uniformly effective in curing the disease, relieving the symptoms, or preventing progression of the airway manifestations. The airway can be maintained by tracheobronchial stents as in the patient described.

Nonsurgical Management Options for Central Airway Obstruction

Treatment is determined by the type and location of the obstruction, pulmonary function, previous treatments, and patient life expectancy. Selection of the therapeutic modality also depends upon its invasiveness because the intended treatment is usually palliative in most of these patients as curative surgical treatment is rarely possible. Palliative treatment modalities that are available for the management of CAO include balloon bronchoplasty, electrosurgery, argon plasma coagulation, brachytherapy, laser photoresection, cryotherapy, radiofrequency ablation, microdebrider, and stent placement.

The majority of these procedures can be performed with either the flexible or a rigid bronchoscope. The flexible bronchoscope can be used under conscious sedation and local anesthesia and can access more distal areas outside the reach of the rigid bronchoscope. On the other hand, rigid bronchoscopy provides better control of the airway either using conventional or jet ventilation, especially during bleeding, and allows placement of silicone stents, when required.

BALLOON BRONCHOPLASTY

Balloon bronchoplasty with or without stent placement is a simple, rapid, and safe method for restoring the airway in tracheobronchial strictures, including anastomotic stenoses after lung transplantation (Chhajed et al, 2001; Lee et al, 2002). It can be performed in an outpatient setting under local anesthesia using bronchoscopic visualization or fluoroscopy.

The balloons used for the bronchoplasty are made of silicone and require high inflation pressures (CRE pulmonary balloon dilatation catheter, Boston Scientific, Natick, MA). These specially designed balloons can be expanded to three different preset diameters corresponding to three different inflation pressures. Inflation is maintained for 30 to 60 seconds. The procedure is repeated until the desired effect is obtained. Long-term success in nonmalignant airway stenoses is between 54 and 71% (Hebra et al, 1991; Ferretti et al, 1995; Sheski and Mathur, 1998). Complications include mucosal laceration and bronchospasm.

ENDOBRONCHIAL ELECTROSURGERY

Endobronchial electrosurgery (EBES) allows resection and debulking of polypoid and sessile lesions, respectively. This is used for both benign and malignant endobronchial processes. It can also be used to cut stenosing scar tissue at a bronchial anastomosis after lung transplantation, and to excise granulation tissue. It is successful in 70 to 95% of patients (Petrou et al, 1993; Coulter and Mehta, 2000).

ARGON PLASMA COAGULATION

Argon plasma coagulation (APC) is used for smaller benign or malignant endobronchial lesions and for coagulation of superficial hemorrhage. It is also used for treating granulation tissue associated with uncovered metallic stents. Although it does not vaporize the tissue, it can be used to reduce the degree of tumor-related airway obstruction (Morice et al, 2001; Ernst et al, 2004). In the presence of high fraction of inspired oxygen (FIO_2) (>40%) it is possible to ignite inflammable materials during APC; hence it should not be used in the presence of covered metallic or silicone stents.

BRACHYTHERAPY

Endobronchial brachytherapy (usually iridium-192) is used for malignant lesions as well as granulation tissue associated with metallic stents and at the site of bronchial anastomoses following lung transplantation (Mulligan, 2001; Halkos et al, 2003). Results vary, with improvement reported in 35 to 100% of patients with endobronchial tumors (Nori et al, 2004).

Other treatment modalities include lasers, photodynamic therapy, cryotherapy, microdebrider, radiofrequency ablation, and laser photoresection (Marasso et al, 1998; Simoni et al, 2003).

Tracheobronchial Stents

Stents play a major role in the management of large airway obstruction due to either malignant or benign diseases. Stents used for reestablishing patency of stenotic central airways are usually the final option after all other therapeutical options for CAO have been exhausted. They are used for supporting weakened cartilages in tracheobronchomalacia, sealing fistulous communication to the esophagus, and managing dehiscence (Phillips, 1998; Freitag, 2000). Self-expandable airway stents have been used successfully in patients with relapsing polychondritis. **Table 8-3** lists the benign tracheobronchial diseases in which the stent placement may be indicated.

Table 8-3   Potential Indications for Stent Placement in Benign Tracheobronchial Diseases

Tracheal Stenosis	Bronchial Stenosis	Tracheobronchomalacia	Tracheobronchial Compression
Congenital	Post–lung and	Generalized or focal	Vascular anomalies
Endotracheal	post–heart-lung	Congenital	and malformations
tube–induced injury	transplantation	Idiopathic	Fibrosing mediastinitis
Tracheotomy-related	Relapsing	Tracheobroncho-megaly	Kyphoscoliosis
Systemic diseases	polychondritis	(Mournier-Kuhn syndrome)	
Wegener's	Postinfectious	Relapsing polychondritis	
granulomatosis	(tuberculosis)	Tracheotomy related	
Relapsing		Post–lung and post–heart-lung	
polychondritis		transplantation	
Amyloidosis		Radiation therapy–induced	

Over the past decades, several stent designs and modifications have surfaced in the market. This diversity attests to an ongoing pursuit of an ideal endobronchial stent, which is not yet available (Rafanan and Mehta, 2000). Based upon the composition material, they are classified as silicone, metallic (covered or uncovered), and hybrid stents. Metal stents are radiopaque and are relatively easy to deploy. They are either fixed-diameter balloon-expandable or self-expanding, made of bare metal or covered with a coating of silicone, nylon, or polyurethane. Silicone stents can be used in all forms of CAO. In malignant obstruction, silicone or covered metallic stents are recommended to prevent tumor ingrowth. Placement of silicone stents requires the use of the rigid bronchoscope, whereas metallic stents can be placed via a flexible bronchoscope, with or without fluoroscopic guidance. **Table 8-4** provides a comparison of tracheobronchial stents.

SILICONE STENT (POLYMER STENT)

This is the most commonly used stent (Freitag, 2000). Its placement requires the rigid bronchoscope under general anesthesia. Its main advantage is that it can be easily repositioned or removed (Wood, 2002). The stent is easily customized according to tracheobronchial anatomy and is free of tumor ingrowth. The disadvantage is that the thick wall of the stent provides a reduced inner diameter. Complications include granuloma formation, migration, and retained secretions.

DUMON STENT

Small studs on the outer wall of the Dumon stent (**Fig. 8-5**) prevent migration. It is used for both malignant and benign lesions and requires the use of a dedicated introducer. The stent provides a relatively narrow airway lumen because of its wall thickness. The Dumon Y stent is designed for carinal lesions. In a multi-institutional study involving 1058 cases, there was a high success rate for immediate palliation (Dumon et al, 1996). Stent migration occurred in 9.5%, mucous obstruction in 3.6%, and granuloma formation in 7.9% (Dumon et al, 1996).

POLYFLEX STENT

These are synthetic, self-expandable stents made of polyester wire mesh with a thin layer of silicone (Freitag, 2000). The wall is thinner, providing a larger airway lumen. The outer wall is smoother than that of the Dumon stent, although a stent with a studded outer wall has been introduced. The Polyflex stent is suitable for most causes of CAOs, including tracheoesophageal fistula. The stent is constrained into a smaller introducer and inserted through a rigid bronchoscope. The overall results are similar to those of the Dumon stent (Bolliger et al, 2004).

METALLIC STENTS

Metallic stents are available as covered and uncovered, self-expanding and balloon-expandable stents. They possess the advantage of easy delivery using a flexible bronchoscope under local anesthesia (Wood, 2002). They have a low potential for migration and retention of secretions. Once epithelialized, they are difficult to reposition or remove. Complications include tumor ingrowth, granulation tissue formation, and airway wall perforation. They have been used to treat bronchial stenosis in selected lung transplant recipients and bronchomalacia.

Table 8-4   Comparison of Commonly Used Tracheobronchial Stents and Their Applications

	Name	Characteristics	Advantages	Disadvantages	Suitable Disorders
Silicone Stents	Montgomery T Tube	T-shaped silicone prosthesis Horizontal limb requires tracheostomy	No excessive pressure against airway wall No migration	Tracheostomy needed Obstruction by secretions	Tracheal stenosis Subglottic stenosis
	Dumon stent	Silicone tube with studs Rigid scope required	Removable No ingrowth Absence of radial force reduces chance of perforation Relatively less expensive	Decreased inner diameter Migration Mucostasis	Extrinsic compression
	Polyflex stent	Polyester wire mesh with thin layer of silicone Self-expandable Rigid scope required	Thin stent wall No perforation of the airways Larger inner diameter	Migration	All airway stenoses Anastomotic stenosis posttransplant
Metallic Stents	Ultraflex stent (nitinol)	Nitinol retains shape memory Self-expanding	Easy delivery with flexible bronchoscope Less mucostasis Reposition and extraction possible after insertion	Ingrowth obstruction Granulation Extraction difficult after epithelialization	Malignant extrinsic compression Anastomotic stenosis posttransplant
	Wallstent	Wire mesh made of woven cobalt-based alloy filaments Self-expanding	Easy delivery with flexible bronchoscope Flexible, compressible, and self-expanding	Shortens after full expansion	Malignant airway stenoses
	Palmaz stent	Balloon expandable	Easy delivery	Sharp borders Easy to collapse	Malignant airway stenoses
	Strecker stent	Woven tantalum wires Balloon expandable	Easy delivery	Easy to collapse	Malignant airway stenoses
Hybrid Stents	Dynamic stent	Silicone, metal hoops Imitates trachea with physiological function	Posterior wall facilitates mobilization of secretions	Difficult insertion	Carinal lesions
	Orlowski stent	Made of vinyl chloride Armored with metal rings	Difficult to collapse	Stiff Mucostasis Requires experience for delivery	Long, and hard stenoses
	Nova stent	Nitinol hoops embedded in silicone sheets Self-expanding Squeezed down in refrigeration	Easy delivery	Migration	Airway stenoses Malacia

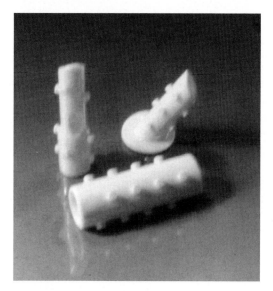

Figure 8-5 Dumon stents.

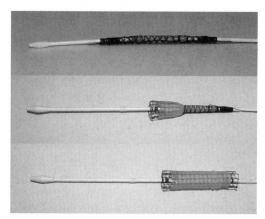

Figure 8-6 Covered Ultraflex stents. Top: constrained, Middle: partially deployed, Bottom: fully deployed stent.

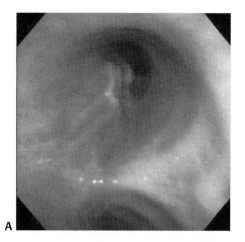

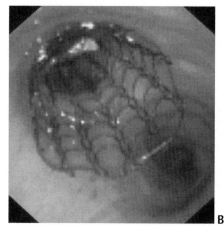

Figure 8-7 Covered Ultraflex stent used to seal a bronchoesophageal fistula. (**A**) Bronchoscopic view before and (**B**) after stent deployment. (See Color Plate 8–7B.)

ULTRAFLEX STENT Ultraflex stents (**Figs. 8-6** and **8-7**) are self-expanding stents composed of a single, woven nitinol wire with good biocompatibility. The uncovered version of the stent does not interfere with ciliary movement of the bronchial mucosa and thus causes less retention of secretions. The covered version has been used to seal fistulas to the esophagus and to prevent tumor ingrowth. The stent can be placed through a flexible bronchoscope over a guide wire using fluoroscopic guidance. This stent can be removed after 6 to 8 weeks, before it epithelializes (Mughal et al, in press).

HYBRID STENT In hybrid stents, metal parts are incorporated in the silicone structure to reinforce certain parts of the prosthesis.

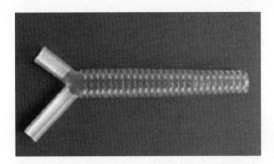

Figure 8-8 Dynamic Y stent.

DYNAMIC Y STENT (RUSCH STENT) The dynamic Y stent (**Fig. 8-8**) imitates the normal structure of the trachea and possibly the physiological function (Freitag et al, 1997). The anterior part of its tracheal leg is horseshoe shaped and is reinforced with metal hoops. The posterior wall consists of a thin, pliable silicone sheet, which bulges inward during coughing, thereby facilitating mobilization of secretions. The stent is most suitable for carinal lesions, including tracheobronchomalacia and esophagotracheal fistula. Its insertion remains challenging, requiring a dedicated forceps and direct laryngoscopic as well as fluoroscopic guidance.

Technique for Metallic Tracheobronchial Stent Deployment

The metallic stent can be deployed as an outpatient procedure with local anesthesia and conscious sedation using a flexible bronchoscope and fluoroscopic guidance (see **Fig. 8-2**). The initial bronchoscopy is performed to (1) confirm the diagnosis, (2) assess the need for stent placement, and (3) gauge the length of airway requiring stenting. The length of the obstructive or collapsible segment is measured as follows: The tip of the flexible bronchoscope is placed at the distal end of the obstruction. The bronchoscope is then withdrawn to the proximal end of the obstruction. The length of the obstruction is determined by measuring the movement of the bronchoscope in relation to the tip of the patient's nose. The stent diameter is estimated by measuring the diameter of the adjacent normal airway on the chest CT.

The stent placement procedure involves repeat flexible bronchoscopy (see **Figs. 8-2** and **8-3**). The distal and the proximal ends of the abnormal airway (as localized by the flexible bronchoscope) are marked on the skin surface by radiopaque markers (straight metal wires or radiopaque ruler) for fluoroscopic guidance. A 180 cm long guide wire is inserted through the working channel of the flexible bronchoscope and passed beyond the obstructed airway segment under bronchoscopic and fluoroscopic guidance. The bronchoscope is then removed, leaving the guide wire in place. The stent delivery system is inserted over the guide wire and the distal end (identified by the distal radiopaque marker band) is positioned beyond the obstruction using fluoroscopic guidance. The stent is gradually deployed under continuous fluoroscopic monitoring. Following deployment, the stent delivery system is removed together with the guide wire. An angioplasty balloon catheter of appropriate size is then used to dilate the obstructed segment and facilitate full expansion of the stent. Patency of the airway lumen is confirmed by repeat bronchoscopy (see **Fig. 8-3**). A chest radiograph is obtained to document stent positioning (see **Fig. 8-4**).

Complications

In general, complications associated with airway stents are uncommon and include stent migration, granulation tissue formation leading to stenosis and obstruction, retention of secretions, bleeding, ulceration, mechanical stent failure, and, rarely, erosion through the tracheobronchial wall into the surrounding structures. A disadvantage of a self-expanding stent is that, once placed, it cannot be removed without significant morbidity.

- Relapsing polychondritis is a rare multisystem disorder that affects cartilage and connective tissue. Clinical features include polychondritis (auricular, nasal, laryngeal, tracheobronchial), polyarthritis, uveitis, and audiovestibular damage.
- Airway obstruction, which is seen in ~50% of patients with relapsing polychondritis, is the most serious complication.
- Airway stents play a major role in the palliative management of large airway obstruction secondary to malignant and benign diseases.
- Self-expandable stents are easy to deploy and have multiple advantages and relatively few complications.

Further Reading

Boiselle PM, Feller-Kopman D, Ashiku S, et al. Tracheobronchomalacia: evolving role of dynamic multislice helical CT. Radiol Clin North Am 2003;41:627–636

Boiselle PM, Reynolds KF, Ernst A. Multiplanar and three-dimensional imaging of the central airways with multidetector CT. AJR Am J Roentgenol 2002;179:301–308

Bolliger CT, Breitenbuecher A, Brutsche M, et al. Use of studded Polyflex stents in patients with neoplastic obstructions of the central airways. Respiration 2004;71:83–87

Britt EJ. Transbronchial needle aspiration. In: Beamis JF, Mathur PN, Mehta AC, eds. Interventional Pulmonary Medicine. New York: Marcel Dekker; 2004:385–410

Burns KEA, Orons PD, Dauber JH, et al. Endobronchial metallic stent placement for airway complications after lung transplantation. Longitudinal results. Ann Thorac Surg 2002;74:1934–1941.

Chhajed PN, Malouf MA, Tamm M, et al. Interventional bronchoscopy for the management of airway complications following lung transplantation. Chest 2001;120:1894–1899

Choi YW, McAdams HP, Jeon SC, et al. Low-dose spiral CT: application to surface-rendered three-dimensional imaging of central airways. J Comput Assist Tomogr 2002;26:335–341

Coulter TD, Mehta AC. The heat is on: impact of endobronchial electrosurgery on the need for Nd-YAG laser photoresection. Chest 2000;118:516–521

Damiani JM, Levine HL. Relapsing polychondritis: report of ten cases. Laryngoscope 1979;89:929–946

Dumon JF, Cavaliere S, Diaz-Jimenez JP, et al. Seven-year experience with the Dumon prosthesis. J Bronchol 1996;3:6–10

Ernst A, Feller-Kopman D, Becker HD, et al. Central airway obstruction. Am J Respir Crit Care Med 2004;169:1278–1297

Ferretti G, Jouvan FB, Thony F, et al. Benign noninflammatory bronchial stenosis: treatment with balloon dilation. Radiology 1995;196:831–834

Freitag L. Tracheobronchial stents. In: Bolliger CT, Mather PN, eds: Interventional Bronchoscopy: Progress in Respiratory Research. Basel: Karger; 2000:171–186

Freitag L, Tekolf E, Stamatis G, et al. Clinical evaluation of a new bifurcated Dynamic airway stent: a 5-year experience with 135 patients. Thorac Cardiovasc Surg 1997;45:6–12

Gadaleta C, Mattioli V, Colucci G, et al. Radiofrequency ablation of 40 lung neoplasms. Preliminary results. AJR 2004;183:361–368.

Gotway MB, Golden JA, LaBerge JM, et al. Benign tracheobronchial stenosis. Changes in short-term and long-term pulmonary function testing after expandable metallic stent placement. J Comput Assist Tomogr 2002;26:564–572.

Grenier PA, Beigelman-Aubry C, Fetita C, et al. New frontiers in CT imaging of airway disease. Eur Radiol 2002;12:1022–1044

Halkos ME, Godette KD, Lawrence EC, et al. High dose rate brachytherapy in the management of lung transplant airway stenosis. Ann Thorac Surg 2003;76:381–384

Hebra A, Powell DD, Smith CD, et al. Balloon tracheoplasty in children: results of a 15-year experience. J Pediatr Surg 1991;26:957–961

Herth F, Becker HD, LoCicero J, et al. Endobronchial ultrasound in therapeutic bronchoscopy. Eur Respir J 2002;20:118–121

Lee KH, Ko GY, Song HY, et al. Benign tracheobronchial stenoses: long-term clinical experience with balloon dilation. J Vasc Interv Radiol 2002;13:909–914

Letko E, Zafirakis P, Baltatzis S, et al. Relapsing polychondritis: a clinical review. Semin Arthritis Rheum 2002;31:384–395

Lunn WW, Feller-Kopman D, Ernst A, et al. Microdebrider bronchoscopy. A new tool for the interventional pulmonologist. Chest 2004;126 (Suppl) 706s–707s

Madden BP, Datta S, Charokopos N. Experience with Ultraflex expandable metallic stents in the management of endobronchial pathology. Ann Thorac Surg 2002;73:938–944

Mair EA, Parsons DS, Lally KP. Treatment of severe bronchomalacia with expanding endobronchial stents. Arch Otolaryngol Head Neck Surg 1990;116:1087–1090

Marasso A, Bernardi V, Gai R, et al. Radiofrequency resection of bronchial tumours in combination with cryotherapy: evaluation of a new technique. Thorax 1998;53:106–109

Mayse ML, Greenheck J, Friedman M, et al. Successful bronchoscopic balloon dilation of nonmalignant tracheobronchial obstruction without fluoroscopy. Chest 2004;126:634–637

Mehta AC, Dasgupta A. Airway Stents. Clin Chest Med 1999;20:139–151

McAdam LP, O'Hanlan MA, Bluestone R, et al. Relapsing polychondritis: prospective study of 23 patients and a review of the literature. Medicine (Baltimore) 1976;55:193–215

Morice RC, Ece T, Ece F, et al. Endobronchial argon plasma coagulation for treatment of hemoptysis and neoplastic airway obstruction. Chest 2001;119:781–787

Mughal MM, Gildea TR, Murthy S. Temporary self-expandable metallic stents in promoting healing of bronchial dehiscence. Am J Resp Crit Care Med. Submitted

Mulligan MS. Endoscopic management of airway complications after lung transplantation. Chest Surg Clin N Am 2001;11:907–915

Nomori H, Kobayashi R, Kodera K, et al. Indications for an expandable metallic stent for tracheobronchial stenosis. Ann Thorac Surg 1993;56:1324–8

Nori D, Ravi A, Parikh S, et al. Endobronchial brachytherapy. In: Beamis JF, Mathur PN, Mehta AC, eds. Interventional Pulmonary Medicine. New York: Marcel Dekker; 2004:181–202

Petrou M, Kaplan D, Goldstraw P. Bronchoscopic diathermy resection and stent insertion: a cost effective treatment for tracheobronchial obstruction. Thorax 1993;48:1156–1159

Phillips MJ. Stenting therapy for stenosing airway diseases. Respirology 1998;3:215–219

Rafanan AL, Mehta AC. Stenting of the tracheobronchial tree. Radiol Clin North Am 2000;38:395–408

Rousseau H, Dahan M, Lauque D, et al. Self-expandable prostheses in the tracheobronchial tree. Radiology 1993;188:199–203.

Saad CP, Murthy S, Krizmanich G, et al. Self-expandable metallic airway stents and flexible bronchoscopy. Chest 2003;124:1993–1999

Sheski FD, Mathur PN. Long-term results of fiberoptic bronchoscopic balloon dilation in the management of benign tracheobronchial stenosis. Chest 1998;114:796–800

Simoni P, Peters GE, Magnuson JS, et al. Use of the endoscopic microdébrider in the management of airway obstruction from laryngotracheal carcinoma. Ann Otol Rhinol Laryngol 2003;112:11–13

Susanto I, Peters JI, Levine SM, et al. Use of balloon-expandable metallic stents in the management of bronchial stenosis and bronchomalacia after lung transplantation. Chest 1998;114:1330–1335

Wood DE. Management of malignant tracheobronchial obstruction. Surg Clin North Am 2002;82:621–642

CHAPTER 9 Esophageal Stricture

Murray Asch and John Kachura

Clinical Presentation

A 72-year-old woman presented with difficulty in swallowing and choking after eating. She had been diagnosed with locally advanced squamous cell carcinoma of the right upper lobe bronchus 3 months earlier. Palliative radiotherapy had been administered. Two weeks prior to this presentation, she had undergone endoscopic dilation, at which time a radiation-induced esophageal stricture was diagnosed.

Radiological Studies

The patient's current complaint of choking was investigated with repeat endoscopy and a barium swallow, which now revealed an irregular stenosis associated with a tracheoesophageal fistula (**Fig. 9-1**).

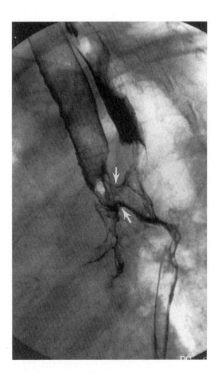

Figure 9-1 72-year-old woman with right upper lobe bronchogenic carcinoma treated with palliative radiotherapy. Oblique view from barium swallow reveals an irregular midesophageal stricture with a large fistula (arrows) extending to the lower trachea.

Diagnosis

Radiation-induced esophageal stricture with esophagorespiratory fistula

Treatment

In preparation for stent placement, the patient was brought to the interventional suite. The pharynx was anesthetized by having the patient gargle with a 2% viscous lidocaine. She was then placed on the fluoroscopy table in the left semiprone oblique position. A 5 French angled multipurpose catheter

44

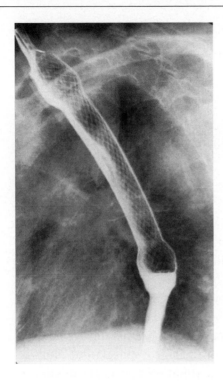

Figure 9-2 Following insertion of a covered Wallstent (20 mm diameter × 90 mm length), the esophagus is widely patent with no opacification of the fistula.

was advanced through the mouth and into the esophagus. The stricture was crossed with the catheter using a 180 cm length 0.038 in. Amplatz extra-stiff guide wire (Boston Scientific, Natick, MA) and was advanced into the stomach. The proximal and distal margins were then delineated by performing a "pull-back" dilute barium injection as the multipurpose catheter was withdrawn. After the location of the stenosis was carefully noted, the catheter was readvanced and the Amplatz wire coiled within the stomach.

A standard protective plastic endoscopic mouth guard was inserted, and a 20 mm diameter by 90 mm length silicone-covered Wallstent (Boston Scientific, Natick, MA) was advanced over the guide wire and deployed across the stricture. The patient was then taken to the recovery room for observation. Once the effect of the topical anesthetic had worn off, a follow-up barium swallow was performed (**Fig. 9-2**). This demonstrated the esophagus to be widely patent with no opacification of the tracheoesophageal fistula. The patient was then discharged home with instructions to remain on a soft diet for 1 week, following which she was converted to a normal diet with instructions to avoid large pieces of solid food, such as meat.

Discussion

Although carcinoma of the esophagus accounts for <1% of all malignancies, it is advanced and incurable in 60% of cases at the time of presentation, with an overall 5-year survival rate of <10%. Therefore, palliation of symptoms is the goal of therapy for these patients. Progressive dysphagia and chest pain are the major symptoms, often leading to malnutrition. Esophageal strictures and dysphagia may also occur with other cancers involving the mediastinum, such as bronchogenic carcinoma and metastases or as a result of radiation treatment of these entities. The degree of dysphagia can be quantified according to the grading scale developed by Mellow and Pinkas (**Table 9-1**). As shown in this chapter, esophagorespiratory fistula is another complication of this disease process that occurs in 15% of patients with esophageal cancer and 5% of patients with other malignancies involving the esophagus. Such a fistula often results in death from aspiration and pneumonia.

Table 9-1   Dysphagia Score

Dysphagia Score	Degree of Dysphagia
0	No dysphagia
1	Ability to eat some solid food
2	Ability to eat semisolids
3	Ability to swallow liquids only
4	Complete inability to swallow

From Mellow and Pinkas, 1985.

Many palliative treatment modalities are available for patients with unresectable esophageal carcinoma, but all have shortcomings. The mortality rate from palliative surgical resection with primary esophagogastric anastomosis may be as high as 40 to 60%, with either recurrence or anastomotic stricture causing further swallowing difficulties in 20% of patients. Chemotherapy alone is usually insufficient for palliation of dysphagia. Radiation therapy improves swallowing in 40% but requires 6 to 8 weeks from initiation of treatment for relief to be achieved. Bougienage or balloon dilation provides only transient relief. Endoscopic tumor ablation with a neodymium:yttrium-aluminum-garnet (Nd:YAG) laser is an effective treatment for malignant dysphagia but must be repeated at regular intervals and is associated with a 6 to 9% perforation rate if pre-dilation is required. In addition, laser ablation does not effectively treat submucosal tumors or those extrinsic to the esophagus. Gastrostomy, gastrojejunostomy, and jejunostomy can alleviate malnutrition but do not address dysphagia as patients may still be unable to tolerate their oral secretions.

Rigid plastic esophageal stents or endoprostheses have been in use for over a century but must be inserted under general anesthesia. Acute procedure-related complications, such as perforation, migration, bleeding, and pressure necrosis occur in up to 20% of cases with a mortality of ~9%.

Metallic esophageal stents have been in clinical use for several years. These devices are an effective, reasonably low-cost palliative treatment modality for malignant dysphagia and esophagorespiratory fistula. They are as effective as rigid endoprostheses in improving dysphagia scores while resulting in significantly less morbidity and mortality. They also represent a more efficient use of hospital resources because hospital stay is substantially reduced.

Cwikiel et al (1998) reported on 100 consecutive patients with malignant dysphagia receiving self-expanding, noncovered nitinol stents. A significant reduction in dysphagia was seen in 97 patients initially. At the time of death (mean survival time 6.2 months), over 75% had either normal swallowing or grade 1 dysphagia. Complications included stent twisting ($n = 4$) and stent migration ($n = 4$). Tumor ingrowth (through the stent struts or wires of this uncovered device) was noted in 17 patients, with tumor overgrowth (extending into the esophageal lumen proximal or distal to the ends of the stent) occurring in three patients. Food impaction ($n = 5$), stent wire fractures ($n = 2$), benign strictures at stent edges ($n = 2$), and tumor bleeding ($n = 3$) were also observed. Recent studies have focused on metal stents covered with a thin membrane because covered stents are much less prone to tumor ingrowth. The various types of expandable esophageal metal stents used in North America are summarized in **Table 9-2** and shown in **Fig. 9-3**. In addition, a thin-walled, flexible silicone stent has become available (Polyflex® Esophageal stent, (Willy Ruesch GMBH, Kernen, Germany/Boston Scientific, Natick, MA).

The perfect stent does not yet exist; thus operator preference determines which device is used. In general, covered stents are most valuable for mucosal lesions because they may offer some protection against tumor ingrowth through the wire mesh. Noncovered metal stents are not suitable for treatment of esophagorespiratory fistulas or esophageal perforations because food, debris, and saliva can easily pass through the mesh and into the defect. Devices differ in unique features for release

Table 9-2 Currently Used Esophageal Stents

Stent Name/Company	Material/Covering	Diameter/Length	Introducer Size
Wallstent/Endoprosthesis Esophageal II/ Boston Scientific	Chromium alloy/ Permalume	20, 28 mm diameter/ 10 and 15 cm length	18 French
Gianturco-Rösch Z Stent/Wilson Cook	Stainless steel/ Polyethylene	18 mm diameter/ 10, 12, and 14 cm length	24 French
EsophaCoil/Medtronic	Nitinol/ No covering	14, 16, 18, and 20 mm diameter/ 75, 100, and 150 cm length	32 French
Ultraflex (Strecker Stent) Microvasive/Boston Scientific	Titanium/ Polypropylene	17, 22 mm diameter/ 10, 12, 15 cm length	24 French
Polyflex Esophageal Stent/Boston Scientific	Silicone		

and the amount of shortening that occurs upon deployment. For example, the Wallstent exhibits a reduction of 30% or more in the overall length. Regardless of the stent used, knowledge of the degree and direction of shortening is essential for positioning the device correctly during deployment.

Technique

Barium esophagography is essential for preprocedural planning. In addition to spot films, large field-of-view thoracic images are extremely helpful in accurately localizing the proximal and distal extent of the stricture. Computed tomography may also provide useful information.

In our institution, esophageal stenting is most commonly performed on an outpatient basis. Careful review of the preprocedure imaging studies is essential. The entire procedure may be performed using fluoroscopic guidance without the need for endoscopy. As with many interventional procedures, the patient should be NPO for at least 4 hours prior to the procedure. Intravenous access is routinely obtained for possible conscious sedation (with midazolam hydrochloride and fentanyl citrate, for example). We have not found it necessary to administer atropine to reduce oral secretions. Oxygen is administered via nasal prongs, and the patient is monitored by means of pulse oximetry. A pharyngeal suction device should be readily available for use.

Generally, the procedure is well tolerated and quicker than diagnostic endoscopy and thus requires minimal sedation. Meticulous topical anesthesia of the oropharynx is essential to patient comfort. We start with the patient sitting up at the side of the fluoroscopy table, gargling with a 2% lidocaine viscous solution. Lidocaine spray can also be used in the pharynx. Following this, we lay the patient in a left side down semiprone oblique position to reduce the risk of aspiration. Reverse Trendelenburg positioning may also help in this regard. Although we do not consider this to be a sterile procedure, we do wear sterile gowns and gloves for our own protection.

Initial access to the esophagus is obtained using an angled multipurpose catheter inserted through the mouth. Our favored guide wire for this procedure is a 180 cm length 0.038 in. Amplatz extra-stiff (Boston Scientific), although a floppy-tipped wire, such as the Bentson wire (Cook Canada, Stouffville, ON), may be helpful. Occasionally, a hydrophilic wire may be necessary to traverse the lesion. Once the catheter has been manipulated beyond the stricture, it is advanced into the stomach. A "pull-back" injection of dilute barium is then done to delineate the proximal and distal aspects of the stricture. We find barium preferable to nonionic water-soluble contrast in that it results in better delineation of the stricture and tends to persist longer, thus providing better "real-time" landmarking during stent deployment. A radiopaque ruler placed under the patient prior to

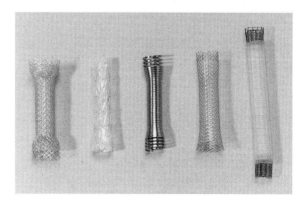

Figure 9-3 From left to right are the self-expanding metal esophagus stents commonly used in North America in their fully expanded configurations: Wallstent I (Boston Scientific), Gianturco-Rösch Z-stent (Wilson-Cook, Bloomington, IN), Esophacoil (Medtronic InStent, Eden Prairie, MN), Wallstent II (Boston Scientific), and Ultraflex stent (Boston Scientific, Natick, MA).

the procedure, or taping small metal beads to the patient's skin can also facilitate accurate positioning.

After careful localization of the stenosis, the catheter is again placed into the stomach and its position confirmed with contrast injection to exclude perforation. The tip of the extra-stiff Amplatz wire is then coiled within the stomach to provide secure purchase. A protective plastic endoscopy mouth guard is placed between the patient's teeth to protect the stent device during insertion. The introducer system is then advanced over the guide wire and the stent deployed across the stricture as per the manufacturer's instructions. It is essential to be familiar with the specifics of the release mechanism of the selected device prior to insertion. It is not necessary to routinely dilate lesions prior to stent placement; in fact, we have never pre-dilated any of our patients prior to stenting. After the stent has been successfully deployed, the patient is taken to the recovery room for observation. Once the effect of the topical oropharyngeal anesthesia has worn off, we perform a limited barium swallow to assess the position and function of the stent. The patient is then discharged home with an information and instruction sheet on esophageal stents and a scheduled follow-up visit.

To reduce the risk of tumor overgrowth and stent migration, stent length should be chosen such that the proximal and distal ends of the expanded device extend beyond the esophageal stricture by at least 2 cm at each end. Esophageal stents should not be placed within 3 cm of the cricopharyngeus owing to possible laryngeal compression and reflux with aspiration.

The metallic tip on the end of the Wallstent mounting catheter may be difficult to pull back, particularly if the stent has not completely expanded. Pulling it back aggressively may displace the stent and should be avoided. Waiting for a minute or so and advancing the outer sheath over the catheter often allows removal of the catheter without displacing the stent.

We have experienced several instances where the immediate poststenting barium study revealed an apparent esophageal obstruction. This occurred even when the distal end of the stent was positioned well below the stricture. In these cases, endoscopy showed no abnormality. This finding may be related to esophageal spasm from expansion of the stent.

On occasion, radiologists may be asked to evaluate an endoscopically placed stent. Intramural lipiodol is often injected by gastroenterologists to mark the site of the stricture. This should not be mistaken for extravasation from an esophageal perforation. Careful evaluation of the scout images prior to contrast injection will clarify this finding.

Post-Procedure Care

Instructions given to the patient following stent insertion are predominantly aimed at avoiding stent obstruction. We advise patients to limit their diet to fluids and soft foods for the first week after stent placement. This allows time for endothelialization to occur, thus reducing the likelihood of stent migration. Subsequently, a normal diet is prescribed, but with avoidance of large pieces of solid food, such as steak or chicken. Chewing solids thoroughly and drinking carbonated beverages after eating may help. For stents placed across the gastroesophageal junction, instructions must include measures to avoid gastroesophageal reflux, which could put the patient at risk of aspiration. Patients are told not to eat just prior to going to bed and that the head of the bed should be elevated. Motility agents may be of value as well. In the event of stent occlusion, endoscopy is ideal for clearing an impacted food bolus and in delineating an underlying problem. An additional stent can usually restore patency if tumor ingrowth, tumor overgrowth, or stent migration has occurred.

Outcome

The technical success in placing metal esophageal stents approaches 100%. Failures have occurred with early experience and have usually been subsequently avoided with device and/or technique modifications. All studies have shown a substantial clinical improvement in dysphagia and in the sequelae of esophagorespiratory fistulas. In malignant dysphagia, esophageal stents provide immediate relief in up to 97% of patients, with the mean dysphagia grade of 3.1 to 3.5 prior to stent insertion decreasing to 0.6 to 0.8 post-stenting. Sustained relief of dysphagia has occurred in over 80% of patients until the time of death. Complete relief of aspiration has been achieved in 67 to 95% of patients with esophagorespiratory fistulas, with partial relief (tolerance of a soft diet but continued aspiration of liquids) observed in the remaining patients.

Complications

Transient chest pain lasting 1 to 5 days following placement of esophageal stents occurs in up to 50% of patients. This pain is usually effectively treated with oral analgesics. Warning the patient of this problem prior to stent placement is of some value in relieving anxiety. Reflux is universal in patients receiving stents that span the gastroesophageal junction; therefore, such patients should have appropriate antireflux therapy.

Stent migration occurs more commonly with covered stents, with a reported incidence of up to 30% of covered Wallstents. In contrast, the rate of migration of noncovered metal stents is 5% or less. Often, stent migration can be easily addressed with standard endoscopic techniques. Although rare, perforations into the pericardium, mediastinum and airway (resulting in esophagorespiratory fistula) have been reported. Tumor overgrowth has been reported as a complication and a cause for recurrent dysphagia in 3 to 9% of patients in most series. Noncovered stents are prone to tumor ingrowth (through the stent "mesh") in 20 to 30%, compared with only 2% of patients treated with covered stents. Tumor ingrowth or overgrowth, however, can be palliated with endoscopic laser therapy or with placement of an additional stent. Food impaction occurs in up to 2% and requires endoscopic treatment. It is usually attributed to the ingestion of large, solid boluses. Upper gastrointestinal hemorrhage has been reported with esophageal stents but has not been shown to be more frequent than would normally be expected in patients with malignant esophageal tumors. Death due to massive gastrointestinal hemorrhage occurs in 5 to 8% of all patients with esophageal carcinoma, usually secondary to tumor erosion into a major vessel.

Optimal management of these patients requires a team approach with open lines of communication among radiologist, thoracic surgeon, and gastroenterologist. Further improvements in this procedure can be expected as more experience is gained and with continued refinement of the devices.

- Fluoroscopically guided insertion of expandable metallic stents in the esophagus is a safe and effective method of palliation in malignant dysphagia and esophagorespiratory fistula.
- With careful preprocedural planning, the procedureis nearly always successful and relatively straightforward.
- The length of the stent should be selected so that the proximal and distal ends of the *expanded* device extend beyond the stricture by at least 2 cm at each end.
- An esophageal stent should not be placed within 3 cm of the cricopharyngeus muscle because of the possibility of laryngeal compression with reflux and aspiration.
- In comparison with other available treatment modalities, esophageal stenting can be performed at low cost and low morbidity in an outpatient setting, with minimum sedation.

Further Reading

Adam A, Ellul J, Watkinson AF, et al. Palliation of inoperable esophageal carcinoma: a prospective randomized trial of laser therapy and stent placement. Radiology 1997;202:344–348

Cwikiel W, Tranberg KG, Cwikiel M, et al. Malignant dysphagia: palliation with esophageal stents-long-term results in 100 patients. Radiology 1998;207:513–518

Gollub MJ, Gerdes H, Bains MS. Radiographic appearances of esophageal stents. Radiographics 1997; 17:1169–1182

Good S, Asch MR, Jaffer N, et al. Radiologic placement of metallic esophageal stents: preliminary experience. Can Assoc Radiol J 1997;48:340–347

Hasan S, Beckly D, Rahamim J. Oesophagorespiratory fistulas as a complication of self-expanding metal oesophageal stents. Endoscopy. 2004;36:731–734.

Knyrim K, Wagner HJ, Bethge N, et al. A controlled trial of an expansile metal stent for palliation of esophageal obstruction due to inoperable cancer. N Engl J Med 1993;329:1302–1307

Langer FB, Wenzl E, Prager G, et al. Management of postoperative esophageal leaks with the Polyflex self-expanding covered plastic stent. Ann Thor Surg 2005;79:398–403

Mellow MH, Pinkas H. Endoscopic laser therapy for malignancies affecting the esophagus and gastroesophageal junction: analysis of technical and functional efficacy. Arch Intern Med 1985;145:1443–1446

Morgan RA, Ellul JPM, Denton ERE, et al. Malignant esophageal fistulas and perforations: management with plastic-covered metallic endoprostheses. Radiology 1997;204:527–532

Nevitt AW, Kozarek RA, Kidd R. Expandable esophageal prostheses: recognition, insertion techniques, and positioning. AJR Am J Roentgenol 1996;167:1009–1013

Saxon RR, Barton RE, Katon RM, et al. Treatment of malignant esophageal obstructions with covered metallic Z stents: long-term results in 52 patients. J Vasc Interv Radiol 1995;6:747–754

Saxon RR, Morrison KE, Lakin PC, et al. Malignant esophageal obstruction and esophagorespiratory fistula: palliation with a polyethylene-covered Z-stent. Radiology 1997;202:349–354

Song HY, Do YS, Han YM, et al. Covered, expandable esophageal metallic stent tubes: experiences in 119 patients. Radiology 1994;193:689–695

SECTION II
Abdomen

CHAPTER 10 Percutaneous Gastrostomy

Stewart Kribs

Clinical Presentation

An 18-month-old male infant with acute lymphocytic leukemia presented with severe oropharyngeal and skull base mucormycosis. This was associated with erosion of the skull base, which precluded oral feeding. Nasogastric tube feeding was instituted. Although the feeds were well tolerated, the patient frequently pulled out the feeding tube. Percutaneous enteral access was requested.

Diagnosis

Oropharyngeal and skull base mucormycosis precluding oral feeding

Treatment

Since the child was tolerating feeds into the stomach, a gastrostomy tube was chosen. The procedure was performed under general anesthesia with the patient supine upon the fluoroscopy table. The location of the left lobe of the liver was marked under ultrasound guidance. A nasogastric tube was inserted and gastric contents aspirated. Air was then insufflated and a suitable site for gastric puncture chosen (usually just below the costal margin and to the left of midline). The surrounding skin was prepped and draped, and local anesthetic was administered along the anticipated tube tract. We have found local anesthetic useful in concert with general anesthesia as it seems to reduce post-procedural pain. A small skin incision was made and the stomach was punctured with a slotted 18 gauge suture anchor needle (Boston Scientific, Watertown, MA). The needle was angled toward the pylorus and advanced into the stomach. Under lateral fluoroscopy the suture anchor was deployed using a guide wire. The anchor was pulled snug and fixed at the skin exit site with a hemostat. An angled catheter (5.5F HBP, Cook Canada, Stouffville, ON) was inserted over the wire and directed toward the gastric fundus. A second suture anchor was placed at the initial puncture site and care was taken not to shear the catheter with the suture anchor needle. A third anchor was then placed ~45 degrees above and to the right of the puncture site. The tract was then dilated and a 12F locking-loop pigtail catheter (Nephrostomycatheter, Cook Canada, Stouffville, ON) placed with its tip in the gastric fundus.

Six weeks later, the child was "sized" for a skin-level, low-profile "button" gastrostomy tube and the radiologically placed catheter was exchanged and upsized for a temporary 14F balloon-retention gastrostomy tube (Kangaroo, Sherwood Medical, St. Louis, MO).

Four weeks later, the balloon-retention tube was exchanged for the button gastrostomy tube (MIC-Key G, Ballard Medical Products, Draper, UT), which also uses a balloon for retention. There were no complications, and the child tolerated gastrostomy tube feeding without difficulty.

Discussion

Percutaneous access to the stomach or jejunum is most commonly requested to provide enteral feeding for patients who are unable to or cannot safely ingest food orally. Another indication is for bowel decompression in patients with gastrointestinal obstruction. Gastrostomy and gastrojejunostomy tube placement may be performed surgically, endoscopically, or radiologically. In general, fluoroscopically guided radiological tube placement is the least invasive of the three options. We perform all our pediatric percutaneous feeding tube insertions under general anesthesia. In adults, however, the procedure is usually performed under local anesthesia and generally requires little or no parenteral sedation.

Percutaneous gastrostomy/gastrojejunostomy under fluoroscopic guidance has a success rate of ~95%. The frequency of major complications, including colonic perforation, peritonitis, and bleeding, is 2%. Minor complications, including tube dislodgment, blockage, or local skin site infection, occur in 3% of cases, with an overall complication rate of ~5%. Procedure-related deaths are uncommon (<1%), but 30-day mortality rates may be as high as 20% depending on the severity of the underlying illness in the population being treated.

Percutaneous feeding tube insertion is contraindicated when the colon or liver is interposed between the stomach and anterior abdominal wall, precluding safe transabdominal access. Under these circumstances, surgical or endoscopic tube placement should be considered. In patients who have had previous gastric surgery (e.g., gastrectomy/gastric pull-up), percutaneous gastrostomy may not be feasible. The presence of portal hypertension with known large gastric varices is also a contraindication due to the risk of hemorrhage. In patients with ascites, percutaneous gastrostomy tube insertion can usually be performed safely with some modifications in technique (described in the following).

Technique for Percutaneous Gastrostomy

Patients are fasted overnight to minimize gastric residue. A nasogastric tube is inserted, and any residue gastric debris is aspirated. The stomach is then insufflated with air. The use of intravenous smooth muscle relaxants (such as glucagons or hyoscine) to facilitate gastric distention is optional. Some centers administer barium the evening before the procedure to opacify the colon; however, we have not found this necessary. We routinely mark the position of the left lobe of the liver under ultrasound guidance prior to choosing the puncture site, to avoid unexpected transgression of this structure. Once the stomach has been inflated, a suitable site for gastric puncture is marked just below the costal margin, to the left of the midline. The surrounding skin is then prepped and draped, and local anesthetic is injected along the intended tube tract. We have found local anesthetic helpful, even in concert with general anesthesia because it seems to reduce post-procedural pain.

A small skin incision is made and the stomach punctured with a slotted 18 gauge suture anchor needle (Boston Scientific). Angling the needle toward the pylorus facilitates subsequent catheterization of the duodenum should conversion to a gastrojejunal feeding tube become necessary. The anchor is deployed under lateral fluoroscopic visualization by advancing the guide wire through the needle. Traction is applied, and the anchor suture is fixed at the skin exit site using a hemostat or similar clamp. An angled catheter (5.5F HBP, Cook Canada) is inserted and the guide wire directed toward the fundus for gastric feeding tubes, or through the pylorus, duodenal "C-sweep" and beyond the ligament of Treitz into the proximal jejunum for gastrojejunostomy tubes. A second suture anchor is then placed at the initial puncture site. We use two suture anchors at the puncture site to distribute force that occurs during tract dilatation and tube insertion, to lessen the likelihood of tearing the gastric wall. We then place the third anchor ~45 degrees above and to the right of the puncture site. The tract is then dilated and the feeding tube inserted. The initial gastrostomy tube is a 12F locking-loop pigtail catheter (Cook Canada) with a tapered tip and can be inserted into the stomach directly over the guide wire (**Fig. 10-1**). For jejunal feeding, we use a 12F, nontapered, end-hole-only gastrojejunal feeding tube (Elliott Feeding Tube, Cook Canada), which must be inserted through a 13F peel-away sheath (**Fig. 10-2A**).

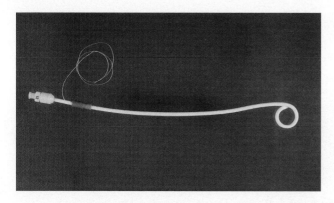

Figure 10-1 12F locking-loop pigtail nephrostomy catheter (Cook Canada, Stouffville, ON) used for initial gastric access.

For gastrojejunostomy tubes, the catheter must be placed distal to the ligament of Treitz in the proximal jejunum (to minimize retrograde passage of tube feeds into the duodenum and stomach) (**Fig. 10-2B**). For gastrostomies, we minimize the length of catheter in the stomach because gastric peristalsis may carry a long gastrostomy tube into the duodenum. This is usually not desirable because a tube in the duodenum prevents comfortable "bolus" feeding.

We secure the catheter to the skin using a retention disc (Molnar Disc, Cook Canada), which prevents distal migration of the tube and provides some security against inadvertent dislodgement. Patients are brought back approximately 10 days following insertion to check position and assess any tube-related problems. If there is no leakage at the insertion site and there are no concerns regarding tissue healing, the suture anchors are cut.

Placement of the Skin-Level (Button) Gastrostomy Tube

Skin-level (button) gastrostomy tubes are low-profile devices for enteral feeding. Less obtrusive and cosmetically more attractive than traditional gastrostomy tubes, they are popular with pediatric patients and their parents. They offer another advantage in that parents or an enteral feeding nurse can carry out catheter exchanges, thereby reducing the time we spend managing tube-related problems. They are designed to be placed through previously created gastrostomy tracts. Care must be taken when placing nontapered percutaneous endoscopic gastrotomy (PEG-type and skin-level) gastrostomy tubes through percutaneous tracts to avoid disrupting the tract.

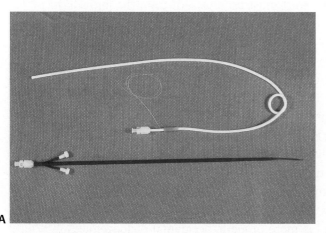
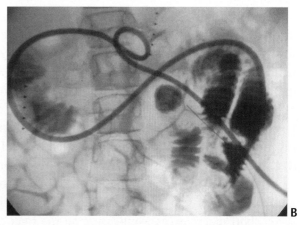

A   B

Figure 10-2 (A) 12F nontapered gastrojejunal feeding tube (Elliott Feeding Tube, Cook Canada, Stouffville, ON), which must be inserted through a 13F peel-away sheath (shown at the bottom). **(B)** Contrast injection through the tube demonstrates the tip distal to the ligament of Treitz.

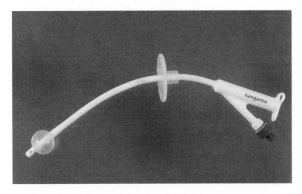

Figure 10-3 14F nontapered balloon-retention catheter (Kangaroo, Sherwood Medical, St. Louis, MO). This is left in place for 4 weeks until the skin-level tube is available.

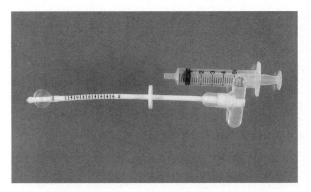

Figure 10-4 MIC-Key Stoma Measuring Device (Ballard Medical Products, Draper, UT).

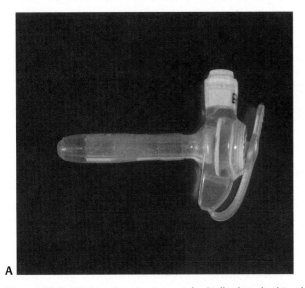

A

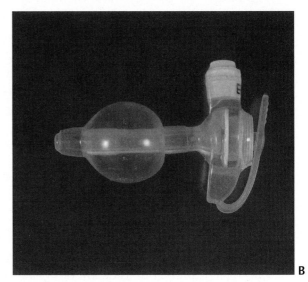

B

Figure 10-5 MIC-Key G gastrostomy tube (Ballard Medical Products, Draper, UT). (**A**) Balloon deflated. (**B**) Balloon inflated. These are "custom-sized" to each patient based on the measured length of the percutaneous tract.

We wait 6 weeks after initial gastrostomy tube placement before making the first exchange. The minimum diameter of the skin-level tube is 14F, so the tract must be "upsized" from the initial 12F catheter. We initially place a 14F, nontapered balloon-retention catheter (Kangaroo, Sherwood Medical) (**Fig. 10-3**), which is left in place for 4 weeks until the skin-level tube is available. Upsizing this small amount is usually easily accomplished, even though the 14F tube is not tapered to a guide wire. The exchange is performed over a stiff guide wire (Amplatz Extra, Stiff, Cook Canada) with the use of topical 2% lidocaine gel to reduce discomfort. It is important to confirm that the 14F tube is appropriately positioned in the stomach because a difficult exchange could disrupt the tract. At this point, the length of the tract is measured either using the device supplied by the button gastrostomy tube manufacturer (MIC-Key Stoma Measuring Device, Ballard Medical Products, Draper, UT) (**Fig. 10-4**) or by the marks on the balloon-retention tube.

The button gastrostomy tubes (MIC-Key G gastrostomy tube, Ballard Medical Products) (**Fig. 10-5**) must be "custom-sized" to each patient based on the length of the percutaneous tract. A tube that is too short places excessive pressure on the tract and is more prone to accidental dislodgement. A tube that is too long tends to move within and enlarge the tract, resulting in pericatheter leakage. It is not practical to stock the many different lengths of the skin-level gastrostomy tubes within the radiology department. Instead, the tube is "custom-ordered" for each patient.

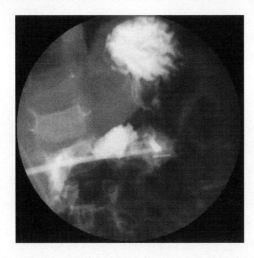

Figure 10-6 Contrast injection through the indwelling skin-level gastrostomy tube demonstrating satisfactory positioning.

We usually wait an additional 4 weeks to make the final exchange to the skin-level tube. Although we make this exchange on the fluoroscopy table, in most cases, neither fluoroscopy nor a guide wire is required. A guide wire should, however, be used if the exchange is difficult or if resistance is encountered. Appropriate positioning of the skin-level tube is confirmed with contrast injection (**Fig. 10-6**).

Borge et al (1995) placed 52 gastrostomy buttons in 27 children and encountered tract disruption in three patients. They concluded that fluoroscopic visualization was critical to avoid incorrect placement of these devices, particularly if there is a long tract length (>4 cm). All three cases of tract disruption in their series occurred with tracts <3 months old. They routinely overdilate the tracts by 2F to facilitate tube placement. Although we convert our patients to skin-level tubes at ~2.5 months, we use smaller caliber tubes than those authors (14F as opposed to 18 or 24F used by Borge et al [1995]).

A radiological technique for placing "pull" type gastrostomy tubes has also been described (Szymski et al 1997, Cahill et al 2001, Maetani et al 2003). Percutaneous access to the stomach is obtained and the wire is brought out through the mouth. This addresses concerns regarding tube size because large caliber tubes (up to 24F) may be placed with this technique. A significant advantage of the pull-type tube is its retention mechanism. Pull-type tubes have an internal disc that is "dragged" through the mouth. It is either very difficult or impossible to pull these tubes out, and they cannot be deflated or unlocked, unlike push-type balloon-retention or locking-loop pigtail gastrostomy tubes. Removal of these tubes, however, usually requires endoscopy. Although some suggest that the catheter may be cut at the skin to allow the internal component to fall into the stomach and be passed through the bowel, there have been reports of these catheter fragments becoming impacted and perforating the bowel. Because the tube passes through the oral cavity, preprocedure antibiotics are given with this technique.

Several specific issues relating to percutaneous enteral feeding tube insertion are addressed in the next sections.

Gastropexy

T-fasteners may be used in the enteric access procedures to fix the anterior gastric wall to the anterior abdominal wall (gastropexy). Their use for radiological gastrostomy or gastrojejunostomy is controversial. Proponents state that gastropexy:

1. facilitates placement of larger caliber (14F or greater) tubes.
2. reduces the frequency of peritonitis from spillage occuring around the catheter
3. facilitates replacement of a catheter that has been inadvertently dislodged before tract maturation (1–3 weeks depending on the patient's healing abilities).

Several studies, however, have shown no difference in patient outcome regardless of whether gastropexy is used. We routinely use gastropexy and believe it is beneficial because many of our patients have impaired tissue healing secondary to malnourishment or chemotherapy.

Patients with Ascites

Large-volume ascites has been considered a contraindication to percutaneous enteral access. Risks include peritoneal fluid contamination from leakage of gastric contents and the prolonged leakage of ascites from the skin site. Studies reporting significantly increased complications and mortality from percutaneous enteral access in patients with ascites led to recommendations for surgical gastrostomies in these patients. However, even surgical gastrostomies have significant complications. Ryan et al (1998) developed a paracentesis/gastropexy protocol for enteral access in patients with massive ascites. Paracentesis was performed immediately before and multiple times after the enteral access procedure for up to 4 weeks. Their goal was to eliminate fluid between the stomach and anterior abdominal wall to allow maturation and healing of the gastrostomy tract. Four-point gastropexy was also performed and the sutures left in place for 4 weeks. Only two of 45 patients (4%) in their series developed peritonitis or leakage of ascitic fluid. They concluded that enteral access in patients with ascites is safe and can be offered to patients with malignant ascites and bowel obstruction requiring gastric decompression.

Management of Gastrostomy or Gastrojejunostomy Tube Leakage

Pericatheter leakage is a common problem with enteral access tubes. Early leakage before tract maturation may result in peritoneal contamination and peritonitis. Gastric contents are very acidic and cause skin breakdown, which can also become a significant problem. In addition, a superficial peri-catheter dermatitis may progress to a serious abdominal wall infection, which can be fatal, if untreated.

For patients with gastric outlet obstruction, it is mandatory to place a gastrojejunostomy as opposed to a gastrostomy tube. Frequently, these patients will require a dual-lumen gastrostomy–gastrojejunostomy catheter or two separate tubes for simultaneous enteral feeding and gastric decompression. Pericatheter leakage may result from unintentional gastric feeding if the gastrojejunostomy tube has migrated back or is leaking into the stomach. If this is the case, the tube should be exchanged or repositioned. It is important to exclude bowel obstruction or ileus as a cause for pericatheter leakage. Some authors advocate gastric motility agents (e.g., metoclopramide) or drugs to reduce gastric secretions (e.g., omeprazole). If these measures fail, upsizing the tube may help, but it is occasionally necessary to remove the tube and place a new tube at a different site once the old site has healed.

PEARLS AND PITFALLS_____

- Enteral access is required for enteral feeding and occasionally for decompression.
- Fluoroscopy-guided techniques for enteral access have success and complication rates of ~95% and 5%, respectively.
- Routine use of T-anchors for gastropexy is controversial, but this technique is recommended for patients with ascites needing enteral access.
- Radiologically placed gastrostomy catheters can be exchanged for "button" gastrostomy devices. Because tract disruption can occur during insertion of these nontapered tubes, this must be undertaen with caution. A guide wire is used if the exchange is difficult or if resistance is encountered, and appropriate positioning is confirmed fluoroscopically with contrast injection.

- The "leaking" enteral tube is a common problem that can usually be managed conservatively. Upsizing the tube may help if conservative measures fail; however, it is occasionally necessary to remove the tube and place a new one at a different site once the old site has healed.

Further Reading

de Baere T, Chapot R, Kuoch V. Percutaneous gastrostomy with fluoroscopic guidance: single-center experience in 500 consecutive cancer patients. Radiology 1999;210:651–654

Barkmeier JM, Trerotola SO, Wiebke EA. Percutaneous radiologic, surgical endoscopic and percutaneous endoscopic gastrostomy/gastrojejunostomy: comparative study and cost analysis. Cardiovasc Intervent Radiol 1998;21:324–328

Bell SD, Carmody EA, Yeung EY. Percutaneous gastrostomy and gastrojejunostomy: additional experience in 519 procedures. Radiology 1995;194:817–820

Borge MA, Vesely TM, Picus D. Gastrostomy button placement through percutaneous gastrostomy tracts created with fluoroscopic guidance: experience in 27 children. J Vasc Interv Radiol 1995; 6:179–183.

Cahill AM, Kaye RD, Fitz CR, et al. "Push-pull" gastrostomy: a new technique for percutaneous gastrostomy tube insertion in the neonate and young infant. Pediatr Radiol 2001;31:550-554

Ho CS, Yeung EY. Percutaneous gastrostomy and transgastric jejunostomy. AJR Am J Roentgenol 1992;158:251–257

Maetani I, Tada T, Ukita T, et al. PEG with introducer or pull method: a prospective randomized comparison. Gastrointest Endosc 2003;57:837–841

McLoughlin RF, So B, Gray RR. Fluoroscopically guided percutaneous gastrostomy: current status. Can Assoc Radiol J 1996;47:10–15

Pien EC, Hume KE, Pien FD. Gastrostomy tube infections in a community hospital. Am J Infect Control 1996;24:353–358

Ryan JM, Hahn PF, Mueller PR. Performing gastrostomy or gastrojejunostomy in patients with malignant ascites. AJR Am J Roentgenol 1998;171:1003–1006

Safadi BY, Marks JM, Ponsky JL. Percutaneous endoscopic gastrostomy: an update. Endoscopy 1998;30:781–789

Szymski GX, Albazzaz AN, Funaki B et al. Radiologically guided placement of pull-type gastrostomy tubes. Radiology 1997;205:669–673

CHAPTER 11 Strictured Enteric Anastomosis

David J.M. Peck and Richard N. Rankin

Clinical Presentation

A 55-year-old obese female presented with a history of recurrent intolerance to solid and liquid food associated with nausea and vomiting. Approximately 3 months earlier she had undergone a transverse stapled gastroplasty with a Marlex-wrapped greater curve stoma. This had been complicated by obstruction, which necessitated two revisions and ultimately required the creation of a second gastrogastrostomy stoma on the greater curve end of the staple line. Despite this, difficulty with retention of high-density foods persisted. At this time, her weight had decreased to 81 kg.

Radiological Studies

An upper gastrointestinal (GI) series showed the previous gastroplasty as well as the gastrogastrostomy, which had a stomal diameter of 5 mm (**Fig. 11-1**).

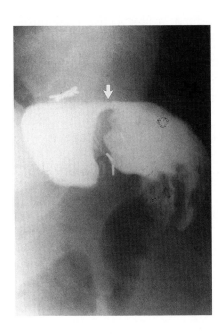

Figure 11-1 Radiograph from an upper gastroinstestinal series showing the gastroplasty and gastrogastrostomy. The diameter of the stoma (arrow) measured 5 mm.

Diagnosis

Gastrogastrostomy stomal obstruction

Treatment

Due to the reduced stomal diameter and persistent symptoms, balloon dilation was performed via a transoral approach following oropharyngeal anesthesia with topical lidocaine spray. The stomach was catheterized with a selective angiographic catheter (Cobra 2, Cook Canada, Stouffville, ON), which

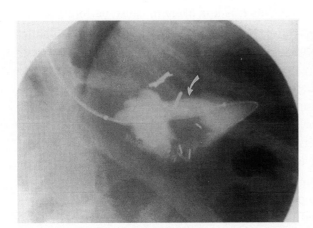

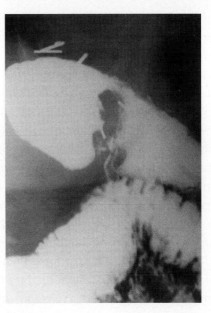

Figure 11-2 Image showing the 12 mm angioplasty balloon catheter across the narrowed stoma (curved arrow). Maximum inflation pressure was required to eliminate the waist on the balloon, which was kept inflated for several seconds.

Figure 11-3 Follow-up upper gastrointestinal series demonstrates a 12 mm stoma.

was coated with lubricating jelly to facilitate oropharyngeal passage and maneuvering. Air was injected into the stomach as a contrast agent and images from the prior upper gastrointestinal (UGI) series were used as a road map. The stoma was identified and traversed using the catheter and a steerable guide wire (Ring-Lunderquist torque guide, Cook Canada). After the catheter was advanced into the distal stomach, it was exchanged for a 12 mm angioplasty balloon catheter. The stoma was dilated using sufficient inflation pressure to eliminate the waist on the balloon (**Fig. 11-2**). The balloon was left inflated for several seconds.

Following dilation of the stoma, there was symptomatic improvement, though occasional vomiting with high-density foods persisted. This was felt to be, at least in part, due to the unusual position of the stoma in relation to the gastric pouch. The patient's weight stabilized at 80 kg and a UGI series demonstrated a 12 mm stoma (**Fig. 11-3**). Long-term radiological follow-up showed the stomal diameter to have stabilized at 11 mm. The patient experienced a steady weight gain despite dietary restrictions with the last recorded weight at 106 kg.

Discussion

Interventional radiologists can facilitate successful treatment of a wide range of enteric strictures by applying to the GI tract techniques used elsewhere in the body. Traditionally, sequential dilation (bougienage) has been the nonoperative method for the management of enteric strictures. Originally described in 1821, this had been the mainstay in therapy but has now been supplanted by balloon dilatation. For both the upper and lower GI tracts, balloon dilatation is now the preferred method for nonoperative management of most GI strictures because of its efficacy and relative safety. It is used for both postoperative as well as nonanastomotic strictures. Fluoroscopy, endoscopy, or a combination of both has provided guidance for balloon dilatation.

The technical success rates for balloon dilatation of enteric strictures are between 77 and 100%. Failures result from an inability to traverse the stricture or are due to patient intolerance. Immediate symptomatic relief is seen in up to 79% of cases. Long-term symptomatic relief is reported in 63 to 83% of cases. Repeat dilatation is not uncommon, with up to 45% of cases requiring two or more dilatations to become asymptomatic.

Balloon dilatation has numerous advantages over the traditional bougienage therapy. The balloon applies a direct radial force against the narrowing and thus it is less likely to cause perforation. The traditional bougie method exerts a longitudinal shearing force through the stricture with a higher risk of perforation. Furthermore, use of the Seldinger technique with steerable catheters and guide wires permits access via tortuous routes previously inaccessible to sequential dilation. It also permits access to severe strictures where bougienage is likely to fail. Often, only a single balloon inflation is sufficient for adequate treatment, resulting in improved patient comfort. In comparison, multiple passes are required for sequential dilation. Fluoroscopic monitoring of the procedure permits assessment of the stricture and also the viscus on either side.

In the stomach, balloon dilatation has been used for anastomotic as well as nonanastomotic strictures. Although described mostly for stomal stenosis following gastric surgery, balloon dilatation has also been used to treat stenosis secondary to peptic ulcer disease. A transoral approach is used and endoscopy, fluoroscopy, or both have provided procedural guidance. Balloon diameters of 12 to 15 mm are routinely used.

Complications

The overall rate of complications for balloon dilatation of enteric strictures ranges from 0 to 4.5%. Complications include mucosal tears and perforations secondary to transmural passage of the guide wire or from balloon expansion. In comparison, complication rates for the traditional bougie techniques are as high as 9%.

PEARLS AND PITFALLS

- Balloon dilation of GI strictures is safe and effective and can be considered as a primary method of treatment prior to surgical intervention.
- Repeat dilatation may be necessary in up to 45% of cases to maintain symptomatic relief.
- Balloon dilatation can be used for anastomotic and nonanastomotic strictures.

Further Reading

Kozarek RA. Hydrostatic balloon dilation of gastrointestinal stenosis: a national survey. Gastrointest Endosc 1986;32:15–19

Lindor KD, Ott BJ, Hughes RW Jr. Balloon dilatation of upper digestive tract strictures. Gastroenterology 1985;89:545–548

McLean GK, Cooper GS, Hartz WH, et al. Radiologically guided balloon dilation of gastrointestinal strictures, II: results of long-term follow-up. Radiology 1987;165:41–43

McNicholas MM, Gibney RG, MacErlaine DP. Radiologically guided balloon dilatation of obstructing gastrointestinal strictures. Abdom Imaging 1994;19:102–107

Whitworth PW, Richardson RL, Larson GM. Balloon dilatation of anastomotic strictures. Arch Surg 1988;123:759–762

CHAPTER 12 Malignant Colonic Obstruction

I.W. Choo

Clinical Presentation

A 70-year-old man presented with a 3-month history of lower abdominal pain and a 10 kg weight loss associated with severe abdominal distension, frequent diarrhea, and intermittent bloody stool.

Radiological Studies

An abdominal radiograph (not shown) obtained in the emergency room demonstrated severe distension of the small and large bowel with multiple air-fluid levels. Barium enema demonstrated complete obstruction of the sigmoid colon and a fistula between the sigmoid colon and proximal jejunum (**Fig. 12-1**).

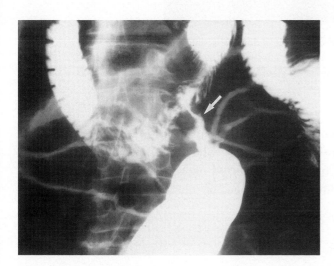

Figure 12-1 Barium enema demonstrates complete obstruction of the sigmoid colon by tumor. A fistulous communication (arrow) is seen between the sigmoid colon and proximal jejunum.

Diagnosis

Intestinal obstruction and jejunocolic fistula from carcinoma of the sigmoid colon

Treatment

A 5 French Kumpe catheter was introduced into the rectum and a 0.035 in. guide wire (Radifocus M wire guide, Terumo, Tokyo, Japan) was advanced to the obstruction. The guide wire was used to cross the stenotic segment, and the catheter was advanced into the proximal descending colon. The length of obstruction was measured with the guide wire as it was withdrawn. The guide wire was then exchanged for an Amplatz super-stiff wire (Boston Scientific, Watertown, MA). A 22 mm diameter covered metallic stent (Choo stent, Solco Intermed, Seoul, South Korea) was then inserted over the guide wire and placed across the stenotic segment and fistula opening. Upon deployment, the stent expanded immediately to >90% of its unconstrained diameter. An upright abdominal radiograph and

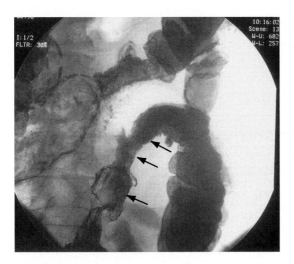

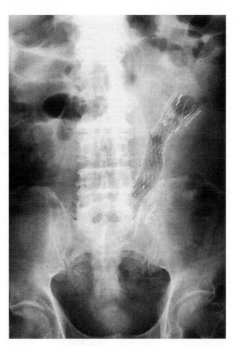

Figure 12-2 Barium study after stent deployment shows relief of intestinal obstruction and occlusion of the fistula. The stent is fully expanded and there is no obstruction to the passage of barium through the stent (arrows).

Figure 12-3 Upright abdominal radiograph shows no evidence for intestinal obstruction and full expansion of the stent in the sigmoid colon.

repeat barium study showed relief of intestinal obstruction and occlusion of the fistula (**Figs. 12-2** and **12-3**). There was no obstruction to the passage of barium through the stent, which was now fully expanded. Three days later, surgery was performed. The tumor was resected and an end-to-end anastomosis of the sigmoid colon was performed. In addition, the segment of jejunum that was involved by fistula was resected.

Discussion

Mechanical obstruction is a common complication of advanced colorectal cancer, particularly if the lesion is located in the left colon. Obstruction is also a rare complication of serosal seeding of advanced rectosigmoid carcinoma. It has been estimated that 8 and 29% of patients with colorectal cancer will have partial or complete intestinal obstruction, respectively.

Acute malignant obstruction of the large bowel is a surgical emergency that carries a poor prognosis. Although there is controversy over the optimal surgical approach, the traditional treatment for patients with distal colonic obstruction consists of a two-stage operative procedure: an initial decompressive colostomy and tumor resection, followed by a second operation for an end-to-end anastomosis. However, surgery is generally not an option for patients who are unfit for general anesthesia, are in poor general condition, or have disseminated neoplastic disease. In such patients, the incidence of postoperative complications is high because of inadequate bowel preparation and the poor general health associated with colonic obstruction. On the other hand, the mortality rate decreases from 15 to 20% to 0.9 to 6.0% when these patients undergo elective surgery.

To decrease the perioperative morbidity and mortality, nonsurgical methods have been used for emergent preoperative decompression of colorectal obstruction. These include dilation (with a bougie or angioplasty balloon), placement of rectal tubes, cryotherapy, electrocoagulation, and insertion of metallic stents. Reports indicate favorable results, emphasizing the usefulness and effectiveness of metallic stents for both preoperative decompression and palliative relief of colonic obstruction.

The Wallstent (Boston Scientific) is one of the commonly used stents in Western hospitals. Several covered stents are now available including the Choo colorectal stent (a self-made Gianturco stent, with design similar to that of the Z-stent), Wallstent, and nitinol stent endoprostheses (Viabahn, W.L. Gore, Flagstaff, AZ). Choo's colorectal stent has evolved from the original design consisting of a polyurethane-covered stainless steel Gianturco stent to the bare nitinol wire stent. The original design was made of 0.4 mm diameter stainless steel wire according to the mesh design of the Gianturco stent. The 3 mm gaps between each segment of body strut, which was made of polyurethane only, provided excellent flexibility. The outer diameter of the delivery system was 7 mm (21 French).

A covered stent is usually not necessary in patients who are to subsequently undergo surgery. Therefore, we now prefer to use the uncovered metallic stent constructed with nitinol wire, which can be introduced through a 12F-diameter introducer system. Covered stents are necessary for patients with enteroenteric fistula and for palliative relief of obstruction where the stent covering prevents tumor ingrowth.

The only absolute contraindication for stent placement is clinical or radiological evidence for intestinal perforation. Complications of colorectal stenting include intestinal perforation, stent migration (especially the covered stents), pain, tenesmus, bleeding, tumor ingrowth or overgrowth, and stent fracture. Post-stenting pain can be severe when the stent interferes with the function of the anal sphincter complex. Therefore, a stent should be placed only in lesions that are located at least 5 cm proximal from the anal verge.

In the patient described, we were able to seal the fistulous tract from the colonic lumen by using the covered metallic stent. Exclusion of the fistula decreases the inflammation around the lesion and also prevents intraoperative spillage of intestinal contents, thereby facilitating the surgery.

PEARLS AND PITFALLS_____

- Metallic stents are useful for preoperative or palliative decompression of acute colorectal obstruction.
- Despite the incidence of migration, the covered stent is both useful and effective for sealing of enteroenteric fistulas.
- Nonsurgical preoperative decompression of colorectal obstruction with a metallic stent reduces the operative morbidity and mortality.
- A colorectal stent should be placed >5 cm above the anal.

Further Reading

Choo IW, Do YS, Suh SW, et al. Malignant colorectal obstruction: treatment with a flexible covered stent. Radiology 1998;206:415–421

Lo SK. Metallic stenting for colorectal obstruction. Gastrointest Endosc Clin N Am 1999;9:459–477

Mainar A, de Gregorio MA, Tejero E, et al. Acute colorectal obstruction: treatment with self-expandable metallic stents before scheduled surgery: results of a multicenter study. Radiology 1999;210:65–69

Saida Y, Sumiyama Y, Nagao J, et al. Stent endoprosthesis for obstructing colorectal cancers. Dis Colon Rectum 1996;39:552–555

Zollikofer CL, Jost R, Schoch E, et al. Gastrointestinal stenting. Eur Radiol 2000;10:329–341

CHAPTER 13 Intussuception

Matthias H. Schmidt and Douglas J. Moote

Clinical Presentation

A 2-year-old boy was brought to the emergency department with a 24-hour history of irritability, vomiting, and drawing up his legs. On examination, no mass was palpable.

Radiological Studies

Abdominal radiographs demonstrated scant bowel gas and a subtle mass outlined by a crescent of air in the right side of the abdomen. The liver edge was indistinct (**Fig. 13-1**). Ultrasound examination confirmed the presence of an abdominal mass to the right of the umbilicus. The mass had a layered appearance, characteristic of an intussusception: a hypoechoic core (the entering portion of the intussusceptum), an outer hypoechoic layer (a combination of intussuscipiens and returning portion of intussusceptum), and an eccentric hyperechoic crescent (mesenteric fat carried along by the intussusceptum) separating the entering portion of the intussusceptum from the intussuscipiens. Ultrasound also demonstrated a trace of fluid trapped between the serosal surfaces of the entering and returning portions of the intussusceptum (**Fig. 13-2**).

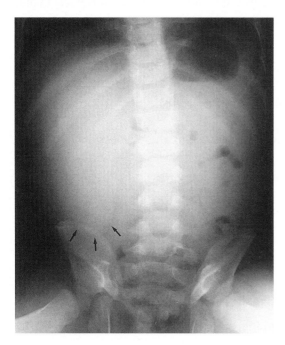

Figure 13-1 Erect radiograph of the abdomen. There is relative paucity of bowel gas on the right side of the abdomen. A mass is delineated by a crescent of air (arrows). The liver edge is indistinct.

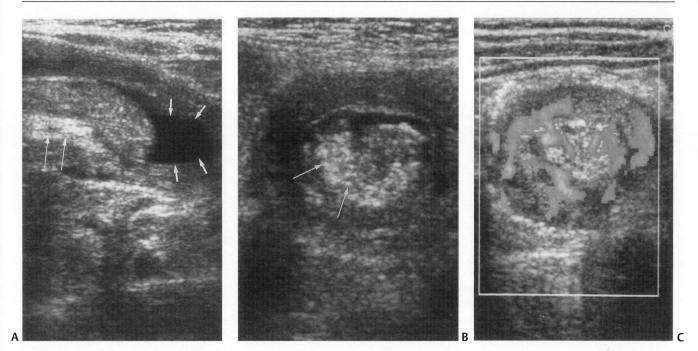

Figure 13-2 Ultrasound examination of the abdomen. (**A**) Longitudinal section through the intussusception. Fluid is trapped between the serosal surfaces of the intussusceptum (short arrows). Long arrows point to the mesenteric fat. (**B**) Transverse section through the intussusception. The eccentric hyperechoic mesenteric fat (long arrows) is characteristic of intussusception. (**C**) Transverse section through the intussusception. Blood flow is identified in the intussusceptum and the intussuscipiens by color Doppler.

Diagnosis

Ileocolic intussusception

Treatment

Following surgical consultation, the patient was taken to the fluoroscopy suite and placed in the prone position. An enema tip with anal occlusion disk was inserted into the patient's rectum and was taped in place. Additional tape was applied across the buttocks to keep them in close apposition. The enema tip was connected to the Shiels Intussusception Air Reduction System (Custom Medical Products Inc., Maineville, OH). This system consists of flexible tubing, a filter, a three-way stopcock for immediate colonic decompression, and an insufflator bulb with a pressure gauge. The leading edge of the intussusception was identified fluoroscopically, and air was insufflated at a resting pressure not exceeding 105 mm Hg. Reduction of the intussusception was monitored fluoroscopically. Reduction was deemed complete when the mass in the colon had disappeared and there was copious reflux of air into the small bowel (**Fig. 13-3**).

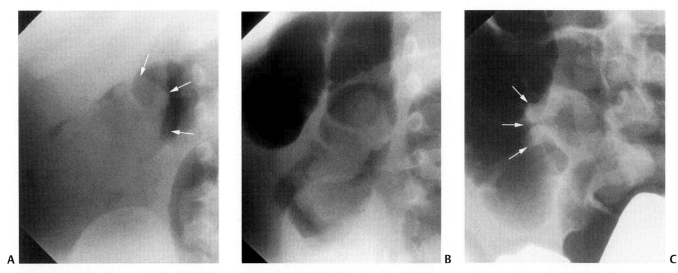

A   B   C

Figure 13-3 Air enema reduction of intussusception. (**A**) The intussusceptum appears as a soft tissue mass (arrows) in the hepatic flexure. (**B**) The intussusceptum has been partially reduced to the ascending colon. (**C**) The intussusception has been completely reduced. The only soft tissue remaining in the region of the cecum is the ileocecal valve (arrows). There is copious reflux of air into the small intestine.

Discussion

Ileocolic intussusception typically affects children between the ages of 6 months and 2 years. It occurs more commonly in autumn and winter, when viral illness is prevalent. Intussusception is thought to be the result of reactive hyperplasia of ileal lymphoid tissue, which acts as a lead point for the invagination of the ileum into the colon. Ileoileal intussusception and colocolic intussusception may also occur, but this is relatively rare. When patients fall outside the typical age range, or when the intussusception is not of the typical ileocolic variety, an unusual lead point, such as a Meckel's diverticulum, hematoma, or neoplasm, may be responsible. Many patients do not present with the classic clinical triad of intermittent abdominal pain, abdominal mass, and "currant jelly" stools. Indeed, the clinical history is often nonspecific, and clinical diagnosis is delayed. Imaging plays a major role in diagnosis and treatment.

The diagnostic and therapeutic sequence of radiographs, sonography, and air enema has gained widespread acceptance. Radiographs are often the first study requested. Their most useful contribution may be the identification of visceral perforation or small bowel obstruction. Typical radiographic findings of ileocolic intussusception include a paucity of bowel gas on the right side of the abdomen, a mass in the right upper quadrant, and an associated crescent of air or mesenteric fat. Indistinctness of the liver edge may also be noted. However, radiographs of the abdomen are often nonspecific and, most importantly, lack sensitivity. They may strengthen the clinical suspicion of intussusception, but they are not considered an appropriate screening test to exclude this diagnosis.

The value of sonography as a screening test has been demonstrated by studies that have consistently reported sensitivities ranging from 92 to 100%. Because false negatives can still occur, an enema should be performed after a negative ultrasound examination if the clinical suspicion is high or if there is a palpable mass that is not adequately explained by ultrasound. False-positive diagnoses are rare and are generally revealed as such by a subsequent enema.

Several sonographic signs of intussusception have been described, including the "donut" or "target" sign (in short axis images) and the "sandwich" or "hay fork" sign (in long axis images). The appearance of intussusception has also been given the designation "pseudokidney." All of these terms reflect the layered arrangement of the intussuscipiens, the intussusceptum, and the accompanying mesenteric fat carried along by the intussusceptum. It is the hyperechoic mesenteric fat that is particularly helpful in distinguishing an intussusception from other abdominal masses. One of the strengths of ultrasound is its ability to demonstrate an unusual lead point or to suggest an alternative diagnosis. Occasionally, the completeness of reduction is uncertain following an enema, and ultrasound can be helpful by demonstrating a residual intussusception.

Patients who present with symptoms of more than 48 hours duration, with dehydration, bloody stool, or small bowel obstruction are less likely to be treated successfully by enema. Also, patients younger than 3 months or older than 5 years are less likely to be reduced in this fashion. Although bowel wall thickening and fluid trapped between the apposed serosal surfaces of the intussusceptum have been touted as sonographic predictors of irreducibility by enema, they are seen not infrequently in intussusceptions that yield to radiological intervention. Their presence should not discourage an attempt at reduction. However, lack of demonstrable blood flow on color Doppler examination is thought to be a predictor of irreducibility by enema and is correlated with the finding of necrotic bowel at surgery. In such cases, attempted enema reduction may still be partially successful and may facilitate subsequent surgical reduction. However, attempts should be made with great caution because of the increased risk of perforation.

The only absolute contraindications to attempted enema reduction of intussusception are shock that has not responded to rehydration, physical findings of peritonitis, and radiographic evidence of perforation. A small amount of free intraperitoneal fluid is seen in uncomplicated intussusception and is not considered a contraindication to enema reduction. Although it was previously considered good practice to follow the "rule of threes" (barium enema bag 3 feet above the table, hydrostatic pressure applied for 3 minutes at a time, maximum of 3 successive attempts), more recent publications advocate a more aggressive approach without specifying exact limits. It seems reasonable to continue with the reduction attempt as long as the intussusception continues to move. If the intussusception moves during an initial reduction attempt but it cannot be reduced completely, it is reasonable to perform delayed, repeated reduction attempts as long as the patient remains stable.

During air enema reduction, it is considered prudent to limit the resting pressure to 105 mm Hg in most patients, or to 80 mm Hg in those patients considered to be at high risk of perforation. An automatic pressure relief device can be added to the Shiels Intussusception Air Reduction System to protect against excessive baseline pressures. Transient pressure spikes, far in excess of baseline, occur when the patient cries or strains. These pressure spikes are not considered to be dangerous because intra abdominal pressure balances intracolonic pressure. Indeed, the ability of the patient to generate a high intra abdominal pressure may protect against perforation. Therefore, premedication with sedatives or muscle relaxants is not advisable.

There has been considerable debate in the literature over the relative merits of air versus barium enema in the treatment of intussusception. Proponents of the air enema cite a higher success rate, lower radiation dose, and less morbidity in the event of perforation. Tension pneumoperitoneum is a recognized, potentially lethal complication of the air enema. However, it is rare, readily recognized fluoroscopically, and effectively treated by 18 gauge needle puncture through the anterior abdominal wall. On the other hand, proponents of the barium enema quote a lower incidence of perforation, better ability to detect pathological lead points, and greater confidence when assessing the completeness of reduction. We favor the air enema, but do occasionally use positive contrast material when marked dilatation of the small bowel is likely to obscure the intussusception.

Ultrasound-guided reduction of intussusception with saline enema has been reported but has not yet gained widespread acceptance in North America. This approach seems appealing because it would be a natural extension of the diagnostic ultrasound examination, would spare the patient the radiation associated with fluoroscopy, and would permit easy identification of residual intussusception after reflux of infusate into the proximal small bowel. Likely, the best method to use in a given chapter depends upon operator experience and comfort with the technique.

PEARLS AND PITFALLS⎯⎯⎯⎯⎯⎯⎯⎯⎯⎯⎯⎯⎯⎯⎯⎯⎯⎯⎯⎯⎯⎯⎯⎯⎯⎯⎯⎯

- The clinical history and physical findings of intussusception are often nonspecific. A high index of suspicion is appropriate.
- Ultrasound is a superior screening tool compared with radiographs.
- The absolute contraindications to attempted enema reduction are refractory shock, clinical evidence of peritonitis, and radiographic evidence of bowel perforation.
- Clinical or radiological risk factors for irreducibility or comprised bowel viability mandate a more cautious approach, using lower resting pressures.
- A pediatric surgeon should be consulted before enema reduction is attempted.
- Tension pneumoperitoneum is a potentially lethal complication of air enema. An 18 gauge needle must be immediately available to treat this complication.
- The choice of method (air versus hydrostatic enema) depends upon local experience and operator comfort. Air enema is favored in most pediatric hospitals in North America.

Further Reading

Daneman A, Alton DJ. Intussusception: issues and controversies related to diagnosis and reduction. Radiol Clin North Am 1996;34:743–756

Del Pozo G, Albillos JC, Tejedor D, et al. Intussusception in children: current concepts in diagnosis and enema reduction. Radiographics 1999;19:299–319

Guo J-z, Ma X-y, Zhou O-h. Results of air pressure enema reduction of intussusception: 6,396 cases in 13 years. J Pediatr Surg 1986;21:1201–1203

Hadidi AT, El Shal N. Childhood intussusception: a comparative study of nonsurgical management. J Pediatr Surg 1999;34:304–307

Kirks DR. Air intussusception reduction: the winds of change. Pediatr Radiol 1995;25:89–91

Navarro OM, Daneman A, Chae A. Intussusception: the use of delayed, repeated reduction attempts and the management of intussusceptions due to pathologic lead points in pediatric patients. AJR Am J Roentgenol 2004;182:1169–1176

Poznanski AK. Why I still use barium for intussusception. Pediatr Radiol 1995;25:92–93

Shiels WE, Bisset GS, Kirks DR. Simple device for air reduction of intussusception. Pediatr Radiol 1990;20:472–474

CHAPTER 14 Abdominal Abscess

Sulaiman Al-Basam and John D. Bennett

Clinical Presentation

A 46-year-old male presented with a 4-day history of malaise, anorexia, and right lower quadrant pain, which had worsened and was associated with fever and chills for 24 hours prior to admission. On physical examination, a tender mass could be palpated in the right lower quadrant associated with mild guarding. Laboratory values revealed an elevated leukocyte count of 19,000 cells/L associated with a "left shift." Hemoglobin, blood chemistry, and coagulation parameters were all within normal limits. The patient was started on intravenous broad-spectrum antibiotics.

Radiological Studies

Computed tomography (CT) of the abdomen demonstrated an 8 cm soft tissue mass in the right lower quadrant containing small bubbles of gas. It indented the superolateral aspect of the bladder with associated soft tissue stranding evident in the adjacent peritoneal fat (**Fig. 14-1**).

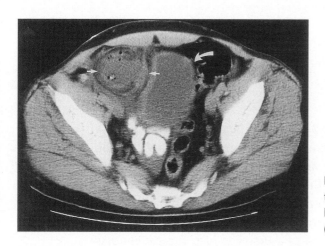

Figure 14-1 Pelvic computed tomography demonstrates an 8 cm soft tissue mass in the right lower quadrant (straight arrows) containing small bubbles of gas and indenting the superolateral aspect of the bladder (curved arrow).

Diagnosis

Right lower quadrant abscess

Treatment

In preparation for drainage, the patient was positioned supine on the CT table. Using the scanner's laser positioning guides, the position of the abscess was noted and marked. A radiopaque bead was placed over the intended puncture site and the patient rescanned to confirm a satisfactory approach.

The skin was cleansed with an antiseptic solution, the patient draped with sterile towels, and local anesthesia (2% lidocaine) infiltrated along the intended tract. A small skin incision was made

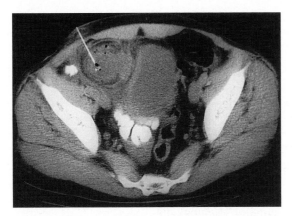

Figure 14-2 An 18 gauge needle has been advanced into the abscess. Purulent liquid was aspirated.

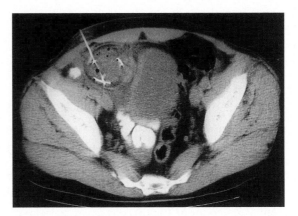

Figure 14-3 A guide wire has been inserted through the needle and is coiled within the abscess cavity.

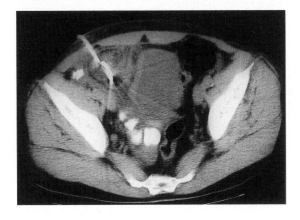

Figure 14-4 A 12F drainage catheter has been inserted over the wire.

and an 18 gauge needle advanced into the abscess (**Fig. 14-2**). Purulent fluid was aspirated and a sample obtained for microbiological evaluation. A guide wire (0.035 in. Amplatz extra-stiff, Cook Canada, Stouffville, ON) was inserted through the needle and coiled within the abscess cavity (**Fig. 14-3**). The tract was dilated and a 12F locking pigtail catheter (Flexima APDL, Boston Scientific, Watertown, MA) advanced over the wire and formed within the cavity (**Fig. 14-4**). The cavity was completely aspirated and repeatedly flushed with small quantities of normal saline until the return was nonpurulent. The tube was sutured in place and attached to a drainage bag. The patient was returned to the ward with instructions to flush the tube every 6 hours with normal saline.

The patient's pain and fever diminished over the next 48 hours. Drainage from the catheter was minimal after the first 24 hours. A follow-up CT scan at 4 days showed no residual abscess cavity, and the catheter was removed.

Discussion

Even as we enter the 21st century with continuing advances in modern antimicrobial therapy, intra-abdominal sepsis remains a significant cause of morbidity and mortality. Surgical drainage has long been established as a standard therapy for patients with infected fluid collections. Antibiotics, while necessary, serve primarily in an adjuvant role. Percutaneous drainage methods have evolved and are now firmly entrenched as a cornerstone of therapy in the management of this problem. With improvements in cross-sectional imaging and advances in catheter technology and drainage techniques, the scope of percutaneous abscess drainage is expanding such that the majority of infected intra-abdominal fluid collections are now amenable to image-guided percutaneous treatment.

Table 14-1 Interpretation of Results for Diagnostic Aspiration of Intra-abdominal Fluid Collections

Leukocytes	Bacteria	Growth	Probable Diagnosis
+	+	+	Abscess
+	+	−	Sterile (treated) abscess
+	−	−	Sterile (treated) abscess
−	+	+/−	Bowel contamination[a]
−	−	−	Noninfected collection

[a]Access route should be carefully reevaluated for possible transgression of bowel.

Ultrasound has gained wide acceptance in the evaluation of abdominal fluid collections and can be used to guide abscess drainage. Its portability allows these procedures to be performed at the bedside when necessary, a distinct benefit when dealing with unstable patients in the intensive care unit. Despite its advantages, ultrasound remains a technique that is highly operator-dependent and will tend to be more successful when performed by those with greater experience. Because sonography is limited by overlying gas and soft tissue, deep pelvic and interloop collections can be difficult to see, particularly in patients who are obese or who have extensive abdominal gas. Overlying incisions and wound dressings also limit sonographic visualization.

Therefore, CT is our preferred modality for the diagnosis and image-guided management of intra-abdominal and retroperitoneal abscesses. Adequate opacification of the bowel is of paramount importance for the accurate recognition of abdominal and pelvic fluid collections. Unopacified loops of bowel can closely mimic or be mimicked by these collections and result in misdiagnosis (and missed diagnoses). We prefer to use a dilute solution of water-soluble contrast (diatrizoate meglumine 1:40), which can be administered orally or through a tube inserted into the rectum, colostomy, or ileostomy. Despite the use of enteral contrast, segments of the gastrointestinal tract may remain unopacified and cause confusion. Repeat scanning following additional contrast or repositioning the patient (prone or decubitus) diminishes this problem.

Despite the contrast resolution of modern ultrasound and CT equipment, neither of these modalities can reliably distinguish infected from noninfected fluid. For this reason, diagnostic needle aspiration may be required to identify those collections requiring drainage. It is our practice to routinely aspirate all collections prior to drainage. If frankly purulent fluid is aspirated, we proceed immediately to catheter drainage. If the fluid obtained appears nonpurulent, Gram staining the aspirate may be useful. Visualizing leukocytes on the smear usually indicates an infected collection even if no organisms can be identified. Visualization of bacteria but no leukocytes on the smear can indicate intestinal contamination and should prompt careful reevaluation of the access route for possible transgression of bowel (**Table 14-1**). If no fluid can be aspirated, a small amount of saline can be injected and then aspirated to obtain material for Gram stain and culture.

Although small, simple collections may be adequately treated by needle aspiration alone, it is our practice to drain most infected collections with a catheter. For most collections, we use the Seldinger technique. For superficial collections where the window of access is large and unimpeded, a trocar ("one-stick") technique may be appropriate. The drainage catheter is back-loaded onto a trocar needle and the assembled unit advanced into the collection in one step. Once positioning is confirmed, the drainage catheter is advanced off the trochar, and the pigtail is allowed to form within the cavity. This technique has the advantage of being very quick; however, because initial access is with a large-diameter device, repeated punctures to get the optimal tube tract are not feasible.

Once the drainage catheter is in place, we immediately aspirate as much of the infected fluid as possible and then irrigate the cavity with multiple aliquots or normal saline, always taking care not to overdistend the cavity (which would precipitate hematological seeding of bacteria and lead to sepsis). The catheter is then sutured to the skin and placed on sealed gravity (bag) drainage. The catheter is flushed with normal saline at least four times per day to maintain patency, and output is documented on a daily basis. The catheter remains in place until output diminishes to ≤10 mL per day. The decision to discontinue catheter drainage is heavily weighted by the patient's clinical condition. Repeat imaging is not always required for uncomplicated cases where drainage steadily diminishes in the setting of clear clinical improvement. If there remains any question as to whether a decrease in drainage is due to resolution of the abscess or to catheter malfunction, we repeat cross-sectional imaging to evaluate the size of the collection and catheter positioning and to determine if any new loculations or collections have developed. Contrast injection into the abscess cavity is helpful in checking for enteric fistulas.

Success rates for percutaneous drainage of most infected abdominal fluid collections are in the 80% range. There is no doubt that percutaneous techniques will have greater success for small, simple collections. Transcatheter drainage is not as likely to be curative for complex collections and cannot obviate the need for surgery to correct an underlying abnormality; however, a beneficial initial effect can be expected in the majority of patients.

PEARLS AND PITFALLS_____

- The majority of infected intra-abdominal and retroperitoneal fluid collections are amenable to image-guided percutaneous treatment.
- We prefer CT for the diagnosis and image-guided management of intra-abdominal and retroperitoneal abscesses because sonography can be limited by overlying gas and soft tissues.
- All collections are initially aspirated. If purulent, a drainage catheter is inserted. If the fluid appears nonpurulent, a Gram stain is obtained (see **Table 14-1**).
- Once the catheter is in place, the abscess is evacuated. The cavity is irrigated with saline. Overdistension of the cavity is avoided to prevent hematogenous bacterial seeding and sepsis.
- Diminishing catheter output may be due to resolution of the abscess or to catheter malfunction. CT may be necessary to evaluate size of the collection and catheter position and to identify loculations or new collections.

Further Reading

Gazelle GS, Mueller PR. Abdominal abscess: imaging and intervention. Radiol Clin North Am 1994;32:913–932

Jeffrey RB Jr, Tolentino CS, Federle MP, et al. Percutaneous drainage of periappendiceal abscesses: review of 20 patients. AJR Am J Roentgenol 1987;149:59–62

Malangoni MA, Shumate CR, Thomas HA. Factors influencing the treatment of intra-abdominal abscesses. Am J Surg 1990;159:167–171

McLean TR, Simmons K, Svensson LG. Management of postoperative intra-abdominal abscesses by routine percutaneous drainage. Surg Gynecol Obstet 1993;176:167–171

van Sonnenberg E, D'Agostino HB, Casola G, et al. Percutaneous abscess drainage: current concepts. Radiology 1991;181:617–626

CHAPTER 15 Ultrasound-Guided Biopsy

Charles O'Malley

Clinical Presentation

A 49-year-old woman with a history of breast carcinoma was referred for liver biopsy. She had undergone abdominal computed tomography (CT) at another hospital, which showed multiple, small liver lesions that were suspicious for metastases. The patient was referred for an image-guided biopsy to confirm the diagnosis.

Radiological Studies

An ultrasound-guided biopsy was considered the most straightforward method for acquiring tissue because of the size and location of the hepatic lesions. The initial ultrasound scans showed multiple small lesions throughout the liver. One readily visible superficial lesion was located in the inferior aspect of the right hepatic lobe (**Fig. 15-1A**). This was targeted for biopsy. Using a 3.5 MHz phase linear array transducer with attached needle guide and color Doppler imaging, a tract to the lesion devoid of large blood vessels was identified (**Fig. 15-1B**). The corresponding skin entry site was identified and marked and the area was prepped and draped in the usual sterile fashion. Local anesthesia was administered and a small (2–3 mm) skin incision was made at the anticipated biopsy

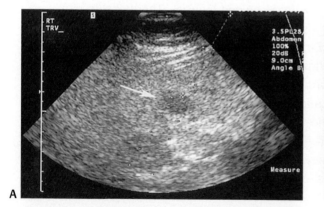

A

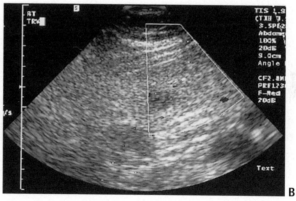

B

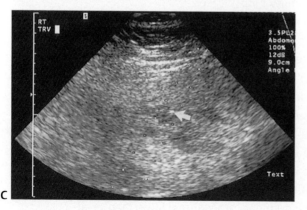

C

Figure 15-1 (**A**) A small (~12 mm), hypoechoic lesion is present in the inferior right hepatic lobe (arrow). The needle guide shows the intended path for the biopsy needle and distance from the skin surface to the lesion. (**B**) Color Doppler shows absence of significant vascular structures along the intended path for the biopsy needle. (**C**) A 22 gauge Chiba needle has been inserted and the tip lies in the lesion (arrow). Needle visualization was more apparent on real-time scanning.

needle entry site. Under direct ultrasound guidance, a 22 gauge Chiba needle (Cook, Incorp., Bloomington, IN) was advanced to the lesion and a sample was obtained by aspiration (**Fig. 15-1C**). The specimen was placed on slides and submitted for cytopathology analysis. Post-procedure color Doppler scans of the lesion and needle tract showed no abnormal blood flow in the tract and no evidence for a developing hematoma.

Diagnosis

Liver metastases from breast carcinoma

Discussion

Liver metastases are far more common than primary malignant liver neoplasms with the liver being the second most common site for metastasis after regional lymph nodes. Although large liver lesions, both benign and malignant, can have a characteristic appearance, many smaller lesions are indeterminate in appearance. With improved technology, more lesions of smaller size are detected with ultrasonography (US), CT, and magnetic resonance imaging (MRI). While these smaller lesions may be visible, further characterization may not be possible with current imaging techniques. Therefore, a biopsy may be required for a definitive diagnosis, especially in patients with a known malignancy. The primary purposes of a biopsy are to confirm or exclude malignancy, stage patients with known malignancy, and to monitor response to therapy. In an effort to better direct patient care, clinicians are increasing their requests for image-guided biopsies of these smaller, indeterminate lesions.

CT and US are the most common modalities employed for image-guided biopsies. The modality chosen for any given case depends upon the size, location, visibility, and accessibility of the lesion, and most importantly, the comfort level of the physician performing the procedure with these modalities. Many lesions may be accessible by either method; however, for small lesions (<1.5–2 cm), successful tissue acquisition is more easily accomplished with US guidance.

There are multiple advantages in using ultrasound for guiding biopsy procedures. These include needle guidance with real-time evaluation of the liver and lesion; real-time confirmation of the needle tip placement during the biopsy; color Doppler imaging for visualization and avoidance of blood vessels; and the potential for relatively simple needle placement in a nonaxial plane. Additionally, US-guided procedures are generally more cost-effective because they usually require less time. Further, the overhead costs for US are lower than those for CT. Lastly, the patient throughput for the CT scanner is not hindered with the more time-consuming biopsy cases.

In preparation for biopsy, any available imaging studies should be reviewed to confirm the presence of a lesion as well as the suitability of the lesion for biopsy. Subsequently, preliminary scans should be obtained at the time of the procedure to reassess the location of the lesion and to determine the shortest, safest needle path. If possible, a subcostal approach is preferred over an intercostal approach to avoid the risk of pneumothorax, injury to intercostal vessels, and contamination of the pleural space with tumor cells or microorganisms. However, we find that many upper hepatic lesions are best biopsied using an oblique intercostal approach.

Prior to the procedure, informed consent is obtained to include possible intravenous sedation, although it is uncommonly required. If intravenous sedation is anticipated or required, patients are kept NPO for at least 4 hours prior to the procedure. No specific, universally accepted guidelines exist regarding evaluation of the hemostatic function prior to image-guided procedures. Silverman et al have proposed preprocedure evaluation of hemostatic function based on the type of procedure to be performed and the patient's medical history. For biopsies, they recommend a screening prothrombin time (PT), partial thromboplastin time (PTT), and platelet count, even in patients who are at low risk for bleeding. In our practice, we will perform a biopsy in patients who do not reveal any risk factors for bleeding, without obtaining any screening tests.

Technique

At the time of biopsy, every attempt should be made to optimize patient comfort with positioning, analgesia, and if needed, sedation. After initial scanning and lesion localization, the skin entry site is marked with a pen. The skin is prepped and sterile draped. Subcutaneous local anesthesia is administered at the skin entry site. A sterile probe cover is then placed over the transducer and the biopsy guide is attached. At this time, using a longer needle (often a 22 gauge spinal needle), additional local anesthesia can be administered directly along the path of the needle guide. Although not required, performing a small (2–3 mm) skin incision at the intended skin entry site can help to avoid resistance or deflection of the needle as it is advanced toward a small lesion. After rehearsing breath-holding instructions with the patient, the biopsy is performed.

Fine needle aspiration (FNA) biopsy is usually done using a 22 gauge Chiba needle or 20 gauge Crown needle (Boston Scientific, Watertown, MA), both of which are end-cutting needles. It is imperative that the tip of the needle is visualized within the lesion to confirm a successful biopsy. Once the needle tip is in position, the stylet is removed and the needle is moved back and forth within the lesion and then removed without replacing the stylet. Using this capillary technique, we do not routinely aspirate during the biopsy. A single drop of "tissue" is placed on the slide, using the stylet. This is then smeared with another slide and placed in absolute alcohol. To facilitate assessment by cytopathology, no more than two slides are smeared. Any remaining tissue is then placed in a transport medium such as Cytolyt (Cytyc, Inc., Boxborough, ME) for cell block processing.

With the availability of an experienced cytopathologist, the reported sensitivity and specificity of FNA for localized, malignant liver lesions is very high (sensitivity, 84–94%; specificity, 80–100%). If a larger tissue sample is necessary, an 18 gauge automated side-cutting core needle with biopsy gun can be employed. The tip of the needle should be advanced to a position ~3 to 5 mm proximal to the lesion before the gun is activated, insuring that there is adequate tissue distal to the tip to accommodate the excursion of the needle.

After completion of the biopsy, the involved area should be rescanned to look for possible hematoma formation. Color Doppler evaluation of the needle tract may be helpful for detection of bleeding. If detected, direct pressure should be applied with the transducer or manually until it stops. If direct pressure is not possible, having the patient lie on the affected side may provide a tamponade effect.

Complications of liver FNA are uncommon. Minor complications include pain, vasovagal reaction, small hematoma, pneumothorax, and bacteremia. Pain and vasovagal reaction are most common and are observed in ~1 to 5% of patients. Fewer than 1% of patients develop a hematoma large enough to require transfusion. A pneumothorax can occur when an intercostal approach is used, due to transgression of the pleural space. However, it is rare unless aerated lung is also traversed. Major complications are very rare. The mortality rate for an image-guided percutaneous biopsy is 0.1%. Tumor seeding of the needle tract is also very rare, with a frequency ranging from 0.003 to 0.009%.

Several factors increase the chances for a successful US-guided biopsy. The most important is optimization of patient cooperation by making the patient physically as comfortable as possible and explaining the biopsy procedure and the steps involved. With appropriate education and assurance, the vast majority of patients will require only local anesthesia. However, for very anxious patients, conscious sedation may be needed. The patient who is comfortable is better able to cooperate with breath-holding instructions and can lie motionless during the procedure.

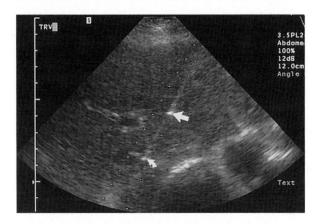

Figure 15-2 Image showing the coaxial technique for biopsy of a small liver metastasis from non–small cell lung carcinoma. The tip of the larger (18 gauge) introducer needle is seen along the path of the needle guide (straight arrow) and the tip (curved arrow) of the smaller, 22 gauge biopsy needle is present inferiorly in the faintly visualized lesion.

Optimal visualization of the lesion is also very important. A transducer that allows good contrast between the lesion and the surrounding liver is essential. For superficial lesions, a 7.5 MHz linear array transducer is usually appropriate, whereas a 3.5 MHz sector or phase linear array transducer is effective for deeper lesions. The sonographic imaging parameters should be optimized, especially the focus and field of view. The focus should be centered at the depth of the near border of the lesion and the field of view should be minimized to allow good visualization of the lesion. The field of view setting should, however, allow for the needle to traverse at least one third of the image diameter. Finally, for subtle lesions, decreasing the dynamic range or employing tissue harmonic imaging may be helpful to more clearly define the lesion from the surrounding parenchyma.

The use of a needle guide usually allows easier and faster visualization and direction of the tip of the biopsy needle into the appropriate location than the freehand technique. Visualization of the needle tip can be difficult using the guide but can be much more difficult without it. Other technical factors that increase the chances of successful US-guided biopsy include the use of a needle with an echogenic tip as well as movement of the needle (and/or stylet in the case of end-cutting needles) back and forth ~1 cm to help localize the tip within the liver when it is not otherwise seen. During advancement of the needle, it is critical to firmly stabilize the hand holding the transducer while keeping the lesion visible within the guides provided on the viewing screen.

If possible, advancing the needle in one steady, continuous motion to the lesion may give a better sense of its location than advancing in short, discontinuous segments while trying to localize the needle after each advance. Finally, rocking the transducer back and forth very slightly may help to localize a needle tip that has been deflected from the plane of scanning; however, the foot plate of the transducer cannot be moved because the needle and guide secure the transducer to the patient. For small lesions that are relatively deep, if the needle has veered from the scanning plane, placing the tip in the lesion may not be possible on that particular pass, and the needle may have to be withdrawn and redirected for a second pass.

If after several attempts the needle tip cannot be directed into the lesion due to the small size of the lesion and/or deflection of the needle, a co-axial technique may be considered before aborting the procedure. The same system is used, and instead of the 22 gauge Chiba, a larger trocar needle is directed toward the lesion. The caliber is selected so that the biopsy needle can easily pass through it. For 20 and 22 gauge biopsy needles, an 18 gauge trocar needle will suffice. When in position, the trocar stylet is removed and the biopsy needle is inserted into the area of interest and a sample is obtained (**Fig. 15-2**). This method often requires an additional person, with one operating the transducer and placing the trocar and the second person performing the biopsy. If the entire procedure cannot be done within a single breath for the patient, consideration should be given to disengaging the trocar needle from the guide once it has been positioned, to decrease the possibility of tearing the liver capsule. While the procedure is essentially converted from "guided" to "freehand," the most crucial step, that of directing the trocar needle to the lesion, is already done. The larger needle is usually more echogenic than the smaller biopsy needle; thus visualization is not difficult.

CT-guided biopsies of small lesions can be very difficult using conventional methods because real-time visualization of the lesion and placement of the needle are not possible, and even slight variations in patient breathing may not allow accurate needle placement. However, with the development of CT fluoroscopy, in which six to eight images of lower resolution and lower milliamperes per second can be obtained with near real-time visualization of the needle tip, CT-guided biopsy of small liver lesions may be considered if they are not visualized by US or accessible with US guidance. Although this technique should be faster than the conventional CT biopsy method and will likely improve needle placement into small lesions, exposure of the patient and radiologist to ionizing radiation has to be considered. We reserve CT for biopsy of lesions not visualized by US.

PEARLS AND PITFALLS

- Small liver lesions (<1.5–2 cm) are best biopsied with US guidance. Advantages include real-time evaluation for confirmation of needle-tip position, color Doppler for visualization and avoidance of intrahepatic blood vessels, and possibility for nonaxial plane biopsy.
- Use of a needle guide allows easier and faster visualization and direction of the biopsy needle tip into the appropriate location.
- Visualization of the needle tip can be enhanced by using an echogenic-tip needle or a minimal back and forth rocking motion of the transducer.
- Adequate visualization of the lesion and appropriate planning, specifically of the intended path of the needle, are essential for a safe and successful procedure.
- A small skin incision may decrease the chance of needle deflection during attempted biopsy of a small liver lesion.

Further Reading

Charboneau WJ, Reading CC, Welch TJ. CT and sonographically guided needle biopsy: current techniques and new innovations. AJR Am J Roentgenol 1990;154:1–10

Dodd GD, Esola CC, Memet DS, et al. Sonography: the undiscovered jewel of interventional radiology. Radiographics 1996;16:1271–1288

Dodd GD, Mooney EE, Layfield LJ, et al. Fine-needle aspiration of the liver and pancreas: a cytology primer for radiologists. Radiology 1997;203:1–9

Hopper KD, Abendroth CS, Sturtz KW, et al. Automated biopsy devices: a blinded evaluation. Radiology 1993;187:653–660

Hopper KD, Grenko RT, Fisher AI, et al. Capillary versus aspiration biopsy: effect of needle size and length on the cytopathological specimen quality. Cardiovasc Intervent Radiol 1996;19:341–344

Matalon TAS, Silver B. US guidance of interventional procedures. Radiology 1990;174:43–47

Middleton WD, Hiskes SK, Teefey SA, et al. Small (1.5 cm or less) liver metastases: US-guided biopsy. Radiology 1997;205:729–732

Paulson EK. Image-guided percutaneous abdominal biopsies. Appl Radiol 1995;24:11–15

Paulson EK, Nelson RC. Techniques of percutaneous tissue acquisition. In: Gore RM, Levine MS, Laufer I. Textbook of Gastrointestinal Radiology. Philadelphia: WB Saunders; 2000:1219–1233

Sheafor DH, Paulson EK, Simmons CM, et al. Abdominal percutaneous interventional procedures: comparison of CT and US guidance. Radiology 1998;207:705–710

Silverman SG, Mueller PR, Pfister RC. Hemostatic evaluation before abdominal interventions: an overview and proposal. AJR Am J Roentgenol 1990;154:233–238

CHAPTER 16 Hepatic Abscess

Robert E. Lambiase

Clinical Presentation

A 68-year-old female on hemodialysis presented with persistent low-grade fever and nonlocalizing abdominal pain. Physical examination elicited diffuse abdominal tenderness without peritoneal signs. Poor dental hygiene with several sites of gingival infection were noted. Oral temperature was 100.2°F and white blood cell count was 17,000 with a moderate increase in bands.

Radiological Studies

A contrast-enhanced computed tomographic (CT) scan of the abdomen was obtained to evaluate the abdominal pain. This revealed a complex hepatic collection with multiple loculations (**Fig. 16-1**). Aspiration under CT guidance revealed tenacious, brownish pus.

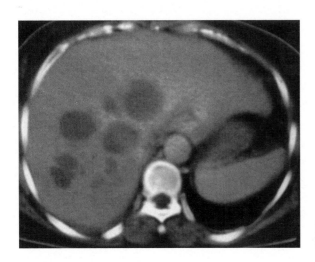

Figure 16-1 Computed tomography of the abdomen demonstrates a complex intrahepatic abscess collection.

Diagnosis

Pyogenic hepatic abscess

Treatment Options

There are three options in the treatment of hepatic abscesses. The first is medical therapy alone. This may be attempted for a single, small (<3.0 cm) abscess in an otherwise stable and immunocompetent patient. Close clinical and radiological follow-up is indicated to avoid potential septic complications if medical therapy fails. The second option is percutaneous drainage under cross-sectional imaging guidance. Imaging allows determination of a safe access route and immediate assessment of the completeness of evacuation. If drainage is not complete, a second drainage catheter may be placed in the same sitting. The procedure can be performed under conscious sedation without general anesthesia. The third option is surgical drainage. The completeness of drainage may be difficult to assess intraoperatively, and additional small collections or loculations may be overlooked. The procedure mandates general anesthesia, is physiologically more stressful than the percutaneous procedures, and requires a significantly longer recuperative period. Multiple collections may require extensive exposure for adequate drainage. For these reasons, percutaneous drainage was selected in this patient.

Treatment

A repeat CT scan was obtained with skin markers in place to localize the site for percutaneous entry. Immediately prior to drainage, ceftizoxime 2 g and gentamicin 80 mg were administered intravenously. Administration of antibiotics immediately before the drainage procedure will mitigate potential septic complications and is not likely to affect the results of the bacterial culture because there is delayed penetration of antibiotics into the abscess. Fentanyl 50 μg and midazolam 1 mg were administered for conscious sedation. Coagulation parameters that had previously been determined were within normal limits (i.e., partial thromboplastin time, International Normalized Ratio (INR), and bleeding time because the patient was on hemodialysis with potential platelet dysfunction).

A safe transhepatic route was mapped and a posterolateral approach was chosen to avoid the pleural space and right kidney. A 20 cm long, 22 gauge noncoring needle was initially placed to mark the anticipated course of the drainage catheter. An 18 gauge sheathed needle was then inserted in tandem. A repeat scan demonstrated a satisfactory needle course with the needle tip in the abscess. A small sample was aspirated and sent for Gram stain, culture, and sensitivity. Subsequently, a 0.038 in. guide wire was placed through the sheath and coiled within the abscess. Serial tract dilatation allowed for the placement of a 14 French sump drainage catheter. Repeat CT scan verified appropriate positioning of the catheter within the collection. Approximately 250 mL of thick, brownish pus was aspirated. The catheter was secured in place to prevent accidental dislodgement. Since the collection was quite complex, dilute contrast was instilled through the catheter to assess completeness of the drainage. Several locules did not opacify in this manner. Therefore, a second drainage catheter was placed into the central portion of these collections. Following aspiration of an additional, ~70 mL of pus, instillation of dilute contrast opacified the remaining locules.

Postdrainage management consisted of daily ward rounds, recording of the drainage output, and irrigation of the drainage catheters each shift (20 mL saline was injected and reaspirated, and subsequently, each catheter was flushed with 10 mL saline). This regimen was continued for 48 hours, then decreased to once every 12 hours for an additional 48 hours, and then once daily. Following irrigation, the catheters were put on low-grade wall suction. Vital signs per shift and daily white blood cell count were obtained.

Following drainage catheter placement, the patient rapidly defervesced, the leucocytosis decreased, and the white blood cell count returned to normal within 96 hours. Drainage tapered to <10 mL per day per catheter within the first 72 hours. The catheters were removed when there was <10 mL of output per catheter for 3 consecutive days. The patient remained well at 1-year follow-up, without recurrence of the abscess. Cultures grew *Actinomyces israelii*, which was believed to be secondary to hematogenous spread from her gingivitis.

Discussion

Four general categories of organisms are responsible for hepatic abscesses; pyogenic, amebic, echinococcal, and miscellaneous including mycobacterial, fungal, and parasitic. Amebic hepatic abscesses are very common worldwide but are rare in the United States. Treatment is almost exclusively medical and the results are excellent. Percutaneous or surgical drainage is rarely necessary. Hepatic echinococcal cysts are relatively common in endemic regions. A large literature documents the efficacy of percutaneous drainage for hydatid disease of the liver (see Chapter 18). The feared risk of anaphylactic shock secondary to intraperitoneal spillage has not materialized to date in the published series.

In the United States, pyogenic organisms are by far the most common cause of hepatic abscesses. Prior to the mid-1970s, mortality was close to 50% and the most common cause of hepatic abscesses was portal seeding from diverticulitis or appendicitis. Improved antibiotic therapy and aggressive drainage have markedly decreased the mortality, which is presently <5%. Today, the majority of hepatic abscesses occur after biliary surgery or manipulation, or biliary inflammatory disease. Other, less common causes include hematogenous spread from sites other than the bowel, following trauma, particularly penetrating injuries, which track contaminated skin or clothing into the liver.

Percutaneous, imaging-guided drainage in combination with appropriate antibiotic coverage is a very safe and effective treatment for hepatic abscesses. The published series report an overall success rate of close to 90%. The pleural space, kidney, large vessels, and surrounding viscera must be avoided to minimize complications. This is easily accomplished with cross-sectional imaging. Bacteremia is common immediately after drainage and sepsis occurs in ~2 to 4% of drainages. Sepsis with hypotension is usually easily controlled with fluid augmentation, and short-term vasopressor therapy is rarely necessary. Death secondary to overwhelming sepsis is extremely rare. Significant bleeding is also uncommon. Hemorrhage secondary to vessel injury is usually tamponaded by the hepatic parenchyma. Bleeding from injury to the hepatic or portal veins usually ceases spontaneously without specific therapy. If venous decompression into the catheter tract is present, this can be tamponaded by upsizing the drainage catheter. Hepatic arterial injury may result in pseudoaneurysm formation or hematobilia and may require transcatheter embolization. However, this is extremely uncommon.

Once the decision is made to percutaneously drain a hepatic abscess, there are two therapeutic options. The abscess collection can be simply aspirated without the placement of an indwelling drainage catheter. This is often successful for smaller, unilocular collections in immunocompetent patients where the collections do not demonstrate ongoing biliary communication. Multiple aspiration sessions may be necessary if there is recurrence of the abscess. The advantage of simple aspiration is that it avoids the discomfort and management requirements of an indwelling catheter. More complex collections, those with a biliary communication and those with multiple recurrences, mandate drainage via an indwelling catheter. Placement of an indwelling catheter also avoids the risks, although small, associated with repeated access to the collection sometimes required when using aspiration alone.

Clinical management following drainage catheter placement is as important as the initial drainage. This includes daily rounds, review of per-shift output, assessment of the persistence and nature of the drainage, as well as overall patient well-being. The white blood cell count should normalize within a week and the patient should defervesce within 72 hours. Persistent leucocytosis or fever should initiate a search for an undrained or incompletely drained collection. A sudden decrease in drainage may indicate either a complete evacuation of the collection or blockage or dislodgement of the drainage catheter. This may require a tube check with contrast opacification of the cavity, cross-sectional imaging, catheter manipulation, or exchange. Persistent drainage or a change in the nature of the drainage may indicate the presence of a communication with the biliary system. As a rule, an intrahepatic biliary communication usually does not preclude successful percutaneous therapy. However, the duration of drainage is prolonged in this setting. Biliary diversion is usually not needed unless the leak is very large, or from a major duct. If prolonged drainage is required, the patient can be discharged home with minimal nursing requirements.

PEARLS AND PITFALLS_____

- Percutaneous drainage is the therapeutic procedure of choice for hepatic abscesses, with a ≥90% durable success.
- Almost all hepatic collections are amenable to percutaneous drainage based on anatomical considerations.
- Complex, loculated collections may also be drained by a single catheter because the loculations are often interconnected, or they may necessitate multiple drainage catheters.
- Intrahepatic communication between the abscess cavity and bile ducts usually does not require biliary diversion for cure, although duration of drainage is prolonged.
- Many drainage regimens can be completed on an outpatient basis.

Further Reading

Barakate MS, Stephen MS, Waugh RC, et al. Pyogenic liver abscess: a review of 10 years' experience in management. Aust N Z J Surg 1999;69:205–209

Bayraktar Y, Arslan S, Sivri B, et al. Percutaneous drainage of hepatic abscesses: therapy does not differ for those with identifiable biliary fistula. Hepatogastroenterology 1996;43:620–626

Giorgio A, Tarantino L, Mariniello N, et al. Pyogenic liver abscesses: 13 years of experience in percutaneous needle aspiration with US guidance. Radiology 1995;195:122–125

Huang CJ, Pitt HA, Lipsett PA, et al. Pyogenic hepatic abscess: changing trends over 42 years. Ann Surg 1996;223:600–607

Lambiase RE, Deyoe L, Cronan JJ, et al. Percutaneous drainage of 335 consecutive abscesses: results of primary drainage with 1-year follow-up. Radiology 1992;184:167–179

McDermott VG. What is the role of percutaneous drainage for treatment of amebic abscesses of the liver? AJR Am J Roentgenol 1995;165:1005–1006

Rintoul R, O'Riordain MG, Laurenson IF, et al. Changing management of pyogenic liver abscess. Br J Surg 1996;83:1215–1218

Seeto RK, Rockey DC. Pyogenic liver abscess: changes in etiology, management, and outcome. Medicine 1996;75:99–113

Tazawa J, Sakai Y, Maekawa S, et al. Solitary and multiple pyogenic liver abscesses: characteristics of the patients and efficacy of percutaneous drainage. Am J Gastroenterol 1997;92:271–274

CHAPTER 17 Cyst Ablation

Tapani Tikkakoski

Clinical Presentation

A 76-year-old woman presented with an 8-month history of epigastric pain without weight loss.

Physical examination of the abdomen was normal. Laboratory tests including hemoglobin, leucocyte and platelet counts, serum albumin, renal, and liver function tests were normal.

Radiological Studies

An ultrasound of the abdomen showed a 13 cm diameter, solitary, anechoic liver mass (**Fig. 17-1**). There was a coexisting cyst in the left kidney. The remainder of the examination was normal.

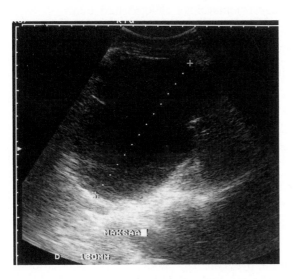

Figure 17-1 Sonogram obtained prior to treatment shows a large, anechoic, solitary hepatic cyst.

Diagnosis

Symptomatic congenital hepatic cyst

Treatment Options

Surgery has been the traditional therapy for symptomatic liver cysts. Surgical options consist of excision, unroofing, fenestration, or partial hepatectomy (Furuta et al, 1990; van Sonnenberg et al, 1994). An effective alternative to surgical treatment is the single-session percutaneous drainage and ethanol sclerotherapy (Bean and Rodan, 1985; Kairaluoma et al, 1989; Tikkakoski et al, 1996; Larssen et al, 1997).

Treatment

The single-session percutaneous drainage and ethanol sclerotherapy treatment option was selected. The patient was premedicated with 50 mg pethidine hydrochloride (meperidine hydrochloride) and 0.5 mg atropine sulfate subcutaneously. Lidocaine 1% was injected at the puncture site and a small

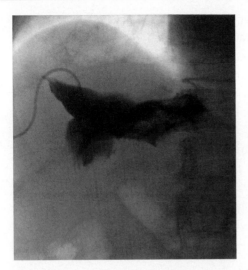

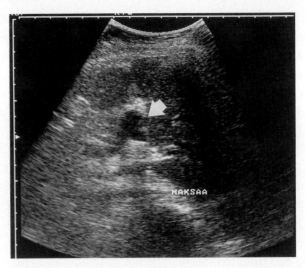

Figure 17-2 Posteroanterior radiograph obtained after injection of contrast shows partially collapsed cavity of the cyst. No contrast extravasation or communication with the biliary ducts is demonstrated.

Figure 17-3 Sonogram obtained 32 months after ethanol sclerotherapy shows a small, residual cyst (arrow). The patient was asymptomatic.

skin incision was made. Under ultrasound guidance, a 15 cm long, 18 gauge needle (PBN Meda, Stenløse, Denmark) was inserted into the cyst. The needle path was chosen to traverse normal liver tissue to prevent leakage of the alcohol at the time of sclerosis. A 0.028 in. stainless steel guide wire with a 7.5 cm long flexible tip (PBN Meda) was inserted through the needle, which was then removed. A drainage catheter was placed in the cyst and 700 mL fluid was aspirated. A fluid sample was sent for cytology. After complete evacuation of the cyst, diluted contrast (Omnipaque 300 mg/mL mixed with an equal volume of saline) was injected and radiographs were obtained in different positions to exclude a communication with the biliary tree or extravasation into the peritoneal cavity (**Fig. 17-2**).

The contrast material was then aspirated completely and 60 mL sterile absolute alcohol (Etanol 99%; Apoteksbolaket, Sweden) was injected into the cyst. The alcohol was left in the cyst for 20 minutes, during which time the patient was rolled from side to side and into various positions at intervals of 5 minutes to ensure that the alcohol came into contact with the entire surface of the cavity. This procedure was repeated three times. The alcohol was then aspirated and the drainage catheter was removed. Following the treatment, the patient became asymptomatic. Follow-up ultrasound examinations were obtained at 2, 4, 8, and 32 months after sclerotherapy. There was a gradual decrease in size of the cavity. The corresponding cyst measurements were 4, 4, 2, and 2 cm (**Fig. 17-3**).

Discussion

Congenital, nonparasitic hepatic cysts arise from malformation of the intrahepatic bile ducts. Symptoms occur when the cyst becomes enlarged from secretion of fluid into the cavity by the epithelium lining the cyst. Small cysts are seldom clinically symptomatic. Larger cysts may cause hepatomegaly, pain, local bulging, early satiety, bile duct and inferior vena cava compression, or acute abdominal symptoms in the case of cyst rupture (Bean and Rodan, 1985; Kairaluoma et al, 1989; Furuta et al, 1990; van Sonnenberg et al, 1994; Larssen et al, 1997).

Aspiration of the fluid alone without destruction of the cyst epithelium has not been effective for the prevention of recurrence. Bean and Rodan (1985) reported that aspiration of fluid and injection of alcohol, which destroys the epithelium and its secretory ability, might be the treatment of choice for symptomatic congenital cysts. Since then ethanol sclerotherapy has replaced hepatic surgery in the treatment of symptomatic hepatic cysts at our hospital.

Although ethanol sclerotherapy is effective treatment for symptomatic solitary hepatic cysts, the results are less satisfactory in polycystic liver disease because of enlargement of untreated cysts (Tikkakoski et al, 1996). Other sclerosing agents that have been used include doxycycline, tetracycline, and minocycline (van Sonnenberg et al, 1994; Cellier et al, 1998). We have no experience with these agents and most of the published reports deal with alcohol as a sclerosing agent (Bean and Rodan, 1985; Kairaluoma et al, 1989; Furuta et al, 1990; van Sonnenberg et al, 1994; Tikkakoski et al, 1996; Larssen et al, 1997).

We have treated as many as three hepatic cysts in a single session using ultrasound guidance. Each cyst was sclerosed up to three times with ethanol. For the instillation of ethanol, a 5F catheter was inserted into the cyst using the Seldinger technique. The catheter was removed upon completion of the procedure. The volumes of the aspirated fluid and ethanol instilled were as follows (Tikkakoski et al, 1996):

100 mL aspirated—30 mL ethanol instilled
200 mL aspirated—50 mL ethanol instilled
300 mL aspirated—75 mL ethanol instilled
400 mL aspirated—100 mL ethanol instilled.

A good result was achieved even after instillation of a smaller volume of ethanol (**Figs. 17-1** and **17-3**). Like Larssen et al, we prefer the single session therapy in which the catheter is removed upon completion of the treatment session. Others have left a catheter in the cyst for several days (up to 10 and 44 days) for sequential sclerotherapy (Furuta et al, 1990; van Sonnenberg et al, 1994). We feel that this increases the risk for secondary infection and causes discomfort to the patient. Although post-procedural reaccumulation of fluid is common, it has proven to be transient and repeat sclerotherapy of the same cyst is usually not necessary (Larssen et al, 1994; Tikkikoski et al, 1996).

Contraindications for ethanol sclerotherapy include coagulation abnormality, cystic neoplasms, communication of the cyst with the bile ducts, and demonstration of contrast extravasation into the peritoneal cavity.

Reported major complications include pleural effusion and secondary infection (van Sonnenberg et al, 1994). Minor complications include pain, fever, inebriation, and hemorrhage into the cyst (Kairaluoma et al, 1989; Furuta et al, 1990; van Sonnenberg et al, 1994; Tikkakoski et al, 1996). An iatrogenic communication with the biliary tract; that is, a cystobiliary fistula, was observed in one of our patients (Oikarinen et al, 1996). A similar complication was reported by Cellier et al (1998). As ethanol sclerotherapy is contraindicated in this situation, a contrast cystogram must be obtained before initiating sclerotherapy.

PEARLS AND PITFALLS_____

- Percutaneous aspiration and ethanol sclerotherapy is a safe and effective, minimally invasive method of treating symptomatic congenital hepatic cysts.
- Iatrogenic communication with the biliary tree is a rare complication and must be excluded by contrast cystography before beginning sclerotherapy.

Further Reading

Bean WJ, Rodan BA. Hepatic cysts: treatment with alcohol. AJR Am J Roentgenol 1985;144:237–241

Cellier C, Cuenod CA, Deslandes P, et al. Symptomatic hepatic cysts: treatment with single-shot injection of minocycline hydrochloride. Radiology 1998;206:205–209

Furuta T, Yoshida Y, Saku M, et al. Treatment of symptomatic non-parasitic liver cysts: surgical treatment versus alcohol injection therapy. HPB Surg 1990;2:269–279

Kairaluoma MI, Leinonen A, Stahlberg M, et al. Percutaneous aspiration and alcohol sclerotherapy for symptomatic hepatic cysts: an alternative to surgical intervention. Ann Surg 1989;210:208–215

Larssen TB, Viste A, Jensen DK, et al. Single-session alcohol sclerotherapy in benign symptomatic hepatic cysts. Acta Radiol 1997;38:993–997

Oikarinen H, Paivansalo M, Tikkakoski T, et al. Radiological findings in biliary fistula and gallstone ileus. Acta Radiol 1996;37:917–922

van Sonnenberg E, Wroblicka JT, D'Agostino HB, et al. Symptomatic hepatic cysts: percutaneous drainage and sclerosis. Radiology 1994;190:387–392

Tikkakoski T, Makela J, Leinonen S, et al. Treatment of symptomatic congenital hepatic cysts with single session percutaneous drainage and ethanol sclerosis: technique and outcome. J Vasc Interv Radiol 1996;7:235–239

CHAPTER 18 Hydatid Disease

Okan Akhan

Clinical Presentation

A 46-year-old woman presented with right upper quadrant pain of 6-month duration. The physical examination and laboratory tests revealed no abnormality. She was referred for upper abdominal ultrasonography (US).

Radiological Studies

Ultrasound examination revealed a 7 × 6 × 6 cm, oval-shaped, cystic mass in the posterior segment of the right lobe of the liver, adjacent to the diaphragm (**Fig. 18-1**). The cyst had a double contour at the wall and contained neither septa nor internal echoes. No other abnormality was seen. Computed tomography (CT) (not shown) confirmed this finding.

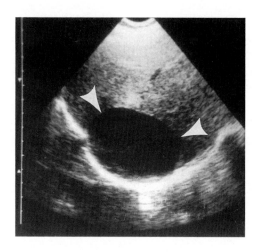

Figure 18-1 Hepatic ultrasound demonstrates a type I hydatid cyst in the right lobe of the liver (arrowheads).

Diagnosis

Hydatid cyst of the liver. Type-I according to the Gharbi classification

Treatment Options

Treatment options included medical treatment, percutaneous aspiration, percutaneous catheter drainage, and surgery. Using the classification of Gharbi et al (1981), type I and II hydatid cysts of the liver are best suited for percutaneous treatment. Therefore, this approach was selected for the treatment of the hydatid cyst in this patient. As the estimated cyst volume was >100 mL, the catheterization technique was used.

Treatment

The patient was started on mebendazole prophylaxis (50 mg/kg/day) 1 week before the procedure and it was continued for 4 weeks thereafter. The drainage was performed after an overnight fast and

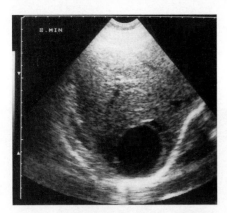

Figure 18-2 Ultrasound image obtained 8 minutes after injection of hypertonic saline shows separation of the endocyst from the pericyst.

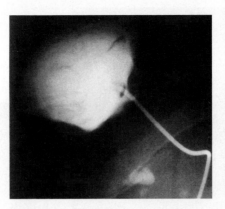

Figure 18-3 Contrast injection into the cavity 1 day after the procedure demonstrates a detached endocyst in the cavity and absence of a cystobiliary fistula.

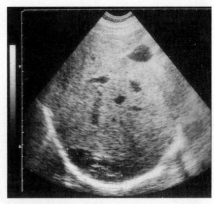

Figure 18-4 Ultrasound image obtained at 3 months shows a substantial decrease in the size, volume, and fluid in the cyst as well as detachment and degeneration of the endocyst.

under conscious sedation. An antibiotic was given for infection prophylaxis. She was monitored for the possibility of an anaphylactic or allergic reaction during the procedure.

The patient was placed on the fluoroscopy table and after a standard skin prep, local anesthesia was injected at the access site. Using ultrasound guidance, an 18 gauge Seldinger needle was inserted into the lesion. Upon removal of the stylet, crystal-clear fluid gushed out as a result of high pressure inside the cyst. This is considered pathognomonic for the diagnosis and viability of hydatid cyst. The fluid was sent to the laboratory for microbiological and cytological examinations to look for the presence and viability of protoscolices and membrane fragments. Subsequently, at least 35% of the estimated volume of the cyst was aspirated. Hypertonic saline (20% NaCl) was then injected into the cavity (injected volume was 10% less than that of the aspirated volume). Subsequently, concentration of the hypertonic saline in the cavity was increased as much as possible by repeating the aspiration and reinjection of fresh hypertonic saline. The injection was monitored by ultrasound and fluoroscopy. Within 10 minutes of the saline injection, there was separation of the endocyst from the pericyst (**Fig. 18-2**). This is another pathognomonic sign for the diagnosis and viability of hydatid cysts.

Following visualization of the separation, a 6F pigtail catheter was inserted into the cavity using the Seldinger technique and fluoroscopic guidance. The cavity was rinsed with hypertonic saline and all contents were aspirated through the catheter. The catheter was affixed to the skin and left to gravity drainage for 24 hours. As the amount of drainage was <10 mL in 24 hours, a contrast cystogram was obtained to confirm the absence of a communication with the biliary system (**Fig. 18-3**). Subsequently, 95% sterile absolute alcohol was injected into the cavity (~35% of the cavity volume). It was left in place for 20 minutes and then reaspirated. After catheter removal, the patient was discharged from the hospital.

She has been followed for 9 years. US was performed once every 3 months during the first year, twice during the second year, and subsequently once a year. CT was obtained every 2 years. These examinations were used to assess the size, volume, content, and wall changes of the cavity, and the findings were correlated with the healing criteria described in an experimental study (Akhan et al, 1993).

Three months after percutaneous treatment, there was a significant decrease in the size, volume of fluid in the cyst as well as detachment and degeneration of the endocyst (**Fig. 18-4**). At 4 years, there was total solidification of the lesion (pseudotumor appearance) and there was no fluid in the cavity, which was barely visible (**Figs. 18-5A,B**). During the entire 9-year follow-up period, this appearance has remained unchanged (**Fig. 18-6**).

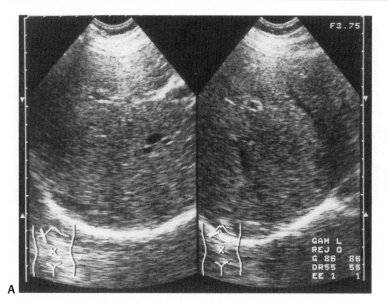
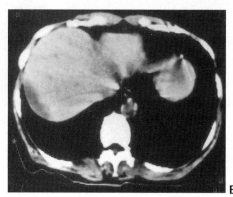

Figure 18-5 (**A**) Ultrasound and (**B**) computed tomography obtained at 4 years show total solidification of the remnant without any fluid component (pseudotumor appearance).

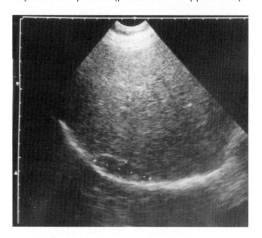

Figure 18-6 Ultrasound image obtained 9 years after percutaneous treatment demonstrates no change in the appearance of the pseudotumor.

Discussion

Hydatid disease caused by *Echinococcus granulosus*, a common health problem in some regions of the Mediterranean, Middle East, South America, and Africa, is uncommon in North America. Serological diagnosis by the Casoni, Weinberg, complement fixation, and indirect hemagglutination tests is unreliable. Although specific antibodies (IgG, IgM, IgA) are used for the diagnosis of exposure or active disease, negative serology does not exclude hydatid disease, and positive serology does not confirm its presence (Harris et al, 1986). Imaging modalities used for diagnosing liver hydatid disease are US, CT, and magnetic resonance imaging. Some cysts may present a diagnostic dilemma even on US, which is the most useful imaging modality and considered the method of choice for classification of hydatid cysts.

The conventional treatment of hydatid liver disease is surgery. This is associated with considerable mortality (up to 6.3%), morbidity (12.5–80%), high recurrence rates, and a long hospital stay (uncomplicated cases 14, complicated cases 30 days) (Sayek, 1983; Dawson et al, 1988). Postoperative recurrence rates are 2.2%, 8.5%, and 11.3%, respectively, in three different series published before 1980 (Barros, 1978; Motaghian and Saidi, 1978; Gilevich et al, 1980). In other series where US and CT were used for follow-up, recurrent disease was found in as many as 10 to 30% of cases (Little et al, 1988; Yalin et al, 1989; Abu Zeid et al, 1998).

Medical therapy with mebendazole or albendazole is still controversial, and low success rates are observed in the series with long-term follow-up. However, these drugs have been used successfully for prophylaxis against spillage before and after surgery or percutaneous treatment. Follow-up criteria for the medical treatment are also controversial.

Classification of Hydatid Disease of the Liver

All the published classifications are based on the morphological appearance of the hydatid cysts and do not reflect all the subtypes, the natural aging process including complications, as demonstrated by ultrasound. Furthermore, these classifications do not provide criteria (based upon the ultrasonographic appearance) for determining the optimal management, (i.e., surgery or percutaneous treatment). Therefore, a new classification is required that addresses the indications for percutaneous and surgical treatments. Despite its limitations in the evaluation of the appropriateness of percutaneous treatment of the liver hydatid cysts, Gharbi's classification is still used (Gharbi et al, 1981).

In Gharbi's classification, the liver hydatid cysts are classified into five groups:

Type I (pure fluid collection)
Type II (fluid collection with a split wall)
Type III (fluid collection with septa)
Type IV (hydatid cysts with heterogeneous echo patterns)
Type V (hydatid cysts with reflecting thick walls).

According to this classification, type I and type II are considered to be most appropriate for both the PAIR (**P**uncture, **A**spiration of cyst content, **I**njection of hypertonic saline solution, and **R**easpiration of all fluid) and catheterization techniques of percutaneous treatment. Other types for which PAIR and percutaneous catheterization techniques may be indicated include some subtypes of type III that do not have nondrainable solid material, some subtypes of type IV that have a considerable fluid component, suspected postoperative fluid collections, and infected hydatid cysts. The size, number, or location of the hydatid cysts in the liver are not contraindications for percutaneous treatment.

Percutaneous treatment is relatively contraindicated in some subgroups of type III that contain nondrainable solid material and in cysts that have ruptured into the biliary system or peritoneum. These cases should be treated either by surgery or by modified catheterization techniques such as percutaneous evacuation (PEVAC). No treatment is necessary in patients with totally calcified liver hydatid cysts (type V) and some subtypes of type IV that do not contain a fluid component.

Several reports of successful percutaneous treatment have been published. In an experimental study in sheep, there was a good correlation between ultrasonographic features and gross and microscopic findings representing the healing process after percutaneous treatment. The criteria indicating healing included a reduction in size and volume of the cyst, thickening and irregularity of the wall, decrease in the fluid component of the cavity, and gradual solidification of the remnant. All these criteria have been used successfully and confirmed by large series with long-term results.

Percutaneous Treatment

Three different techniques are used for percutaneous treatment of liver hydatid cysts.

The **PAIR** technique was described by Ben Amor et al in 1986. The catheterization technique with hypertonic saline and alcohol was described by Akhan et al in 1993 in an experimental study in sheep. In both techniques, hypertonic saline (20%) is used to irrigate and inactivate the cyst. This should remain in the cavity for ~10 minutes to destroy all the viable protoscolices. Hydatid cysts <6 cm in diameter (volume < ~100 mL) should be treated by the PAIR technique, whereas cysts >6 cm in diameter (volume > ~100 mL) should be treated by the catheterization technique so that cyst can be safely sclerosed using 95% sterile alcohol. The aim of the sclerosis is to prevent formation of a post-procedure cavity with the potential risk of infection or fistulization into the biliary system. Sclerosis by alcohol minimizes this risk. In addition to having scolecidal and sclerotic effects, absolute alcohol also destroys daughter cysts. Therefore, its use is also appropriate when the hypertonic saline is not sufficient to destroy daughter cysts.

Modified catheterization techniques such as PEVAC are used for the complicated cases such as some subgroups of type III that contain nondrainable solid material and the cysts that have ruptured into the biliary system (Schipper et al, 2002). In this technique, a 14F catheter is inserted into the cavity whose nondrainable content is also evacuated via the catheter, besides the cystic component.

The aim of surgical treatment of hydatid cysts is to inactivate the parasites, aspirate the crystal-clear fluid, remove the germinative membrane, and obliterate the residual cavity. PAIR and catheterization techniques of percutaneous treatment fulfill these aims of treatment except for removing the germinative membrane. With hypertonic saline, these membranes are inactivated and the process of degeneration is initiated. Absolute alcohol also serves the same function. In addition, alcohol helps to obliterate the residual cavity by its sclerotic effect. Observations of the long-term changes in the wall of the hydatid cyst and cavity after PAIR and catheterization techniques of percutaneous treatment suggest that inactivation of the germinative membrane and sclerosing the cavity may be sufficient, eliminating the need for removing the germinal layer. The contents of the cavity may be evacuated by modified catheterization techniques whenever indicated.

Complications

Hydatid cyst puncture was contraindicated because of two potential, major complications: anaphylaxis and spillage of scolices with peritoneal seeding and dissemination. Although anaphylaxis from rupture of a hydatid cyst has been documented, its occurrence is rare. Anaphylactic shock resulting in death during percutaneous treatment was reported in two cases (Akhan and Ozmen, 1999; Men et al, 1999). When the number of hydatid cysts treated percutaneously is taken into consideration, the mortality rate from anaphylactic shock is between 0.1 and 0.2%. It can be safely stated that percutaneous aspiration of a hydatid cyst is not necessarily followed by an anaphylactic reaction. Allergic reactions may appear during or after surgery or percutaneous treatment. Therefore, appropriate preparations to treat such a complication are necessary. Abdominal dissemination after percutaneous treatment was not reported in any published series but is not rare after surgery.

Urticaria, itching, and hypotension are minor complications that may occur during or several hours after the procedure. These symptoms can be treated by antihistamines. In some patients, fever (<38.5°C) may be observed, and, generally, this does not require any medication.

More serious complications are cavity infection, fistula between the cavity and the biliary system, and a serious anaphylactic reaction. In larger series, such complications are reported in 10% of cases. Abscess formation in the cavity is treated by percutaneous drainage and appropriate antibiotics. A cystobiliary fistula in the absence of biliary obstruction is treated by continued catheter drainage of the cavity, which leads to closure of the fistula. If there is biliary obstruction, biliary drainage is necessary for decompression.

Serious clinical symptoms such as dyspnea, cyanosis, and hypotension should be treated immediately. To cope with such complications, necessary equipment and medication should be readily available and the procedure should be performed with the assistance of an anesthesia team (Akhan and Ozmen, 1999).

If there are no complications after percutaneous treatment, the hospitalization period is ~1 day. In the complicated cases, hospitalization is ~17 to 20 days. The mean hospitalization period in the larger series was ~2.5 to 4.2 days. The recurrence rates reported after percutaneous treatment are between 0 and 4%. Recurrent cysts may also be treated percutaneously (Akhan and Ozmen, 1999).

Percutaneous treatment plays an important role in the management of liver hydatid cysts. It is an effective and reliable interventional procedure with the successful results of long-term follow-up (Gargouri et al, 1990; Akhan et al, 1996; Khuroo et al, 1997; Akhan and Ozmen, 1999; Men et al, 1999; Ustunsoz et al, 1999). In appropriate cases, it should be treatment of first choice (Akhan and Ozmen, 1999; Men et al, 1999).

PEARLS AND PITFALLS_____

- Type I and II liver hydatid cysts are best suited for either the PAIR or the catheterization technique.
- Cysts <6 cm in diameter (volume ≤100 mL) should be treated by the PAIR technique and cysts >6 cm in diameter (volume ≥100 mL) should be treated by the catheterization technique with subsequent sclerosis of the cavity.
- Modified catheterization techniques such as PEVAC are used for the complicated cases, such as some subgroups of type III that contain nondrainable solid material and the cysts that have ruptured into the biliary system.
- Percutaneous treatment of liver hydatid cysts is a safe and effective procedure with low recurrence rates (<4%).
- In the appropriate patient, percutaneous treatment should be considered the treatment of first choice.

Further Reading

Abu Zeid M, El-Eibiedy G, Abu-El-Einien A, et al. Surgical treatment of hepatic hydatid cysts. Hepatogastroenterology 1998;45:1802–1806

Akhan O, Ozmen MN. Percutaneous treatment of liver hydatid cysts. Eur J Radiol 1999;32:76–85

Akhan O, Dinçer A, Gokoz A, et al. Percutaneous treatment of abdominal hydatid cysts with hypertonic saline and alcohol: an experimental study in sheep. Invest Radiol 1993;28:121–127

Akhan O, Ozmen MN, Dinçer A, et al. Liver hydatid disease: long-term results of percutaneous treatment. Radiology 1996;198:259–264

Barros JL. Hydatid disease of the liver. Am J Surg 1978;135:597–600

Ben Amor N, Gargouri M, Gharbi HA, et al. Traitment du kyste hydatique du foie du mouton par ponction sous echographie. Tunis Med 1986;64:325–331

Dawson JL, Stamatakis JD, Stringer MD, et al. Surgical treatment of hepatic hydatid disease. Br J Surg 1988;75:946–950

Gargouri M, Amor NB, Chehida FB, et al. Percutaneous treatment of hydatid cysts (*Echinococcus granulosus*). Cardiovasc Intervent Radiol 1990;13:169–173

Gharbi HA, Hassine W, Brauner MW, et al. Ultrasound examination of the hydatid liver. Radiology 1981;139:459–463

Gilevich IuS, Ataev BA, Vafin AZ, et al. Relapses in echinococcal disease. Vest Khir Im I I Grek 1980;124:39–45 (Russian)

Harris KM, Morris DL, Tudor R, et al. Clinical and radiographic features of simple and hydatid cysts of the liver. Br J Surg 1986;73:835–838

Khuroo MS, Wani NA, Javid G, et al. Percutaneous drainage compared with surgery for hepatic hydatid cysts. N Engl J Med 1997;337:881–887

Little JM, Hollands MT, Eckberg H. Recurrence of hydatid disease. World J Surg 1988;12:700–704

Men S, Hekimoglu B, Yücesoy C, et al. Percutaneous treatment of hepatic hydatid cysts: a justified alternative to surgery. AJR Am J Roentgenol 1999;172:83–89

Motaghian H, Saidi F. Postoperative recurrence of hydatid disease. Br J Surg 1978;65:237–242

Sayek I. Hydatid disease of the liver. Hacettepe Med J 1983;16:84–92

Schipper HG, Lameris JS, van Delden OM, et al. Percutaneous evacuation (PEVAC) of multivesicular echinococcal cysts with or without cystobiliary fistulas which contain nondrainable material: first results of a modified PAIR method. Gut 2002;50:718–723

Schipper HG, Kager PA. Diagnosis and treatment of hepatic echinococcosis: an overview. Scand J Gastroenterol Suppl 2004;241:50–55.

Ustunsoz B, Akhan O, Kamiloglu MA, et al. Percutaneous treatment of hydatid cyst of the liver: long-term results. AJR Am J Roentgenol 1999;172:91–96

Yalin R, Aktan O, Açikgozlu S. Computed tomography and sonography of hydatid cysts of the liver after surgical management. J Med Imaging 1989;3:301–305

CHAPTER 19 Laser Ablation

Thomas J. Vogl and Martin G. Mack

Clinical Presentation

A 49-year-old man who had undergone resection of a rectal carcinoma 2 years earlier presented with a solitary liver metastasis (stage pT3, pN1). After failure of chemotherapy, percutaneous magnetic resonance-guided laser-induced thermotherapy (LITT) was undertaken, to ablate the tumor.

Radiological Studies

Pre- and post contrast magnetic resonance imaging (MRI) studies were performed to define the extent of the tumor in hepatic segments 7 and 8. These revealed a 20 mm solitary metastasis adjacent to the ascending hepatic veins. No further hepatic involvement was demonstrated and extrahepatic spread was excluded.

Diagnosis

Solitary hepatic metastasis from rectal carcinoma

Treatment

After placement of two cannulas (9 French, 20 cm length; Somatex, Berlin, Germany), using the Seldinger technique, two thermostable catheters and sheaths (9 French, Somatex) were placed in the metastasis in anterior and posterior positions (**Figs. 19-1** and **19-2**). MR thermometry was performed using FLASH two-dimensional (2D) gradient echo sequences in a transverse and coronal slice orientation. Laser treatment was performed using a neodymium:yttrium-aluminum-garnet (Nd:YAG) laser (1064 nm) and was completed when MR thermometry showed the lesion with a signal loss

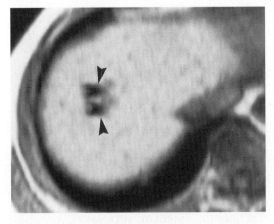

Figure 19-1 Gradient echo sequence, FLASH two-dimensional, T1-weighted, transverse orientation. The two magnetite markers (arrowheads) are seen anterior and posterior to the lesion, which appears as a hypointense structure.

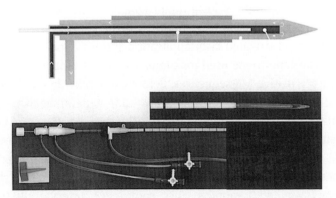

Figure 19-2 Image showing the instruments used for the procedure.

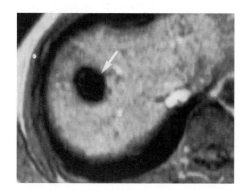

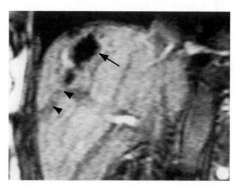

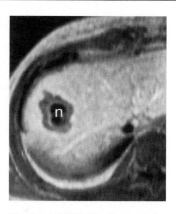

Figure 19-3 Magnetic resonance (MR) thermometry via gradient echo sequence, FLASH two-dimensional, T1-weighted. Twenty-two minutes after laser application, MR thermometry reveals a homogeneous signal loss within the lesion and the surrounding normal hepatic parenchyma (arrow).

Figure 19-4 Gradient echo sequence, FLASH two-dimensional, T1-weighted coronal image shows the cranial extension of the laser-induced necrosis during magnetic resonance thermometry. Arrowheads point to the transhepatic tract whereas the arrow points to the lesion.

Figure 19-5 Gradient echo sequence, FLASH two-dimensional, T1-weighted, gadolinium-enhanced. There is complete destruction of the metastasis (n) and peripheral flow reduction in the safety margin.

including the 10 mm safety margin surrounding the lesion (**Figs. 19-3** and **19-4**). This safety margin is necessary because clinical as well as experimental studies show that residual tumor foci might be located up to a distance of 5 mm in the periphery of tumors. The total laser irradiation period was 18 minutes. At the completion of the treatment, another contrast-enhanced MR T1-weighted sequence scan was obtained. Twenty-four hours after the laser treatment, pre- and postcontrast T1- and T2-weighted spin echo sequences were obtained to define the extent of laser-induced necrosis and to exclude the presence of possible side effects and complications (**Fig. 19-5**). Follow-up at 3-month intervals over a period of 5 years using MRI showed that there was no local recurrence and there was absence of metastatic spread.

Discussion

Tissue-ablating techniques are of increasing interest in oncology. The minimal invasiveness of these procedures as well as the high effectiveness of local tumor control may allow them to replace invasive resective techniques. MR-guided LITT is a newly developed, locally ablative technique that demonstrates a high rate of local tumor control combined with a low incidence of side effects and complications. The procedure is performed on an outpatient basis under local anesthesia with specially designed irrigated laser application systems. Special laser applicators and an Nd:YAG laser (1064 nm wavelength) are used for tumor ablation. Guidance and monitoring of the therapy employ temperature-sensitive MR sequences. Before each individual ablation procedure, coagulation parameters are checked. Contraindications are poor general health status of the patient, coagulation abnormalities, and elevated bilirubin.

Percutaneous MR-guided LITT achieved a local tumor control rate of 98.1% at 3 months follow-up and 97.3% at 6 months follow-up in metastases <5 cm in diameter. The mean survival rate (Kaplan-Meier method) in a total of 411 patients with 1154 metastases that were treated with 3415 laser applications was 45.0 months (95% confidence interval: 40.9–49.2 months, median survival 39.8 months, maximum survival 74.6 months). No statistically significant differences have been observed in the survival rates for patients with liver metastases from colorectal cancer versus metastases from other primary tumors. The overall incidence of side effects and complications was 9.5%. However, the incidence of clinically relevant side effects and complications requiring a second procedure was only 2.7%.

A broader application of MR-guided LITT is justified in patients with liver metastases from colorectal and breast cancer. In addition, this treatment may also be applicable to carefully selected patients with liver metastases from other primary tumors.

PEARLS AND PITFALLS

- MR-guided LITT is a highly successful, locally ablative technique that uses Nd:YAG laser for ablation of focal hepatic tumors. It has a low incidence of side effects and complications.
- It is an outpatient procedure performed under local anesthesia using specially designed irrigated laser application systems. Temperature-sensitive MR sequences are used to guide and monitor the therapy.
- MR-guided LITT is indicated in patients with liver metastases from colorectal and breast cancer. It may also be indicated in some patients with liver metastases from other primary tumors.

Further Reading

Doci R, Gennari L, Bignami P, et al. One hundred patients with hepatic metastases from colorectal cancer treated by resection: analysis of prognostics determinants. Br J Surg 1991;78:797–801

Germer CT, Albrecht D, Roggan A, et al. Experimental study of laparoscopic laser-induced thermotherapy for liver tumors. Br J Surg 1997;84:317–320

Herfarth C, Heuschen UA, Lamade W, et al. Resections of recurrence in the liver of primary and secondary liver cancers [in German]. Chirurg 1995;66:949–958

Hohenberger P, Schlag P, Schwarz V, et al. Leberresektion bei Patienten mit Metastasen colorektaler Carcinome: Ergebnisse und prognostische Faktoren. Chirurg 1988;59:410–417

Nordlinger B, Guiguet M, Vaillant JC, et al. Surgical resection of colorectal carcinoma metastases to the liver: a prognostic scoring system to improve case selection, based on 1568 patients. Association Francaise de Chirurgie. Cancer 1996;77:1254–1262

Scheele J, Altendorf-Hofmann A, Stangl R, et al. Surgical resection of colorectal liver metastases: gold standard for solitary and completely resectable lesions [in German]. Swiss Surg 1996;Suppl 4:4–17

Smith EH. Complications of percutaneous abdominal fine-needle biopsy. Radiology 1991;178:253–258

Soyer P, Pelage JP, Dufresne A-C, et al. CT of abdominal wall metastases after abdominal percutaneous procedures. J Comput Assist Tomogr 1998;22:889–893

Stangl R, Altendorf-Hofmann A, Charnley RM, et al. Factors influencing the natural history of colorectal liver metastases. Lancet 1994;343:1405–1410

Sugihara K, Hojo K, Moriya Y, et al. Pattern of recurrence after hepatic resection for colorectal metastases. Br J Surg 1993;80:1032–1035

van Ooijen B, Wiggers T, Meijer S, et al. Hepatic resections for colorectal metastases in the Netherlands: a multiinstitutional 10-year study. Cancer 1992;70:28–34

Vogl TJ, Mack MG, Roggan A, et al. Internally cooled power laser for MR-guided interstitial laser-induced thermotherapy of liver lesions: initial clinical results. Radiology 1998;209:381–385

Weiss L, Grundmann E, Torhorst J, et al. Hematogenous metastatic patterns in colonic carcinoma: an analysis of 1541 necropsies. J Pathol 1986;150:195–203

CHAPTER 20 Radio-Frequency Ablation

Tito Livraghi

Clinical Presentation

A 63-year-old man with asymptomatic chronic hepatitis C underwent an ultrasound (US) examination for evaluation of abnormal liver function tests (bilirubin 1.5 mg/dL; albumin 3.2 g/L; AST 112 IU; PT 68%). He also had endoscopy, which detected esophageal varices. Subsequent to the radiographic evaluation, additional tests were obtained and revealed abnormal levels of α-fetoprotein (AFP, 126 ng/mL [normal: <2]) and des-gamma-carboxy-prothrombin (DCP, 40 ng/mL [normal: <20]).

Radiological Studies

US detected an 8.6 cm diameter hypoechoic hepatic nodule with apparent encapsulation, located in the right lobe (**Fig. 20-1**). Biphasic spiral computed tomography (CT) confirmed the sonographic findings. The nodule appeared relatively hyperdense during the arterial phase and hypodense during the portal phase. Changes typical of cirrhotic disease were seen in the liver (**Fig. 20-2**).

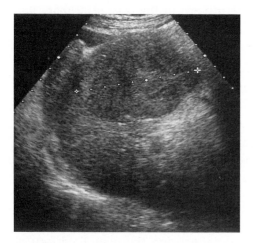

Figure 20-1 Transcostal sonogram shows an 8.6 cm hypoechoic mass.

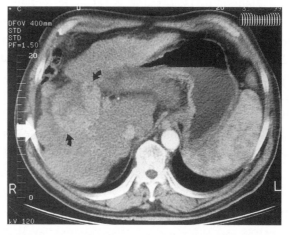

Figure 20-2 Image from the arterial phase of a computed tomographic scan shows a densely enhancing nodular tumor (curved arrows). Liver surface nodularity typical for cirrhosis is present (straight arrow).

Diagnosis

Hepatocellular carcinoma arising in Child's class A cirrhosis

Treatment Options

The diagnosis was based upon the clinical history, abnormal DCP values, and typical findings on the imaging studies. Therefore, a biopsy was considered unnecessary. In such cases, there are several treatment options: surgical resection, transarterial chemoembolization (TACE), percutaneous ethanol injection (PEI), and percutaneous ablation with radio frequency (RF).

Surgery was not considered because the abnormal liver function placed this patient at a higher risk for postoperative complications. TACE was excluded because it would cause additional damage to the liver. Furthermore, Lipiodol uptake would have been insufficient in the large tumor volume. Conventional multi-session PEI was excluded because the volume of tumor would have required too many sessions (Livraghi et al, 1995), and the "one-shot" PEI technique was excluded to avoid possible side effects (i.e., transient increase in portal hypertension with consequent risk of variceal bleeding) because of the large amount of ethanol required (Livraghi et al, 1998). Therefore, percutaneous ablation with RF was chosen for treatment of this lesion.

Treatment

RF ablation was performed under general anesthesia, with endotracheal intubation. Electrode placement was guided by US using a 3.5 MHz convex probe (CA B411, Hitachi, Tokyo, Japan) with an incorporated guide device. The skin was cleansed with iodized alcohol, which also served as contact medium. An intercostal approach was used for the placement of a 20 cm long, 18 gauge, internally cooled electrode with 3 cm of exposed tip (Radionics, Burlington, MA). For grounding, two dispersive pads were placed on the patient's thighs. The RF electrode was attached to a 500 KHz generator capable of producing 200 W of power. A peristaltic pump was used to infuse cooled (0°C) normal saline solution into the lumen of the electrode at a rate sufficient to maintain the tip temperature at 20 to 25°C.

As RF energy was applied, a hyperechoic focus developed around the uninsulated portion of the electrode due to tissue vaporization and cavitation. The appearance and progression of the size of this hyperechogenicity were used to guide additional insertions. In this case, two additional electrode insertions were performed, and their placement was directed to an area of the tumor without hyperechogenicity. Each insertion lasted for 10 minutes and the entire treatment session was completed in less than 1 hour. Treatment was considered sufficient when the entire tumor appeared completely hyperechoic. Following RF therapy, the patient was hospitalized for 2 days (3 nights in total). No side effects or complications occurred. Biphasic spiral CT and serum tumor markers (AFP and DCP) were obtained 1 month after treatment. Arterial and portal phases showed absence of contrast enhancement within the tumor, indicating complete necrosis. AFP and DCP levels had normalized. The appearance of the lesion remained unchanged at follow-up studies obtained 6 and 12 months after treatment (**Fig. 20-3**).

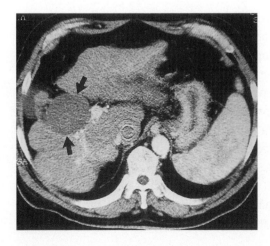

Figure 20-3 Image from the arterial-phase of a computed tomographic scan obtained 1 year after radio-frequency ablation shows absence of contrast enhancement in the tumor (arrows), which is consistent with complete necrosis.

Discussion

In countries where hepatocellular carcinoma (HCC) occurs frequently because of the high incidence of hepatitis B or C virus infection, the population at risk is submitted to sonographic screening. When screening is performed regularly (i.e., every 6 months), there is a high possibility of detecting an early-stage tumor (and thus a potentially curable tumor). HCC has a multicentric organ pathology and, although a single lesion may be present initially, in due time, other lesions will appear. For this reason, the only treatment providing a definitive cure is orthotopic liver transplantation (OLT), which also eliminates the chronic hepatic disease. All the other treatments are palliative. However, because of the shortage of donors and various contraindications, OLT can only be offered to a few patients. For example, in Italy only 100 to 200 patients are transplanted each year, whereas the number of new patients diagnosed with HCC each year is estimated to be around 10,000 to 12,000. In Japan the number is estimated at around 25,000.

For many years, surgical resection was considered the only curative treatment. PEI was proposed in 1986, initially only for inoperable patients (Livraghi et al, 1986). As long-term results of surgery and PEI became available, although based on historical data, the results were similar. The 5-year survival of patients with a single HCC <5 cm in size in Child's A cirrhosis was 48% for PEI and 49% for surgery (Livraghi et al, 1995). Such comparable results were probably due to a balance between the advantages and disadvantages of the procedures. Surgical resection assures complete removal of the tumor (compared with 70–80% for patients treated with PEI) but it is also associated with a mean perioperative mortality of 7% (vs 0% for PEI). Furthermore, PEI does not damage nonneoplastic parenchyma (some resections include a wide margin of normal tissue), can be repeated when new lesions appear, can also be performed in nontertiary care centers, and is relatively inexpensive.

In recent years, several factors have been identified that adversely affect surgical outcomes (The Liver Cancer Study Group of Japan, 1994). When present, these factors also alter the prognosis in untreated patients as well as those treated by other methods. At univariate analysis, in patients presenting with such adverse factors, survival after surgery was always shorter than that of patients treated with PEI. We can therefore argue, that the overall surgical survival was affected by the liberal enrollment and therefore mandatory implementation of very strict selection criteria is necessary according to the identified prognostic factors. The candidates for surgery should meet the following criteria: Child's A class, age <70 years, bilirubin <1.5, transaminases no more than three times the normal value, absence of portal hypertension or without risk of esophageal variceal bleeding, AFP <400 ng/mL, a single lesion and resectable by an anatomical resection, without portal vein thrombosis. In all the other patients, PEI should be considered, at least if the disease is not too far advanced.

Tumor ablation with RF demonstrates some advantages over PEI. In a randomized study performed in 86 patients with HCC <3 cm in size, RF obtained complete necrosis in 90% of cases versus 80% for PEI, using a mean of 1.2 treatment sessions versus 4.8 for PEI (Livraghi et al, 1999). In another study performed in medium (3–5 cm) to large (5–10 cm) HCC, local efficacy was roughly comparable, but RF demonstrated fewer side effects and complications than PEI used as a "one-shot" technique for larger tumors. Our initial data clearly show that RF has a higher local efficacy than TACE, without causing damage to normal tissue (Livraghi et al, 2000).

In the patient described, treatment with RF was successful. Complete necrosis was obtained in <1 hour without side effects. In case of a partial necrosis, management would depend on the assessment of the residual neoplastic tissue. If there is residual viable tumor, another RF session would be performed. Residual viable tumor is usually easily recognized on the arterial phase of the CT and also on the US examination. If the residual tumor is not recognizable with US, segmental TACE should be performed.

PEARLS AND PITFALLS

- Chronic hepatitis B or C virus infection predisposes to hepatocellular carcinoma.
- Regular sonographic screening can detect the tumor at an early, potentially curable stage.
- RF tumor ablation has some advantages over PEI in small (<3 cm) HCCs, by providing a higher incidence of tumor necrosis using fewer treatment sessions.
- In larger tumors, up to 10 cm in diameter, efficacy was comparable, but RF demonstrated fewer side effects and complications than PEI.

Further Reading

The Liver Cancer Study Group of Japan. Predictive factors for long term prognosis after partial hepatectomy for patients with hepatocellular carcinoma. Cancer 1994;74:2772–2780

Livraghi T, Benedini V, Lazzaroni S, et al. Long-term results of single-session PEI in patients with large hepatocellular carcinoma. Cancer 1998;83:48–57

Livraghi T, Festi D, Monti F, et al. US-guided percutaneous alcohol injection of small hepatic and abdominal tumors. Radiology 1986;161:309–312

Livraghi T, Giorgio A, Marin G, et al. Hepatocellular carcinoma and cirrhosis in 746 patients: long-term results of percutaneous ethanol injection. Radiology 1995;197:101–108

Livraghi T, Goldberg N, Lazzaroni S, et al. Radiofrequency ablation vs ethanol injection in the treatment of small hepatocellular carcinoma. Radiology 1999;210:655–661

Livraghi T, Goldberg N, Lazzarono S, et al. Hepatocellular carcinoma: radio-frequency ablation of medium and large lesions. Radiology 2000;214:761–768

CHAPTER 21 Cryoablation of Hepatic Masses

Josef Tacke and Rolf Günther

Clinical Presentation

A 34-year-old woman underwent a left mastectomy and axillary node dissection for breast carcinoma. A lymph node metastasis was found in the left axilla. Breast histology revealed an invasive intraductal tumor. Radiological evaluation including computed tomography (CT) of the thorax and abdomen revealed no distant metastases. She underwent chemo- and radiation therapy: three cycles of chemotherapy with epirubicine and cyclophosphamide followed by radiation to the left thoracic wall and axilla (cumulative dose 60.4 Gy) and an additional three cycles of chemotherapy with cyclophosphamide, methotrexate, and 5-fluorouracil. A subsequent radiological evaluation, which included 18 flourodeoxyglucose positron emission tomography (18FDG-PET) and abdominal ultrasonography revealed a mass lesion in the left lobe of the liver. A solitary liver metastasis was suspected, which was believed to have developed during the course of the chemotherapy. She was referred for percutaneous biopsy and assessment for ablation using a minimally invasive procedure. Laboratory data including red and white blood cell counts, liver enzymes, coagulation parameters, and blood chemistry were normal.

Radiological Studies

The suspected liver metastasis was evaluated by three-phase spiral CT (Tomoscan AV, Phillips Medical Systems) using 5 mm collimation, 7 mm table increment, and 5 mm reconstructions. Intravenous nonionic contrast (100 mL Isovist 300, Schering, Germany) was injected at 2.5 mL/sec, followed by an injection of 20 mL saline. CT confirmed the presence of a 2.5 cm, poorly enhancing mass in the left lobe of the liver (**Fig. 21-1**). No other lesions were found. On multiplanar T2-weighted turbo spin echo magnetic resonance imaging (MRI) (1.5 T Gyroscan ACS NT), the mass was oval shaped and showed a subcapsular location (**Fig. 21-2**). The cranial border of the lesion was directly beneath the left portal vein, and caudally the lesion abutted the pancreas and gastric antrum. An MR-guided biopsy was performed and histology confirmed the diagnosis.

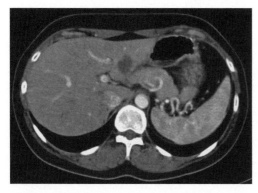

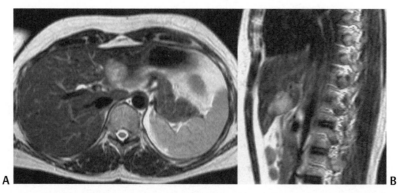

Figure 21-1 Portal venous phase of contrast-enhanced CT of the liver. A 2.5 cm, poorly enhancing lesion is seen in the left lobe of the liver.

Figure 21-2 Axial (**A**) and sagittal (**B**) images from a T2-weighted turbo spin echo sequence demonstrate subcapsular location of the metastasis. In addition, proximity to the left portal vein and antrum is demonstrated.

Diagnosis

Solitary liver metastasis from breast carcinoma

Treatment Options

Under the assumption that the liver metastasis had grown during chemotherapy and therefore would be insensitive to further chemotherapy protocols, a palliative treatment was chosen and surgical resection was not considered an option. Because of the palliative intention, the procedure-related risk was to be kept as small as possible and the treatment as effective and radical as possible. Thus both hyperthermal and hypothermal ablation techniques were considered. To avoid thermal damage to the adjacent structures and organs, precise planning and thermal mapping during ablation are necessary. As MRI is generally sensitive to temperature changes and offers multi-planar imaging capabilities, an MR-guided and MR-monitored procedure was chosen. Hyperthermal techniques such as laser- or radio-frequency-induced hyperthermia require dedicated software to visualize temperature-related changes. Because the quality of thermal mapping is affected by motion artifacts, information about the actual temperature gradients with a sufficiently high temporal and spatial resolution is difficult to achieve, especially in the abdominal region. Cryotherapy does not have these limitations and allows precise delineation of the frozen tissues during the ablation procedure using standard or interventional MR pulse sequences. Thus percutaneous cryoablation of the metastasis was selected.

Treatment

Prior to ablation, the lesion was biopsied with an 18 gauge cutting needle (Biopsy Needle, Daum, Schwerin, Germany) (**Fig. 21-3**). For planning of the percutaneous approach, dynamic gradient echo sequence images with inversion prepulse (TR 16 msec, TE 6 msec, inversion time 100 msec, flip angle 20 degrees, matrix 256 × 179 mm, 5 mm slice thickness) were obtained with a gadolinium-filled grid to mark the skin entry point. Subsequently, local anesthesia was injected and a small skin incision was made. Using the trocar technique, two MR-compatible cryotherapy probes (tapered tip, 3.4 mm diameter, 12 cm length) were placed in the lesion through 10F angiographic introducer sheaths (Terumo, Tokyo Japan). Because of the oval shape of the anticipated ice formation along the probe axis, a craniocaudal orientation of the probes was chosen to cover the entire lesion. Probe placement as well as the cryoablation were monitored by an interactive, ultrafast, T2-weighted, single-shot,

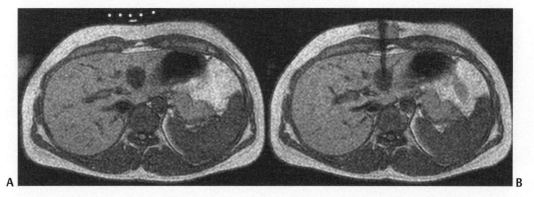

Figure 21-3 (**A**) Prebiopsy T1-weighted gradient echo image shows the gadolinium grid. (**B**) Scan obtained for confirmation of the biopsy needle tip position, which is in the center of the lesion.

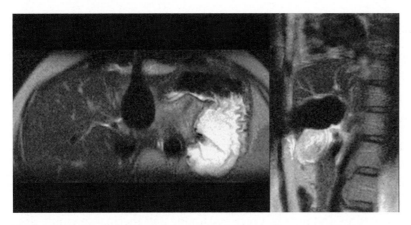

Figure 21-4 Interactive, multiplanar local look sequence magnetic resonance scan obtained during cryoablation shows a signal-free area representing ice that has completely covered and extends beyond the tumor margin by ~5 to 10 mm. Note the indentation of the ice by the left portal vein (white arrow) and the common hepatic artery (black arrow). A, water-filled antrum.

turbo spin echo sequence using the zoom imaging method (LoLo, *local look,* TR 800 msec, TE 77 msec, echo train length 46, matrix 256 × 256, 7 mm slice thickness, 800 msec/image acquisition time). This allowed precise monitoring and extension of the sharply marginated, signal free tissue ice relative to the liver capsule, antrum, and vascular structures. When the ice extended more than 1 cm beyond the tumor margin, the process was stopped and the ice was allowed to thaw passively. The cryoprocedure was then repeated. The maximum diameter of the ice was 4 cm (perpendicular to the probe) by 4.5 cm (along the shaft axis). An indentation of the ice was seen as a result of heat transfer from the left portal vein and common hepatic artery (**Fig. 21-4**). The ice extended beyond the liver capsule to the antral wall. The latter was protected from significant cryoinjury by having the patient drink warm water during the procedure. Upon completion, the probes were removed and the transhepatic tract was occluded by injection of a two-component tissue glue (Tissucol Duo S, Baxter, Germany) as the sheaths were retracted. There was no pain associated with the ablation. Scans obtained immediately after the intervention showed no bleeding complications (**Fig. 21-5**).

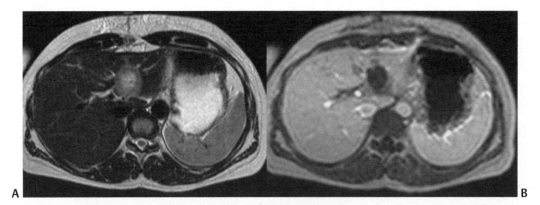

Figure 21-5 (A) Axial T2-weighted scan obtained immediately after cryoablation shows the metastasis surrounded by cryoinduced edema. **(B)** T1-weighted scan after gadolinium injection shows no tumor contrast enhancement. There is no thermal injury to the vascular structures, antrum, or pancreas.

Cryoinduced edema was observed that covered the tumor in its entirety. On contrast-enhanced, T1-weighted gradient echo sequence, the tumor appeared avascular. A contrast-enhanced CT obtained 3 days later (not shown), demonstrated a large, nonenhancing necrotic lesion. There was mild edema of the gastric antral wall but the patient remained clinically asymptomatic.

Discussion

During the past decade, various percutaneous tumor ablation techniques have been developed. Transarterial chemoembolization (TACE) is used preoperatively for hypervascular metastases or as palliative treatment in hepatocellular carcinoma. It is rarely used for the treatment of metastases and can only be recommended for palliation. Percutaneous ethanol injection (PEI) has been shown to be effective in encapsulated hepatocellular carcinoma. Due to the poor predictability of ethanol distribution in nonencapsulated lesions, it is of limited use in metastases. Moreover, if ethanol comes into contact with the liver capsule, it can be severely painful, requiring intensive pain management.

Thermal ablation can be accomplished by hyper- or hypothermia. Hyperthermal ablation, which is commonly used, is based on heat mediated tissue denaturation at temperatures between 50° and 100°C resulting in coagulation necrosis. Established hyperthermal techniques are laser induced thermal therapy (LITT) and radio–frequency-induced thermal ablation (RF). During LITT, optical fibers (7F, with or without saline-cooled introducer catheters) emit laser energy, which heats the target tissue. The process is influenced by multiple factors such as duration of laser emission, laser fiber cooling, carbonization, and blood perfusion. By using temperature-sensitive MR sequences, heat distribution within the target lesion can be monitored. If multiple laser fibers are used simultaneously, metastases of up to 5 cm in diameter can be treated.

RF induces heat as a result of rapidly alternating current passing RF energy through a shielded electrode with an exposed tip. Both an active and a dispersive probe are connected to the RF generator and form a complete electrical circuit through the patient's body. The heat is generated in the target tissue as a result of the resistance to the passage of electrical current and not by the probe itself. Depending on the RF probe design and generator capacity, a zone of hyperthermal damage 3 to 5 cm in diameter can be achieved. As harmonics and digital circuits interfere with the resonant frequencies of an MR system, simultaneous RF ablation and MR monitoring is difficult and is not yet possible clinically. Thus precise monitoring of the heat extension is not possible and has to be estimated during ablation. However, both techniques have been shown to be effective in the treatment of primary and secondary liver lesions. A drawback of all hyperthermal ablation procedures is pain due to heat distribution, especially in paraportal and subcapsular regions. Depending upon the location of the target lesion, deep analgesia and sedation or general anesthesia may be required.

Cryotherapy or cryosurgery is the irreversible damage to tissue by the application of deep (subzero) temperatures. Damage to the target tissue occurs by direct or indirect contact with a cryo source. As the tissue temperature falls, regional freezing occurs and extends outward from the cryo source. When the target tissue is frozen, the freezing process is stopped and the tissue is allowed to thaw. The damaged tissue becomes necrotic and scarring occurs soon afterward. Because the treated tissue is left in situ, cryotherapy is considered an interstitial, nonresective ablation technique.

Cryotherapy has been available for some time. There has been renewed interest in this procedure with the availability of ultrasound for real-time monitoring of the ice extension. Until recently, cryoprobes were available only in diameters >5 mm and therefore cryotherapy was only used intraoperatively. For a long time, liquid nitrogen (−195.6°C) was the only available coolant. Nitrous oxide and argon gas have been found to be as effective and have now replaced liquid nitrogen. According to the Joule-Thomson effect, a rapid temperature drop occurs if a highly pressurized gas suddenly expands. Thus modern gas expansion systems allow cooling capacities between −150°C and

−180°C, depending upon the probe design and diameter. The greatest advantage of the currently used system over the liquid nitrogen based systems is that the deep temperatures "arise" at the probe tip, and, unlike the liquid nitrogen based systems, the supply tubings remain at room temperature and the probe shaft does not require thermal insulation. This makes it possible to have smaller-diameter probes for percutaneous application. Another advantage of the modern gas expansion systems is a more rapid cooling rate (temperature drop per minute) because no precooling of the supply tubings is necessary.

The system that we used is argon-based and has a system pressure of 300 bar (600 psi). To the best of our knowledge, this was the first MR-compatible cryotherapy device available that allowed MRI for both planning and monitoring the cryoablation. The greatest advantage of combining cryoablation and interventional MRI is the possibility for precise delineation of frozen tissue by the multiplanar imaging capabilities of MRI. Due to an extreme shortening of T2- and T1-relaxation times, there is virtually no high-frequency signal from the frozen tissue on conventional MR pulse sequences. Consequently, frozen tissue is signal free and allows a high contrast relative to the untreated tissue. The use of modern ultrafast pulse sequences like the LoLo sequence (800 msec acquisition time) increases patient comfort and safety during the intervention because no breath-holding is necessary during imaging. Thus optimal information about the actual extent and size of the ice is available at any time during the intervention. This was the most important reason for choosing cryotherapy for ablation of the lesion in this anatomically difficult location.

Another characteristic of cryotherapy is that deep temperatures are intrinsically analgesic. With the exception of percutaneous insertion of the probes, which required local anesthesia, no analgesic drugs are necessary. This makes cryotherapy suitable for tissue ablation in sensitive locations such as subcapsular or paraportal regions. With cryotherapy, it is also possible to ablate target tissues in proximity to large blood vessels. Due to the heat transfer from flowing blood in the arteries and veins, significant damage to the vessel wall is unlikely because of the temperature balance between the ice on the one and the warm blood on the other side of the vessel wall. This is demonstrated in **Fig. 21-4**, where the left portal vein and common hepatic artery cause an indentation on the ice without any intrinsic vascular damage.

PEARLS AND PITFALLS_____

- Cryotherapy is ideally suited for percutaneous treatment of liver lesions in anatomically critical regions.
- The combination of percutaneous cryotherapy and interventional MRI enables precise and safe tissue ablation with a high temporal and spatial resolution for monitoring the procedure.
- In contrast to hyperthermal ablation techniques, imaging of frozen tissue does not require dedicated temperature-sensitive sequences and can be performed on all interventional MR systems.
- Due to its intrinsic analgesic effects, cryotherapy does not require specific pain management and is ideally suited for treatment of lesions in sensitive regions of the liver.

Further Reading

Solbiati L, Goldberg SH, Ierace T, et al. Hepatic metastases: percutaneous radio-frequency ablation with cooled-tip electrodes. Radiology 1997;205:367–373

Tacke J, Adam G, Haage P, et al. MR-guided percutaneous cryotherapy of the liver: in vivo evaluation with histologic correlation in an animal model. J Magn Reson Imaging 2001;13:50–56

Tacke J, Speetzen R, Heschel I, et al. Imaging of interstitial cryotherapy: an in vitro comparison of US, CT and MRI. Cryobiology 1999;38:250–259

Vogl TJ, Mack MG, Roggan A, et al. Internally cooled power laser for MR-guided interstitial laser-induced thermotherapy of liver lesions: initial clinical results. Radiology 1998;209:381–385

Weaver ML, Atkinson D, Zemel R. Hepatic cryosurgery in treating colorectal metastases. Cancer 1995;76:210–214

CHAPTER 22 Obstructive Jaundice

Saadoon Kadir

Clinical Presentation

An 83-year-old woman was evaluated for a 2-week history of painless jaundice. Bilirubin was 13 mg/dL.

Radiological Studies

Abdominal computed tomography (CT) demonstrated dilated intra- and extrahepatic ducts and a mass in the region of the pancreatic head (**Fig. 22-1**). Endoscopic retrograde pancreatocholangiography (ERCP) was performed and revealed a common bile duct (CBD) stricture (**Fig. 22-2**).

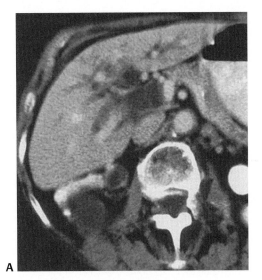
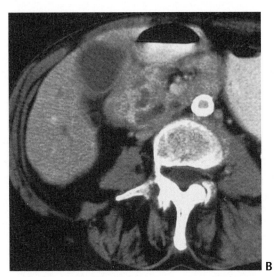

Figure 22-1 (A,B) Contrast-enhanced abdominal computed tomography shows dilated intra- and extrahepatic ducts and a pancreatic head mass.

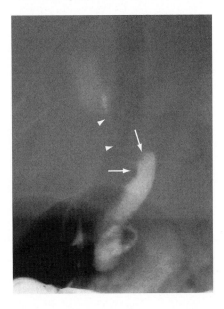

Figure 22-2 Image from the endoscopic retrograde cholangiopancreatography shows a severe stenosis (arrowheads) and mass effect (arrow).

Differential Diagnosis

Painless jaundice in an elderly individual without a prior history of hepatobiliary-pancreatic disease or injury is highly suspicious for ductal obstruction from a malignancy. The stricture seen on ERCP involves the proximal–CBD, and the distal duct is normal appearing. Although the duct proximal to the stricture is only faintly opacified, there appears to be an abrupt transition. The distal transition is also abrupt, the lumen is eccentric, and there is a mass effect. On CT, the proximal extrahepatic duct is markedly dilated and redundant with a Courvoisier gallbladder. These findings are indicative of a slowly progressing obstruction of some duration. Carcinoma of the pancreas is the most frequent cause of a malignant stricture and can involve any segment of the CBD. Other causes for a stricture in this location include chronic pancreatitis, sclerosing cholangitis, and cholangiocarcinoma, or the cause may be iatrogenic (surgery, instrumentation, or injury). Rare causes include collagen vascular diseases, retroperitoneal fibrosis, and lymphoma. A rare cholangiocarcinoma may develop in a duct affected by sclerosing cholangitis, giving rise to a mass. However, none of the other features of sclerosing cholangitis are seen.

Diagnosis

Obstructive jaundice due to carcinoma of the pancreas

Treatment Options

Most patients with obstructive jaundice undergo diagnostic ERCP. If the obstruction can be crossed, a stent is placed to decompress the ducts. If the obstruction cannot be crossed, the patients are referred for transhepatic cholangiography and drainage. This sequence of procedures is of significance to the interventional radiologist because the attempts at retrograde (transduodenal) CBD cannulation and injection of contrast introduce organisms into the obstructed ducts, increasing the risk of septic complications from the percutaneous transhepatic procedures.

In this patient, ERCP was performed and showed a CBD stricture (see **Fig. 22-2**). As the lesion could not be crossed, the patient was referred for transhepatic cholangiography. She was not considered for surgery because of advanced age and surgical risks. Palliative treatment was undertaken.

Treatment

A right transcostal transhepatic cholangiogram was performed with a 22 gauge Chiba needle. A suitable duct was then selected for the insertion of a catheter (**Fig. 22-3**). Because it was difficult to manipulate and advance a catheter or guide wire through the markedly dilated and redundant common hepatic duct, a drainage catheter was placed proximal to the obstruction and left to gravity drainage (**Fig. 22-4**). Three days later, the patient was returned to the interventional suite. The obstruction was crossed and an internal drainage catheter was placed.

To overcome the difficulty posed by the redundant common hepatic duct, a 10F nontapered catheter was inserted into the duct to serve as a guiding catheter (alternatively, a long 8-10F sheath can be used for this purpose). A 5F multipurpose (hockey-stick shape) catheter was then inserted coaxially and used to negotiate the obstruction with a torqueable guide wire, followed by placement of the percutaneous biliary drainage (PBD) catheter (**Figs. 22-5** and **22-6**). A single episode of fever (100°F) occurred after the percutaneous transhepatic cholangiogram (PTC) and drainage. A few days later, she underwent placement of a self-expandable stent (**Fig. 22-7**) and was subsequently discharged home.

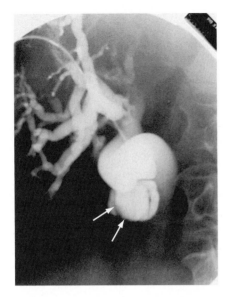

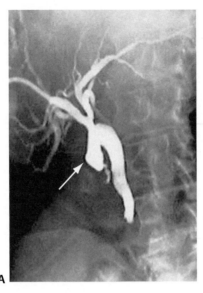

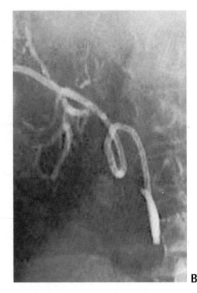

Figure 22-3 Cholangiogram after insertion of the Teflon sheath (of three-part needle) shows a markedly dilated and redundant common hepatic duct and dilated cystic duct (arrows).

Figure 22-4 (**A**) Cholangiogram after external drainage catheter placement and decompression of the ducts shows a persistent looping of the common hepatic duct (arrow). (**B**) Image shows the catheter course. The catheter is coiled in the distal CBD.

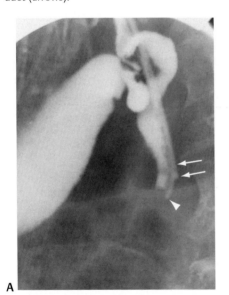

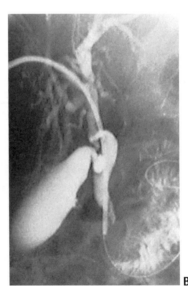

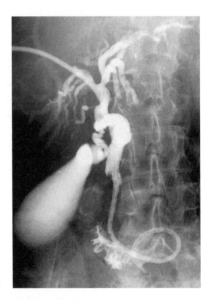

Figure 22-5 (**A,B**) A 10F nontapered guiding catheter (arrows) has been advanced to the obstruction and a multipurpose angiographic catheter (arrowhead) is used to guide the crossing of the stricture. Note that the common duct redundancy has diminished considerably after several days of biliary decompression.

Figure 22-6 A percutaneous biliary drainage catheter has been inserted over a heavy-duty guide wire.

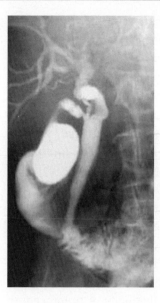

Figure 22-7 Cholangiogram after Wallstent placement shows unobstructed contrast flow.

Discussion

Elective PBD is indicated for:

- Palliation in patients with obstructive jaundice due to an unresectable malignancy
- Preoperative catheter placement in patients undergoing hepatojejunostomy for benign or malignant disease. These catheters can then be used by the surgeon to guide placement of Silastic tubes for stenting the anastomoses.
- Preintervention, for example, for retrieval of calculi and stricture dilatation
- Postendoscopy, after a failed procedure, or for the management of complications associated with endoscopic manipulation or stent placement. This often necessitates emergency PBD.

The indications for emergency PBD are:

- Obstructive cholangitis
- Postoperative or postendoscopic complications

Contraindications for PBD include:

- Abnormal clotting parameters: international normalized ratio (INR) >1.2, partial thromboplastin time >45 sec, platelets <80,000. Abnormal clotting parameters may be corrected as needed, by fresh frozen plasma, Factor 7a, or platelets given immediately before and during the procedure.
- Ascites. If severe, this is often associated with technical problems; in particular, difficulty in maintaining access. Such patients should undergo endoscopic drainage. If this is unsuccessful or not possible because of anatomy (Billroth II, large duodenal diverticulum, antral stenosis) surgery should be considered. In some cases, the left hepatic ducts may provide a safer alternative to the right transcostal approach.
- Diffuse hepatic metastases. Multiple ducts are obstructed and frequently isolated, or diffuse parenchymal disease may be responsible for the jaundice.

Patient Preparation

In preparation for the drainage procedure, patients are placed on clear liquids after midnight before the day of the procedure. Intravenous access is obtained for administration of fluids and medication. Laboratory data are reviewed, including renal function and clotting parameters. Significant volumes of contrast may be injected and deterioration of renal function can occur. Patients at risk for renal failure should be hydrated, contrast load kept at a minimum, and nephrotoxic medication avoided. If other contrast studies such as computed tomography (CT) have been performed in the preceding hours, PTC–PBD may be postponed for a few hours to avoid contrast nephrotoxicity or consideration be given to administration of nephroprotective medication such as fenoldopam mesylate or acetylcysteine.

Patients with known contrast allergy are prepped with corticosteroids and antihistamines: 40 mg prednisone PO and 50 mg benadryl PO every 6 hours for three consecutive doses, with the last dose taken shortly before the procedure. In addition, nonionic contrast is used in all patients. Alternative strategies should be exercised for patients who have suffered severe contrast reactions.

Patient comfort and cooperation are necessary, therefore, a satisfactory level of analgesia and sedation must be obtained prior to beginning the procedure. Premedication may be given on the patient floor or preferably after the patient arrives in the department. In either case, premedication should be given after consent has been obtained. I prefer an intramuscular injection of Demerol (meperidine) 70 to 100 mg given before prepping. During the procedure, intravenous meperidine is given in combination with Versed (midazolam) or Valium (diazepam) as the need arises. Alternatively, fentanyl and Versed can be used. Maximal safe dosage is determined individually. A preprocedure intercostal nerve block may decrease the analgesia requirement.

All patients are monitored for oxygen saturation (continuous), EKG (continuous), and noninvasive blood pressure (every 5–10 minutes and as needed). All patients receive an intravenous dose of a broad spectrum cephalosporin prior to PTC–PBD. The antibiotic is administered within an hour of the procedure. Patients who are already on antibiotics should also receive a dose within 1 hour of the procedure to provide maximal blood levels.

Technique

PBD can be performed as a one- or two-puncture procedure. The former is used if a suitable duct (for catheter placement) is entered with the 22 gauge PTC needle. More commonly, the two-puncture approach provides the flexibility to choose the most suitable duct for drainage catheter placement. For the right ductal system, I prefer fluoroscopic guidance. For the left-sided drainage, fluoroscopy or ultrasound guidance is used.

A wide area of the skin, from the lower right lateral ribs to the left upper quadrant, is prepped with Betadine or Hibiclens and sterile draped. The skin, subcutaneous tissues, and rib periosteum at the anticipated access site are infiltrated with local anesthetic (lidocaine 2%, 10–15 mL). A small skin incision is made with a no. 11 blade, and a 20 cm long 22 gauge Chiba needle is used for PTC. For the second puncture, a three-part needle is used (metal cannula with trocar and Teflon sheath).

Right Hepatic Ducts

For the right hepatic ducts (**Fig. 22-8**), the anterior to midaxillary line is chosen for entry. The needle is inserted staying above the rib, at least one to two intercostal spaces below the costophrenic sulcus as seen on deep inspiration. This avoids the pleural space. The needle is advanced in the direction of the cardiophrenic angle in suspended midrespiration in one smooth forward stroke. Subsequently, shallow respiration is permitted. The stylet is removed and a syringe with undiluted nonionic contrast on an extension tubing is attached to the needle hub. Under fluoroscopic observation, while continuously injecting contrast, the needle is gradually withdrawn until a duct is opacified. If a duct does not opacify on the first pass, the needle is withdrawn to the liver periphery and is redirected and readvanced in suspended respiration. The needle is not removed completely, to avoid multiple punctures of the liver capsule. Should a different intercostal space become necessary to redirect the

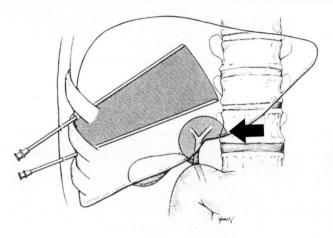

Figure 22-8 Diagram illustrating area for percutaneous transhepatic cholangiography needle insertion. Dotted area (arrow) represents the extrahepatic segments of the central ducts and should be avoided. (From Kadir S, Diagnostic Angiography, WB Saunders, 1986. With permission.)

needle, the first needle is left in place and a new needle is used. Violation of the capsule more than once may result in severe pain (due to capsular distention from leakage of bile, blood, or contrast) or peritonitis (from bile leakage).

Left Duct Puncture

If a left duct is to be used as the primary access (**Fig. 22-9**), ultrasound guidance is helpful. If left duct puncture is to be performed subsequent to PBD of the right hepatic ducts and contrast injected through the indwelling catheter opacifies the left ducts, a three-part needle is used for cannulation. In other cases, a 22 gauge PTC needle cholangiogram is obtained, via the right transcostal or the left subxiphoid approach.

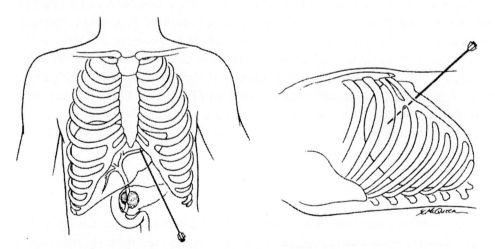

Figure 22-9 Diagram illustrating needle position and angulation for left hepatic duct percutaneous transhepatic cholangiography–percutaneous biliary drainage. (From Kadir S, Current Practice of Interventional Radiology, BC Decker, 1991. With permission.)

Single-Puncture PBD

Once a duct is opacified with the 22 gauge needle, an additional 5 to 7 mL contrast is injected. Topography of the duct is assessed for feasibility of catheter placement by placing a marker at the

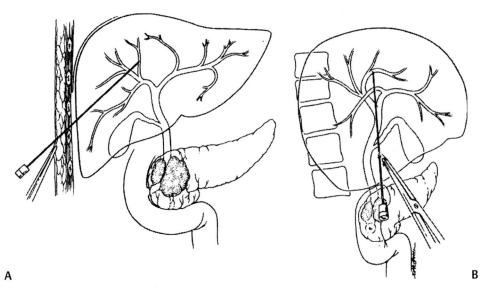

Figure 22-10 Diagram illustrating the single puncture approach for percutaneous biliary drainage. (**A**) In the anteroposterior projection, the 22 gauge needle tip is in a duct that is amenable to this technique. Location of the duct, transhepatic needle course, and angle of needle entry into the duct appear acceptable for catheter placement. (**B**) Lateral projection. A Kelly clamp placed at the skin entry site shows alignment of the duct and needle entry point. (From Kadir S, Current Practice of Interventional Radiology, BC Decker, 1991. With permission.)

skin puncture site and turning the C-arm to the lateral position (**Fig. 22-10**). If the duct is relatively aligned with the puncture site, an 0.018 in. coathanger wire (Cope, Cook Incorp., Bloomington, IN) is inserted and passed into the common hepatic or common bile duct. The needle is removed and a coaxial dilator system (Cook, Incorp., 4.2F inner and 6F outer catheter) is inserted. The inner catheter is removed. A bile sample is aspirated and sent for Gramstain and culture. Bile samples for cytology are rarely diagnostic. Catheter tip position in the common duct is confirmed by contrast injection. The duct is then decompressed by removal of some bile, and contrast is reinjected to delineate the anatomy. A torqueable guide wire is inserted and an attempt made to traverse the obstruction. If this is successful, the catheter is advanced beyond the obstruction. It is then exchanged for a PBD over a heavy-duty guide wire (e.g., Amplatz super stiff wire, Boston Scientific, Natick, MA). From the right transcostal approach, an 8 or, 10F, 32 or 45 side-hole Ring- or Cope-type catheter is used; from the left ducts, a 45 or 65 side-hole catheter is used. If the liver consistency is hard, the tract is first dilated with 7 to 9F dilators before catheter insertion.

Two-Puncture PBD

If the 22 gauge needle has entered a duct that does not lend itself to easy catheter insertion, lateral fluoroscopy (or an image) is used to determine the plane of the more appropriate duct. For reference, a metal clamp or other radiopaque marker is placed at the 22 gauge needle skin entry site (**Fig. 22-11**). A three-part needle is inserted through a second access site. With the C-arm in the anteroposterior projection, the needle is advanced into the duct in a single, slow, continuous thrust, in suspended respiration. As it enters, the needle displaces the duct. Once in the duct, the stylet is removed (leaving the metal cannula and Teflon sheath in place) and a bile sample is obtained for bacteriology. Contrast is injected to confirm needle tip position and define anatomy for guide wire manipulation. A torqueable guide wire is inserted and advanced into the common duct, and if possible, into the bowel. While holding the metal cannula in place, the Teflon sheath is advanced over the guide wire. The metal cannula and guide wire are removed and again contrast is injected to assess the position of the Teflon sheath tip.

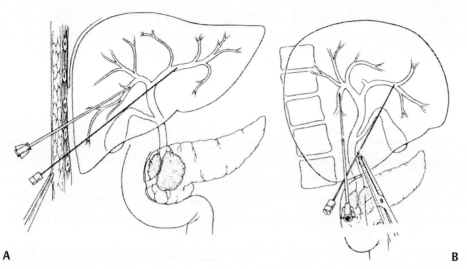

Figure 22-11 Diagram illustrating the two-puncture approach for percutaneous biliary drainage (PBD). (**A**) In the anteroposterior projection, the 22 gauge needle tip is in a duct that does not lend itself to easy PBD catheter placement. (**B**) In the lateral projection, a clamp placed at the skin entry site shows the 22 gauge needle tip in an anterior duct. Using the clamp as a guide, a suitable duct is selected for the second puncture and drainage catheter insertion. (From Kadir S, Current Practice of Interventional Radiology, BC Decker, 1991. With permission.)

If the obstruction has been crossed, a stiff shaft guide wire (e.g., Amplatz super stiff wire) is inserted for placement of a drainage catheter. If the common duct obstruction cannot be easily crossed, a heavy-duty J guide wire is inserted for placement of a catheter proximal to the obstruction. If the common duct is dilated, a nephrostomy catheter is used. Alternatively, a straight catheter with multiple side holes is used (e.g., 8.3F, 16 side-hole, Cook Incorp.). The latter is not left in place for longer than 24 hours because it tends to dislodge with respiratory excursions.

Single Versus Bilateral PBD

A single PBD catheter is placed if both left and right ductal systems communicate freely. If one lobar duct is completely obstructed and isolated without communication with the remaining ducts, this maybe left undrained. If the obstructed duct drains a significant portion of the liver, this should be decompressed electively by the placement of a second catheter. A second catheter is also necessary in the presence of severe stenosis of the contralateral ducts.

Stent Placement

Self-expanding stents play an increasing role in patients with an unresectable malignant biliary obstruction. Removal of the drainage catheter not only provides a psychological benefit for the patient but also eliminates the catheter management related problems. As a result, there may be a tendency for the insertion of self-expandible stents early in the course of management. Although there is no real advantage to early stent placement (within 5–7 days of the decompression), experience shows that there is a higher incidence of stent obstruction by viscous bile and debris. Therefore, stent deployment should be delayed for 2 to 3 weeks. This also allows the patient to recuperate and liver functions to stabilize, and permits management of problems and reassessment of the treatment plan. Furthermore, as maturation of the transhepatic tract occurs, fewer complications such as bleeding and cholangitis can be expected upon removal of the catheter.

Stent patency seems to vary with the type of underlying malignancy and location of the stent. The reported median patency for biliary stents placed for all malignancies was 135 days (1 week to over a year). Stent occlusion occurred in up to 19% of patients, usually due to tumor overgrowth.

Post-Procedure Care

The PBD catheter is secured by skin suture. The patients remain on external drainage for 24 to 48 hours after PBD. In septic patients, external drainage is maintained until sepsis has cleared. Subsequently, a cholangiogram through the catheter delineates the anatomy and permits determination of the course of management (internal drainage, retrieval of calculi, endoprosthesis, stricture dilatation, surgery, etc.). If there is free flow of contrast with the catheter through the obstruction, it is converted to internal drainage by placing an injection-site adapter or stopcock at the catheter hub.

For the duration of external drainage, the catheter is flushed once or twice a day with 5 to 10 mL saline. Aspiration is avoided because this draws bowel contents into the catheter, predisposing to obstruction and infection. Antibiotics are continued for at least 24 hours for routine PBD and longer in the presence of sepsis or cholangitis. Routine access site care and dressing change is recommended every 3 to 4 days. Outpatient catheter exchange is performed every 2 to 3 months or sooner if necessary (for obstruction or bile leakage). In asymptomatic patients, antibiotic coverage is not necessary for routine catheter exchange. For those with fever or cholangitis, a single intravenous dose of a broad spectrum cephalosporin is given before catheter exchange.

Results

In the presence of dilated ducts, a 22 gauge needle cholangiogram can be obtained in all patients. In unobstructed ducts, the success rate for PTC is ~85%. Drainage catheter placement is possible in all patients with successful PTC, although several sessions maybe required for tract dilatation and catheter advancement through a severe obstruction or fibrotic liver. Relief of symptoms usually occurs immediately after decompression of the ducts. With a catheter in the bowel, there is bacterial seeding of the biliary tract in >95% of patients within 2 to 3 days. Presence of intestinal air in the intrahepatic ducts is not uncommon after internal drainage.

Complications

Serious complications, such as sepsis or severe bleeding occur in less than 6% of patients undergoing PTC–PBD. Overdistention of ducts, prolonged catheter and guide wire manipulation, insufficient antibiotic coverage, and presence of infection (PBD following failed ERCP, acute obstructive cholangitis, CBD calculus) predispose to septic complications. A transient increase in intrabiliary pressure >20 cm H_2O occurs during contrast injection and can lead to biliovenous or biliolymphatic reflux and sepsis. In such patients, excessive manipulation should be avoided.

Bile leakage can be a difficult management problem. Potential causes are:

- Malpositioned catheter with proximal side holes either distal to an obstruction or outside the duct (in liver parenchyma or at the skin)
- Damaged catheter
- Increased intra-abdominal pressure (e.g., ascites)
- Small bowel obstruction
- Posterior (dependent) duct access of PBD catheter

Management consists of repositioning or replacement of the catheter. Most efforts fail in the presence of increased intra-abdominal pressure and bowel obstruction.

- Appropriately planned and executed PTC–PBD is successful in virtually all patients with biliary obstruction.
- Indications for PBD include palliation in malignant obstruction, preoperative catheter placement for hepaticojejunal anastomoses, after endoscopy (failed procedure or complications), and obstructive cholangitis.
- Many of the underlying problems leading to obstructive jaundice can be managed by interventional radiological methods (e.g., calculi, strictures, or palliation of malignant obstruction).
- Patients undergoing PTC–PBD following ERCP are at increased risk for septic complications.

Further Reading

Binkley CE, Eckhauser FE, Colletti LM. Unusual causes of benign biliary strictures with cholangiographic features of cholangiocarcinoma. J Gastrointest Surg 2002;6:676–681

Crist DW, Kadir S, Cameron JL. The value of preoperatively placed percutaneous biliary catheters in reconstruction of the proximal part of the biliary tract. Surg Gynecol Obstet 1987;165:421–424

Kim HS, Lee DK, Kim HG, et al. Features of malignant biliary obstruction affecting the patency of metallic stents: a multicenter study. Gastrointest Endosc 2002;55:359–365

Lascarides CE, Bini EJ, Newman E, et al. Intrinsic common bile duct stricture: an unusual presentation of retroperitoneal fibrosis. Gastrointest Endosc 1999;50:102–105

Oberholzer K, Pitton MB, Mildenberger P, et al. The current value of percutaneous transhepatic biliary drainage [in German]. Rofo 2002;174:1081–1088

Rieber A, Brambs HJ. Metallic stents in malignant biliary obstruction. Cardiovasc Intervent Radiol 1997;20:43–49

Stoker J, Lameris JS. Complications of percutaneously inserted biliary Wallstents. J Vasc Interv Radiol 1993;4:767–772

Tumlin JA, Wang A, Murray PT, et al. Fenoldopam mesylate blocks reductions in renal plasma flow after radiocontrast dye infusion: a pilot trial in the prevention of contrast nephropathy. Am Heart J 2002;143:894–903

Winick AB, Waybill PN, Venbrux AC. Complications of percutaneous transhepatic biliary interventions. Tech Vasc Interv Radiol 2001;4:200–206

CHAPTER 23 Malignant Hilar Obstruction

Saadoon Kadir

Clinical Presentation

An 84-year-old woman was evaluated for diminished appetite, weight loss, pruritus, and obstructive jaundice.

Radiological Studies

Abdominal computed tomography (CT) demonstrated a mass at the left and right hepatic duct junction with dilatation of intrahepatic ducts (**Fig. 23-1**). The patient was referred for cholangiography and biliary decompression. The percutaneous transhepatic cholangiogram (PTC) showed narrowing of the common hepatic duct with an apple core appearance (**Fig. 23-2**). There dilatation of the right hepatic ducts and no contrast opacification of the left hepatic ducts is shown. The common bile duct was of a normal caliber.

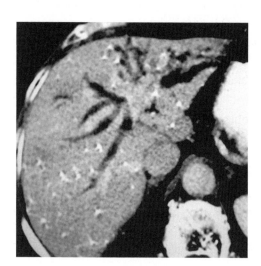

Figure 23-1 Image from the contrast-enhanced abdominal computed tomography shows dilatation of intrahepatic ducts and an obstructing mass.

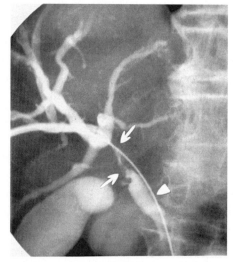

Figure 23-2 Right transhepatic cholangiogram shows a common hepatic duct stricture. The lumen is irregular and narrowed with an apple core appearance (arrows). The right hepatic ducts are dilated and the left hepatic ducts do not opacify. A guide wire has been inserted through the obstruction (arrowhead).

Differential Diagnosis

Causes of hilar biliary obstruction include gallbladder carcinoma, metastases, cholangiocarcinoma, lymphoma, sclerosing cholangitis, benign postoperative or traumatic strictures, Mirizzi syndrome, benign and some rare primary malignant tumors of the bile ducts, and an occasional carcinoma of the pancreas. In malignant disease, frequently a distinction cannot be made between gallbladder carcinoma, metastases, and cholangiocarcinoma. With the exception of the rare multicentric papillary tumors, benign tumors and sclerosing cholangitis rarely lead to isolation of lobar ducts. In sclerosing cholangitis, skip lesions and intrahepatic duct strictures are present and there is usually a lesser degree of intrahepatic ductal dilatation. In addition, longer segments are affected.

118

Diagnosis

Hilar cholangiocarcinoma (Klatskin's tumor)

Treatment Options

For obstructive jaundice, the initial treatment consists of biliary decompression via a percutaneous transhepatic or endoscopic approach. Hilar tumors obstructing both the left and the right hepatic ducts may necessitate placement of drainage catheters in both ducts. Subsequent management depends upon patient age, clinical status, comorbid conditions, and extent of disease.

Surgical management: In the absence of extrahepatic spread (beyond the hepatic pedicle nodes), surgical management consists of tumor excision with or without hepatic resection and hepaticojejunostomy or liver transplantation. The hepaticojejunostomy may be stented with Silastic tubes. To facilitate placement of such tubes, some surgeons may prefer preoperatively placed transhepatic drainage catheters.

Palliation: In the presence of advanced disease or high operative risk, the options are percutaneous or endoscopic drainage and subsequent placement of metallic stents. In patients managed percutaneously, transcatheter brachytherapy is also possible with iridium (Ir^{192}).

In this patient, surgery was not a consideration because of her age and extent of disease. Therefore, palliative intervention was undertaken.

Treatment

Percutaneous right and left hepatic duct drainage catheters were placed. After normalization of liver function tests, the patient underwent hilar reconstruction with metallic stents.

Coagulation parameters and renal function were evaluated and were normal. Ancef 1 g was given intravenously prior to the procedure and antibiotic coverage was continued for several days after each biliary drainage (PBD) catheter placement. Initially, an 8F right transhepatic PBD catheter was inserted. Because there was persistent jaundice and pruritus and slow clinical and laboratory improvement, the left hepatic ducts were drained via the subxiphoid approach (**Fig. 23-3**).

Two weeks later, she was brought back for hilar reconstruction with metallic stents. As the tumor extended further along the left hepatic duct, this access was chosen for the placement of the initial stent. Both PBD catheters were removed over exchange length guide wires. An 8F sheath was placed in the left duct and a 10 × 42 mm Wallstent (Boston Scientific, Watertown, MA) was deployed across the

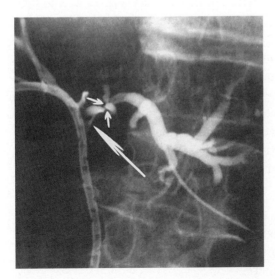

Figure 23-3 Subxiphoid transhepatic cholangiogram of the left hepatic ducts shows severe narrowing of the central segment of the main left hepatic duct (long arrow). The smaller branches are also narrowed at their junction with the left hepatic duct (small arrows).

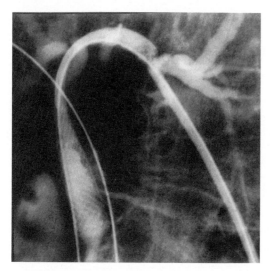

Figure 23-4 A 10 × 42 mm Wallstent has been deployed across the strictured segments in the left and common hepatic ducts. The stent was subsequently balloon dilated to facilitate maximal expansion.

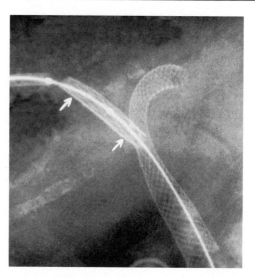

Figure 23-5 Image shows the Palmaz stent (arrows) in the central right hepatic duct, reconstructing the hilar confluence.

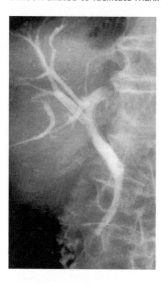

Figure 23-6 Cholangiogram obtained at the time of catheter removal shows unobstructed drainage and decompression of the intrahepatic ducts.

ductal confluence with the proximal end extending well into the left hepatic duct (**Fig. 23-4**). The stent was balloon dilated to 8 mm using a standard angioplasty balloon (Cook Incorp., Bloomington, IN). A second stent was placed from the right side to reconstruct the hilar confluence. A multipurpose catheter was advanced through the Wallstent mesh and the opening was dilated with an 8 mm angioplasty balloon. A long vascular sheath was advanced through the opening into the common duct. A 20 mm length Palmaz stent loaded onto an 8 mm balloon was then inserted through the sheath and deployed across the stricture. The distal end of the Palmaz stent was positioned in the Wallstent and balloon dilated to 8 mm (**Fig. 23-5**). An 8F PBD catheter was then inserted and placed to internal drainage. A cholangiogram was obtained the next day which showed free passage of contrast (**Fig. 23-6**).The catheter was removed over a guide wire There was complete resolution of symptoms and normalization of liver tests.

Discussion

Cholangiocarcinoma is the most common primary malignant bile duct tumor. It is a rare tumor with an autopsy incidence of <0.5% (Sako et al, 1957; Akwari et al, 1975). The peak occurrence is in the sixth to seventh decades, with a slight male preponderance.

The tumor is also seen in younger patients (third–fourth decades), usually in those with preexisting diseases (see following discussion). It is less common in individuals of African descent (Lees et al, 1980).

Although the etiology is not known, there is an unusually high incidence of biliary malignancies in patients with chronic ulcerative colitis (Akwari et al, 1975). In these patients, cholangiocarcinoma occurs at a much younger age and the initial symptoms may be nonspecific. The latency period between onset of ulcerative colitis and cholangiocarcinoma is ~20 years (Akwari et al, 1975). Others at a higher risk of developing cholangiocarcinoma include individuals with preexisting biliary diseases such as choledochal cysts, chronic sclerosing cholangitis, chronic cholangitis following biliary–enteric anastomoses, and parasite infestation (liver flukes, clonorchiasis, *Clonorchis sinensis*) (Flanigan, 1977; Lim, 1990; Campbell et al, 1998; Tocchi et al, 2001). There may also be an increased propensity in Caroli's disease, polycystic liver disease, and congenital hepatic fibrosis.

Cholangiocarcinoma can occur at any location (i.e., in the intra- or extrahepatic ducts). In decreasing order of frequency, it occurs at the junction of left and right hepatic ducts (45%), common bile duct (40%), common hepatic, intrahepatic, and cystic ducts (Okuda et al, 1977; Lees et al, 1980). Occasionally, the tumor is multicentric. Cholangiocarcinoma involving the confluence of the left and right hepatic ducts is also referred to as a *hilar* or Klatskin's tumor and is essentially an extrahepatic tumor. Those arising from intrahepatic ducts are also referred to as *peripheral* cholangiocarcinomas.

The majority of tumors are slow-growing adenocarcinomas with varying grades of differentiation. Tumor spread is via perineural lymphatics in the bile ducts and by direct extension into the liver (Ross et al, 1973). Hilar tumors frequently invade the portal vein and hepatic artery leading to stenoses or occlusions. Splenomegaly may be seen in portal vein obstruction. Hematogenous spread with distant metastases is uncommon.

Presentation

The mode of presentation is determined by the location of the tumor. The common clinical presentation is an insidious onset of jaundice associated with little or no pain, pruritus, fatigue, and loss of appetite and weight. Painless jaundice is more common in distal choledochal tumors. Jaundice with pain (chronic dyspepsia or acute colic-like) and gallbladder distention are seen in tumors that involve the hepatic–cystic duct junction or arise in the cystic duct. Jaundice may fluctuate in intensity, especially in intraductal tumors (Ross et al, 1973). Pain, which may be right upper quadrant, epigastric, or diffuse abdominal, is more frequent in proximal tumors and is believed to result from portal-periportal neural invasion. An occasional tumor may present with an acute onset of fever, chills, jaundice, and right upper quadrant tenderness or pain, simulating acute cholecystitis (Braasch, 1973). The less frequent intrahepatic cholangiocarcinoma may obstruct a segmental or lobar duct and present with fever, cholangitis, and hepatic abscess with or without jaundice. Tumor obstructing a single major hepatic duct may not manifest with clinical jaundice but the laboratory tests (e.g., alkaline phosphatase) are usually abnormal.

Gallbladder distention is often present in distal duct obstruction. The gallbladder is not distended if the tumor is located proximal to the hepatic-cystic duct junction (i.e., intrahepatic, common hepatic duct, or hilar tumor).

Laboratory tests show elevated levels of bilirubin, transaminases, and alkaline phosphatase. Associated findings include biliary calculi (30–40% of patients), ulcerative colitis (5–8%), sclerosing cholangitis, previous biliary surgery (gallbladder, biliary stricture, choledochal cyst), and unrelated previous malignancy (Sako et al, 1957; Ross et al, 1973; Akwari et al, 1975; Flanigan, 1977; Lees et al, 1980; Tocchi et al, 2001).

Diagnosis and Classification

Accurate staging for determination of resectability is often difficult because of the patterns of growth and spread. Although noninvasive imaging studies contribute significantly to the diagnosis, determination of the level of obstruction, and regional spread, this information may be inaccurate for determination of resectability (Triller et al, 1994; Cha et al, 2000). Similarly, laparoscopy has been shown to be inaccurate for determination of tumor resectability in 46% of cases (Tilleman et al, 2002).

If small or the infiltrating type, the tumor may not be demonstrated by ultrasound or CT. On the other hand, duplex sonography and multislice CT angiography can provide valuable information on vascular invasion and obstruction (i.e., of the portal vein and hepatic artery). Endoscopic retrograde cholangiopancreatography (ERCP) (with or without endosonography) and transhepatic cholangiography also provide valuable information in infiltrating and intraductal tumors. There are several advantages of percutaneous cholangiography: (1) the proximal extent of an obstructing tumor can be determined. On ERCP, contrast may not get past an obstruction. (2) Drainage catheters can be placed to aid the surgeon should resection with hepatojejunal anastomosis be a consideration.

Cholangiocarcinoma may be classified according to location (intrahepatic, extrahepatic) or pathology (infiltrating, nodular, polypoid).

Intrahepatic Tumors

These are mostly nodular, masslike, infrequently infiltrating, poorly differentiated, or undifferentiated adenocarcinomas. They arise from the left or right hepatic ducts or their branches, are uncommon, and are often large at the time of diagnosis. Symptoms are nonspecific (epigastric or right upper quadrant pain or discomfort, fever, malaise, weight loss) and jaundice is usually absent unless the tumor extends into the hilar region to obstruct a major duct. If the tumor involves only a single larger hepatic duct, it may remain undetected for some time in the absence of jaundice and pruritus.

On CT, they appear as large, well defined, low attenuation masses, occurring anywhere in the liver. There is peripheral contrast enhancement and delayed enhancement of the more central portions. There may be lobulation, capsular retraction, and dilatation of ducts peripheral to the mass. Hepatic metastases from colon carcinoma and hepatocellular carcinoma may have a similar appearance. The presence of lobar or segmental liver atrophy indicates long-standing obstruction by the tumor that has invaded and occluded the bile duct (usually the central portion of a hepatic duct) or portal vein of the affected segment (or both).

Extrahepatic Tumors

The hilar and perihilar tumor is of the infiltrating type in >75% of cases. It is a poorly differentiated adenocarcinoma that spreads along the duct in a linear fashion, inciting an intense fibrotic reaction. There is thickening of the duct wall involving all layers resulting in encircling, with narrowing or occlusion of the lumen over a longer segment. Often there is no identifiable mass. The classic sign in hilar tumors is dilatation of intrahepatic ducts and a normal-diameter common bile duct. The gallbladder is collapsed unless the tumor extends to obstruct the cystic duct, in which case, it is often distended. In some cases, the tumor extends into the surrounding tissues, giving rise to a small, round mass that circumferentially constricts a segment of duct (**Fig. 23-7**).

Fig. 23-8 shows the modified Bismuth-Corlette classification of hilar cholangiocarcinoma. This classification is based upon the relationship (i.e., extension) of the tumor to the ductal confluence and major branches. It is derived from cholangiography findings and observations at surgery. The Type III and IV lesions occur most commonly.

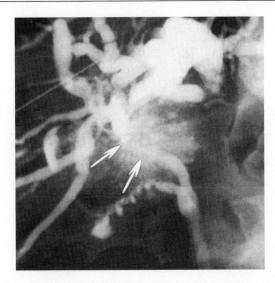

Figure 23-7 Incidental tumor opacification at the time of 22 gauge needle cholangiography demonstrates a periductal mass encasing and severely constricting the common hepatic duct (arrows). (From Kadir, S, Diagnostic Angiography, WB Saunders, Philadelphia, 1986. With permission.)

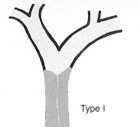

Type I

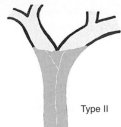

Type II

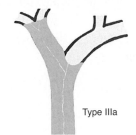

Type IIIa

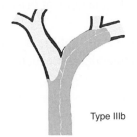

Type IIIb

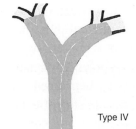

Type IV

Type I: Tumor does not involve
ductal confluence.
Type II: Tumor obstructs the left and right
hepatic duct junction (hilus).
Type III: Tumor extends to a first
order branch on one side.
Type IIIa - right side
Type IIIb - left side
Type IV: Tumor extends to a first
order branch on both sides.

Figure 23-8 Line drawings showing the modified Bismuth-Corlette classification of hilar cholangiocarcinoma. This classification establishes the location of the tumor and its extension with respect to the major ductal confluence and first order branches. (Adapted from Bismuth H, Corlette MB. Intrahepatic cholangioenteric anastomosis in carcinoma of the hilus of the liver. Surg Gynecol Obstet 1975;140:170–178 and Bismuth H, Nakache R, Diamond T. Management strategies in resection for hilar cholangiocarcinoma. Ann Surg 1992;215: 31–38.)

Table 23-1   Diseases and Conditions That May Mimic Cholangiocarcinoma

Malignant diseases	Other benign diseases
Common	Strictures
Gallbladder carcinoma	Postsurgical
Metastases	Posttraumatic
Uncommon	Chronic pancreatitis
Hepatoma	Postradiation
Lymphoma	Inflammatory
Pancreatic carcinoma	Sclerosing cholangitis
Benign tumors	Calculi
Carcinoid	Papillary stenosis
Cystadenoma	Heterotopic pancreas
Fibroma	Collagen vascular diseases
Granular cell tumor	Retroperitoneal fibrosis
Neurofibroma	Vascular causes
Papillary adenoma	Aberrant vessel
	Abdominal aortic aneurysm
	Visceral artery aneurysm

Frequently, the infiltrating tumor is difficult to differentiate from sclerosing cholangitis on cholangiography and also on histology. Cholangiography shows a variable-length stricture with an irregular lumen and stenoses or occlusion and isolation of ducts that join this segment (see **Figs. 23-2** and **23-3**). On sonography, the duct wall is thickened. The thickened duct may show contrast enhancement on CT. If the tumor involves both hepatic ducts (hilar or Klatskin's tumor), ductal isolation (nonunion) may be seen. Tissue diagnosis is often difficult because of the presence of extensive fibrosis. Thus the diagnostic yield of transluminal brushing is low. Needle biopsy, on the other hand, provides a higher yield.

In common duct tumors, most of which are also infiltrating-type lesions, there is dilatation of the intra- and extrahepatic ducts, and the gallbladder is frequently distended.

Intraductal Tumors

Occasionally, an adenocarcinoma may have predominantly intraluminal growth and present as a polypoid intraductal mass. Such tumors are quite uncommon, although in one series, the reported incidence was around 13% (Nichols et al, 1983). Intraductal tumor may occur at any location as a single lesion or as multiple masses. Larger tumors can be visualized on sonography (Marchal et al, 1984). The involved section of the duct is usually widened and filled with the tumor, which may be localized to a segment or extend some distance in the duct. The obstructed peripheral ducts are dilated. In these patients, the jaundice is often fluctuating in intensity. The symptoms are otherwise similar to those of other obstructive lesions. Diseases that may simulate intraductal polypoid cholangiocarcinoma include mucin-producing tumors (mucinous carcinoma metastases), hepatocellular carcinoma that has invaded the bile duct and presents as an intraductal mass, calculi, clot, oriental cholangiohepatitis, and benign tumors (e.g., papillary tumors, cystadenoma). Diseases and conditions that may mimic cholangiocarcinoma are listed in **Table 23-1.**

Nonsurgical Management

Advanced-stage tumors of the hepatic duct confluence necessitate long-term palliation through interventional radiological or endoscopic methods. Although endoscopic management is attractive,

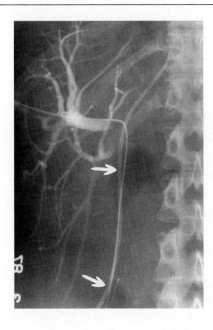

Figure 23-9 Patient with hilar stricture and endoscopically placed left duct stent. Cholangitis due to obstruction of the right hepatic duct by the endoscopically placed stent (arrows) necessitated percutaneous transhepatic drainage catheter placement. Cholangiogram shows dilatation of the right ducts with no contrast passage into the common duct. A guide wire has been inserted in preparation for drainage catheter placement.

it is associated with less than adequate results and significant morbidity, especially if unilateral drainage is undertaken (Liu et al, 1998). Usually, both sides are catheterized and only the dominant ductal system is drained. The contralateral system remains obstructed and cholangitis develops as a result of bacterial introduction from the transduodenal catheterization (**Fig. 23-9**). To avoid this complication, magnetic resonance (MR) cholangiography has been used to guide placement of a single internal stent for drainage of the dominant lobe, and catheterization of the contralateral ducts is avoided (Hintze et al, 2001).

The interventional radiological management consists of placement of two PBD catheters for the drainage of both lobes. If a lobar duct is completely occluded and does not opacify on the initial cholangiograms, it may be left undrained (i.e., only a single PBD catheter is inserted). The undrained lobe subsequently atrophies. If the patient later develops cholangitis, the obstructed system must be drained or sepsis and abscess formation ensue. Pruritus may persist after unilateral drainage and is an indication for drainage (and stenting) of the obstructed lobar duct, as in the patient described.

Hilar tumors can be managed by PBD catheters alone (without metallic stent placement). These catheters then provide access for brachytherapy. The disadvantages are that the catheters cross the papilla, and side-hole occlusion from encrustation of duodenal secretions, bile leakage around the catheter, and ascending cholangitis may necessitate frequent catheter exchange. Therefore, metallic stents are preferred and can be deployed to reconstruct the hilar confluence to provide optimal drainage.

METALLIC STENTS

For the management of hilar obstruction, metallic stents can be placed in several configurations through either a single transhepatic access or separate right and left lobe accesses: two parallel stents, one for drainage of each lobe, Y- or T-configuration or sidearm configuration. Among others, self-expanding Wallstents and Gianturco stents and balloon-expanded Palmaz stents have been used. A combination of the Wallstent with a Palmaz stent (or short Wallstent) in a sidearm con-figuration provides an unobstructed lumen. When a second Wallstent is deployed through the initial stent in a Y-configuration, the mesh of the second stent can potentially obstruct the contralateral duct. The hilum can also be reconstructed with Gianturco stents at a higher cost as multiple stents are required.

From a single access, often there is difficulty in inserting the inflexible Palmaz stent into the contralateral hepatic duct, especially if there is acute angulation at the ductal confluence. Instead, a short Wallstent (8 × 20 mm) can be deployed through the initial stent. The latter is also preferred if bilateral access is available. From the ipsilateral approach, the distal segment of the Wallstent can be anchored in the mesh of the initial Wallstent, lessening the risk of stent migration. From a single access, accurate deployment of a short Wallstent in the contralateral duct may be a challenge because of its shortening and straightening as it fully expands. This problem can be circumvented by using other self-expanding stents that do no shorten upon reexpansion.

Proper stent positioning is important because it is associated with better patency rates. The Wallstent is positioned such that the obstruction lies close to the midsection, so that the tumorous area is not uncovered as the stent shortens while expanding to its unconstrained diameter. Additionally, if the stent margin is close to the tumor, overgrowth may occlude the lumen. Stent slippage is uncommon and has been observed when deployed into an existing stent (Lee et al, 1993).

WHEN SHOULD METALLIC STENTS BE PLACED?

It is prudent to wait at least 2 to 3 weeks after biliary decompression. This has several advantages: it allows the patient to recuperate and the liver functions to stabilize, and permits management of problems (e.g., cholangitis, if present) and reassessment of the treatment plan. In addition, tract maturation occurs, and as a result, there are fewer complications such as bleeding (including minor bleeding) and cholangitis. The stents can placed during a second admission with overnight observation.

Prognosis and Survival

By the time the diagnosis is made, the tumor has usually spread beyond the bile ducts. Most patients have regional nodal metastases (periportal, celiac, hepatoduodenal ligament) whereas a smaller number have hepatic, omental, pancreatic, splenic, and pulmonary metastases. The latter are usually an autopsy finding (Okuda et al, 1977). The prognosis of proximal tumors is poor even after resection. Extrahepatic duct tumors are usually discovered earlier because of onset of symptoms. Intrahepatic tumors are detected later because the symptoms are often nonspecific.

Overall mean survival time after surgery was 28 months in one series and the overall 1-, 3-, and 5-year survival was 70%, 27.5%, and 12.5%, respectively (Launois et al, 1999). Survival after operative treatment depends upon tumor location and is better in type I and II early-stage tumors and improved short-term results are also seen in those undergoing aggressive treatment for advanced disease (Launois et al, 1999). In advanced disease, the prognosis is poor with palliative treatment (median survival 6 months) and there are very few long-term survivors (Born et al, 2000). Although macroscopically the tumor may have been removed in its entirety, histological examination frequently demonstrates tumor at the surgical resection margin (Bismuth et al 1992). Thus only a small percentage of patients may be tumor free even after resection. Survival rates are best in patients with tumor-free excision margins.

Biliary stents placed for all types of malignancies have a median patency of 135 days (1 week to >1 year). In patients with cholangiocarcinoma, the results are variable, with longer stent patency reported by some (average 10 months) and a higher occlusion rate for hilar tumors by others (Stoker and Lameris, 1993; Rieber and Brambs, 1997). Occlusion is due to tumor, and in the majority, this is from tumor overgrowth at the ends. Tumor ingrowth through the struts is uncommon. Less frequently, inspissated secretions may occlude the stent. Endoscopically placed metal stents had a 41.2% reported occlusion rate (Kim et al, 2002). The occlusion rates for endoscopically placed exchangeable stents are significantly higher.

Table 23-2 Complications Associated with Biliary Stent Placement for Obstructive Jaundice

Early[a]	Late
Intrahepatic hematoma	Jaundice from stent obstruction
Bleeding (hemobilia) from biliovenous or arteriobiliary fistula	Stent migration/malpositioning
	Duodenal ulceration
Cholangitis	Cholangitis
Cholecystitis (due to cystic duct obstruction)	Cholecystitis (due to cystic duct obstruction)
Sepsis	
Hepatic abscess	
Duct/duodenal perforation	
Stent obstruction	
Stent malpositioning	
Pleural effusion/empyema	

[a]1–30 days

From Stoker and Lameris, 1993; Rieber and Brambs, 1997; Salomonowitz et al, 1992.

Complications

Procedure-related complications are reported in 7 to 25% of patients (Salomonowitz et al, 1992; Stoker and Lameris, 1993; Rieber and Brambs, 1997). Most are minor and related to the transhepatic cholangiogram and drainage catheter placement. **Table 23-2** lists the stenting-related complications. Some of these, notably those due to bleeding and infection, can be severe. A 2% mortality has been reported (Stoker and Lameris, 1993). The procedures used to manage complications from the initial PBD and stent deployment (reintervention) may also be associated with complications. For example, cholangitis, abscess, and bleeding may complicate PBD for treatment of stent occlusion (Stoker and Lameris, 1993).

MANAGEMENT OF COMPLICATIONS

Complications are managed according to the underlying causes. Infection is treated by appropriate antibiotics. Acute cholecystitis may necessitate ultrasound-guided percutaneous gallbladder aspiration or cholecystostomy. Hemobilia due to a portobiliary or arteriobiliary fistula can often be managed by tamponading the tract with a larger-diameter catheter or arteriography and embolization may be necessary in severe arterial bleeding.

Stent occlusion from tumor overgrowth usually necessitates placement of another stent to cover the segment occluded by tumor. Alternatively, the occlusion can be managed by endoscopic placement of an exchangeable stent or long-term PBD. As overgrowth is the most common cause for tumor-progression-related stent occlusion, it is unlikely that the use of covered stents will provide significantly improved patency rates.

For stent occlusion from debris, after establishing PBD, the stent is cleared with the help of balloon catheters and saline flush. Overdistention of the ducts is avoided because this may cause cholangitis and sepsis. PBD catheters are left in place until stent patency is confirmed, or if symptomatic, then until symptoms have cleared.

PEARLS AND PITFALLS

- Cholangiocarcinoma is the most common primary malignant bile duct tumor.
- It occurs at the junction of left and right hepatic ducts in ~45% of cases.

- Accurate tumor staging for determination of resectability is often difficult. The prognosis of proximal tumors is poor even after resection because histological examination frequently demonstrates tumor at the resection margin.
- Metallic biliary stents can be used to reestablish hilar junction patency for palliative relief of obstructive jaundice.

Further Reading

Akwari OE, van Heerden JA, Foulk WT, et al. Cancer of the bile ducts associated with ulcerative colitis. Ann Surg 1975;181:303–309

Bismuth H, Nakache R, Diamond T. Management strategies in resection for hilar cholangiocarcinoma. Ann Surg 1992;215:31–38

Born P, Rosch T, Bruhl K, et al. Long-term outcome in patients with advanced hilar bile duct tumors undergoing palliative endoscopic or percutaneous drainage. Z Gastroenterol 2000;38:483–489

Braasch JW. Carcinoma of the bile duct. Surg Clin North Am 1973;53:1217–1227

Campbell WL, Ferris JV, Holbert BL, et al. Biliary tract carcinoma complicating primary sclerosing cholangitis: evaluation with CT, cholangiography, US and MR imaging. Radiology 1998;207:41–50

Cha JH, Han JK, Kim TK, et al. Preoperative evaluation of Klatskin tumor: accuracy of spiral CT in determining vascular invasion as a sign of unresectability. Abdom Imaging 2000;25:500–507

Flanigan DP. Biliary carcinoma associated with biliary cysts. Cancer 1977;40:880–883

Hii MW, Gibson RN, Speer AG, et al. Role of radiology in the treatment of malignant hilar biliary strictures 2: 10 years of single-institution experience with percutaneous treatment. Australas Radiol 2003;47:393–403

Hintze RE, Abou-Rebyeh H, Adler A, et al. Magnetic resonance cholangiopancreatography guided unilateral endoscopic stent placement for Klatskin tumors. Gastrointest Endosc 2001;53:40–46

Kim HS, Lee DK, Kim HG, et al. Features of malignant biliary obstruction affecting the patency of metallic stents: a multicenter study. Gastrointest Endosc 2002;55:359–365

Launois B, Terblanche J, Lakehal M, et al. Proximal bile duct cancer: high resectability rate and 5-year survival. Ann Surg 1999;230:266–275

Lee MJ, Dawson SL, Mueller PR, et al. Percutaneous management of hilar malignancies with metallic endoprostheses: results, technical problems and causes of failure. Radiographics 1993;13:1249–1263

Lees CD, Zapolanski A, Cooperman AM, et al. Carcinoma of the bile ducts. Surg Gynecol Obstet 1980;151:193–198

Lim JH. Radiologic findings of clonorchiasis. AJR Am J Roentgenol 1990;155:1001–1008

Liu CL, Lo CM, Lai EC, et al. Endoscopic retrograde cholangiopancreatography and endoscopic endoprosthesis insertion in patients with Klatskin tumors. Arch Surg 1998;133:293–296

Marchal G, Gelin J, Van Steenbergen W, et al. Sonographic diagnosis of intraluminal bile duct neoplasm: a report of 3 cases. Gastrointest Radiol 1984;9:329–333

Nichols DA, MacCarty RL, Gaffey TA. Cholangiographic evaluation of bile duct carcinoma. AJR Am J Roentgenol 1983;141:1291–1294

Okuda K, Kubo Y, Okazaki N, et al. Clinical aspects of intrahepatic bile duct carcinoma including hilar carcinoma: a study of 57 autopsy proven cases. Cancer 1977;39:232–246

Rieber A, Brambs HJ. Metallic stents in malignant biliary obstruction. Cardiovasc Intervent Radiol 1997;20:43–49

Ross AP, Braasch JW, Warren KW. Carcinoma of the proximal bile ducts. Surg Gynecol Obstet 1973; 136:923–928

Sako K, Seitzinger GL, Garside E. Carcinoma of the extrahepatic bile ducts: review of the literature and report of six cases. Surgery 1957;41:416–437

Salomonowitz EK, Adams A, Antonucci F, et al. Malignant biliary obstruction: treatment with self-expandable stainless steel endoprosthesis. Cardiovasc Intervent Radiol 1992;15:351–355

Stoker J, Lameris JS. Complications of percutaneously inserted biliary Wallstents. J Vasc Interv Radiol 1993;4:767–772

Takamura A, Saito H, Kamada T, et al. Intraluminal low-dose-rate 192Ir brachytherapy combined with external beam radiotherapy and biliary stenting for unresectable extrahepatic bile duct carcinoma. Int J Radiat Oncol Biol Phys 2003;57:1357–1365

Tilleman EHBM, de Castro SMM, Busch ORC, et al. Diagnostic laparoscopy and laparoscopic ultrasound for staging of patients with malignant proximal bile duct obstruction. J Gastrointest Surg 2002; 6:426–431

Tocchi A, Mazzoni G, Liotta G, et al. Late development of bile duct cancer in patients who had biliary-enteric drainage for benign disease: a follow-up study of more than 1,000 patients. Ann Surg 2001;234:210–214

Triller J, Looser C, Baer HU, et al. Hilar cholangiocarcinoma: radiological assessment of resectability. Eur Radiol 1994;4:9–17

Waisberg J, Corona A, de Abreu IW, et al. Benign obstruction of the common hepatic duct (Mirizzi syndrome): diagnosis and operative management. Arq Gastroenterol 2005;42:13–18

CHAPTER 24 Sclerosing Cholangitis

Saadoon Kadir

Clinical Presentation

A 30-year-old woman with long-standing chronic ulcerative colitis and sclerosing cholangitis presented with increasing jaundice.

Radiological Studies

Transhepatic cholangiography performed as part of the jaundice workup revealed a segmental common hepatic duct narrowing with shelflike margins, dilatation of intrahepatic ducts, and multiple nonconfluent stenoses (**Fig. 24-1**).

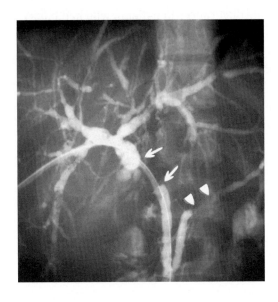

Figure 24-1 Cholangiogram following drainage catheter insertion shows segmental common hepatic duct obstruction with shelflike margins (arrows). Intrahepatic ducts are mildly dilated and multiple nonconfluent stenoses are present. Beading is seen in some smaller intrahepatic ducts. There is mural irregularity in the common bile duct and stenoses are present in the pancreatic duct (arrowheads).

Differential Diagnosis

The intrahepatic bile duct abnormalities are consistent with those of sclerosing cholangitis. In this setting, obstruction of the extrahepatic duct could be due to a stricture, tumor, or calculus. In benign strictures, the margins are tapered. A sharp, shelflike margin is due to a benign or malignant tumor mass or, rarely, from a calculus. With the latter, the lumen of the involved duct segment would be widened and not narrowed. Tumors that occur in this location are cholangiocarcinoma, metastases, pancreatic and gallbladder carcinoma, and rare benign biliary tumors. The likelihood of a neoplastic process is high because of the history of long-standing ulcerative colitis and sclerosing cholangitis.

Diagnosis

Primary sclerosing cholangitis and cholangiocarcinoma

Discussion

Primary sclerosing cholangitis (PSC) is characterized by a slowly progressive inflammation, fibrosis, and obliteration of intra- and extrahepatic bile ducts. It may occur as an isolated illness or in association with other diseases. The latter include inflammatory bowel diseases, pancreatitis, Riedel's (fibrous) thyroiditis, chronic active hepatitis, and retroperitoneal fibrosis.

Improved methods and defined criteria for diagnosis now permit an earlier recognition of this relatively uncommon disease. The estimated prevalence of PSC is between six and nine per 100,000 inhabitants (Lee and Kaplan, 2002). Its prevalence in patients with extensive ulcerative colitis is 5.5% (Olsson et al, 1991). Conversely, up to 79% of patients with PSC have inflammatory bowel disease. Most have ulcerative colitis (~87%), whereas a small number have regional enteritis (Crohn's disease). The course of the inflammatory bowel disease does not correlate with the severity of PSC. Males are affected more commonly (70%) and the mean age at the time of diagnosis is around 40 years.

The clinical course is variable. Patients may be asymptomatic but have a cholestatic liver function test pattern. Absence of clinical symptoms does not necessarily mean early disease; cholangiography and histology in some patients without clinical symptoms have shown severe abnormalities. Patients who are symptomatic at the time of diagnosis usually have a shorter survival.

Symptoms are usually nonspecific and include pruritus, jaundice, abdominal pain, weight loss, and fatigue. Jaundice is usually of insidious onset and may be episodic (intermittent jaundice). Fever and hepatosplenomegaly are present in up to 30% of cases. In a few patients, the initial presentation may be ascites or variceal bleeding. Fever is more frequent in patients with predominantly intrahepatic disease (Olsson et al, 1991). Intermittent fever, which probably represents bacterial cholangitis, is seen in patients who have had prior biliary tract surgery (Cameron et al, 1984).

Small Duct Primary Sclerosing Cholangitis

In a small subset of patients (6%) with or without inflammatory bowel disease, cholestasis, and normal cholangiograms, hepatic biopsies have demonstrated histological changes of sclerosing cholangitis (Angulo et al, 2002; Broome et al, 2002). Long-term follow-up of these patients has shown that a very slow progression to the characteristic cholangiographic manifestations of PSC occurs in only a few cases. Although demographics and symptoms are similar, disease course is usually benign and development of cholangiocarcinoma has not been described. According to some authors, this is an early manifestation of PSC, whereas others believe it to be a separate disease entity (Angulo et al, 2002; Broome et al, 2002).

Etiology, Diagnosis, and Staging

Although the exact etiology remains uncertain, there are indications that PSC is the result of an autoimmune process. Elevated immunoglobulin M (IgM), antimitochondrial, smooth muscle, and antinuclear antibodies are found in up to 20% of patients. In addition, human leukocyte antigen (HLA)-B8, -DR3, and -DR2 as well as autoantibodies against biliary epithelial cells have been detected (Ichimura et al, 2002; Xu et al, 2002).

The diagnosis is based upon cholangiographic and histological findings. Laboratory tests alone are nonspecific and may occasionally be misleading. A cholestatic pattern is present with elevated alkaline phosphatase and aminotransferases and fluctuating jaundice. In some cases, elevated levels of alkaline phosphatase may precede the clinical diagnosis by several years or may be normal in the presence of PSC (Olsson et al, 1991).

Table 24-1   Classification of Cholangiographic Abnormalities in Primary Sclerosing Cholangitis

Type of Ductal Involvement/Classification	Cholangiographic Appearance
Intrahepatic ducts	
0	No visible abnormality
I	Multiple strictures
	Normal caliber or minimally dilated ducts
II	Multiple strictures
	Saccular dilatation, decreased arborization
III	Severe pruning
	Only central branches opacified
Extrahepatic ducts	
0	No visible abnormality
I	No strictures
	Slight duct contour irregularity
II	Segmental stricture
III	Almost entire duct strictured
IV	Extremely irregular duct margin
	Saccular outpouchings

Adapted from Majoie CB, Reeders JW, Sanders JB, et al. Primary sclerosing cholangitis: a modified classification of cholangiographic findings. Am J Roentgenol 1991;157:495–497.

For disease staging, the severity and distribution of the cholangiographic abnormalities are used (**Table 24-1**). Histology is also used to some extent, but there may be considerable variability in the tissue samples because disease distribution may not be uniform and a biopsy may miss the typical lesions.

Pathology

The affected extrahepatic ducts are diffusely thickened and cordlike. Fibrous adhesions may be present between the gallbladder, extrahepatic ducts, duodenum, and liver. On microscopy, there is extensive nonspecific fibrosis. For intrahepatic disease, four histological stages occur in the portal triads (Lee and Kaplan, 2002):

Stage 1 is the initial lesion, which shows degeneration of bile duct epithelium. There is enlargement of the portal triads, a predominantly mononuclear inflammatory reaction, and scarring. Bile duct proliferation may be present demonstrating the characteristic onionskin lesion consisting of concentric layers of connective tissue surrounding bile ducts.

Stage 2 abnormality is more widespread with the inflammation and fibrosis extending to the periportal parenchyma. There is fibrous obliteration (and absence) of ducts and the onionskin lesion is less obvious.

Stage 3 shows bridging fibrous septae, fibrous obliteration of bile ducts, and cholestasis in surrounding hepatocytes.

Stage 4 represents end stage disease (cirrhosis).

Cholangiographic Features

Transhepatic cholangiography has largely been replaced by endoscopic retrograde cholangiopancreatography (ERCP) and cross-sectional imaging. Magnetic resonance cholangiopancreatography and computed tomography are used for evaluation of complications and detection of tumors.

There is a wide range of cholangiographic abnormalities. Strictures are the most common abnormality and are usually multifocal. In ~10% of cases, a dominant (localized, severe) stricture is present (May et al, 1985). In the vast majority of patients, both intra- and extrahepatic ducts are affected. The junction of the left and right hepatic ducts (so-called hilum) is involved in most patients and often most severely. Severe disease of the intrahepatic ducts is usually accompanied by extrahepatic disease of lesser severity (Li-Yeng and Goldberg, 1984). Isolated intrahepatic duct disease is very uncommon but in 20% there is intrahepatic and proximal extrahepatic duct involvement (MacCarty et al, 1983). Diffuse dilatation of intra- or extrahepatic ducts is also very uncommon.

One of the potential pitfalls of transhepatic cholangiography is the nonopacification of the smaller ducts as a result of underfilling, which may suggest pruning or obliteration. In most cases, the presence of centrally located obstructing strictures provides for satisfactory opacification of the smaller radicles. Overdistention of the bile ducts with contrast is known to cause cholangitis and sepsis and is therefore avoided.

INTRAHEPATIC DUCTS (FIGS. 24-2 TO 24-4)

Diminished arborization or pruning is the most common finding and is characterized by obstruction/ obliteration of the smaller peripheral ducts while the larger more central ducts remain patent. Diffuse narrowing, focal stenoses, or mild dilatation of the larger ducts may be present. Short and annular strictures alternating with normal or slightly dilated segments may give the duct a beaded appearance. Skip lesions are common because of the uneven distribution of the disease process. Unlike in other forms of obstructive jaundice, the restrictive nature of the disease permits only some intrahepatic duct dilatation. Occasionally, the extrahepatic sections of the proximal perihilar ducts are markedly dilated.

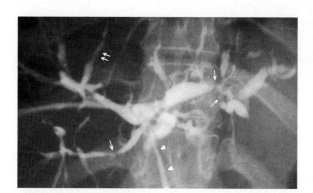

Figure 24-2 Diminished arborization and pruning of smaller peripheral ducts (double arrows), focal stenoses (arrows), and skip lesions. The common hepatic duct is severely narrowed (arrowheads) and the larger central ducts are mildly dilated.

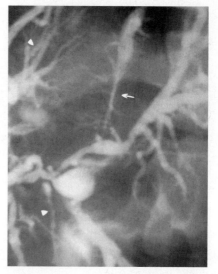

Figure 24-3 Magnification image from a cholangiogram shows pruning of smaller ducts (arrow) and scattered stenoses. Some branches have a beaded appearance (arrowheads).

EXTRAHEPATIC DUCTS (FIGS. 24-5 TO 24-8)

The junction of the left and right hepatic ducts is most frequently affected. The most common feature is a variable-length stricture causing a smooth or irregular narrowing. Strictures may be focal (annular, bandlike), short (1–2 cm), or long. Complete extrahepatic ductal obstruction is uncommon. The ducts central to strictures are either not dilated in the presence of diffuse intrahepatic disease

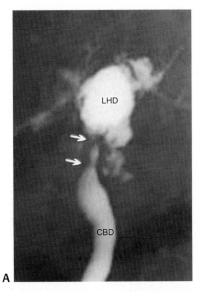
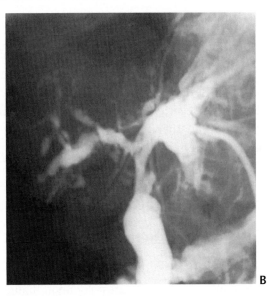

A   B

Figure 24-4 Ductal dilatation. (**A**) Pre- and (**B**) postdrainage images show a severe common hepatic duct stricture (arrows) and marked dilatation of the central left hepatic duct (LHD) and dilatation of the common bile duct (CBD). Pruning of the intrahepatic ducts is also present. This is an uncommon manifestation of PSC.

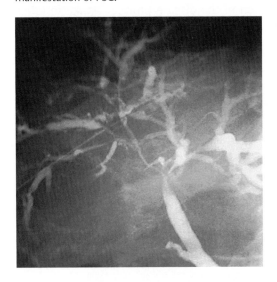

Figure 24-5 Strictures of the hepatic duct confluence and intrahepatic ducts. Transhepatic cholangiogram shows severe strictures of the central left and right hepatic ducts and several intrahepatic ducts.

or only mildly dilated. Occasionally, there is diffuse dilatation of the extrahepatic ducts, including the hepatic duct junction (hilum).

Mural irregularities may give the duct a "shaggy" appearance, varying from fine serrations to coarse nodularity and small outpouchings (sacculations, diverticula) are observed in about one third of the patients (MacCarty et al, 1983). These may occur with or without associated, annular strictures. Their etiology is uncertain but they may represent mucosal herniations between strictures, similar to colonic diverticula.

CYSTIC DUCT AND GALLBLADDER (FIG. 24-8)

Cystic duct abnormalities may be present in up to 18% of cases, although involvement by the disease may be difficult to determine because of the valves of Heister (MacCarty et al, 1983). Mural irregularities, diverticula, ectasia, and stenoses may occur. The true incidence of gallbladder involvement by PSC is unknown. Abnormalities have been demonstrated in a small number of patients.

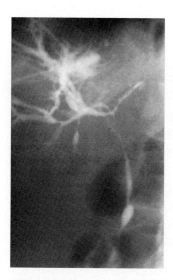

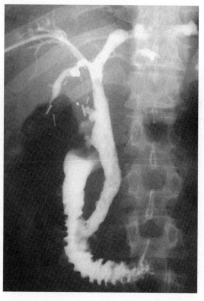

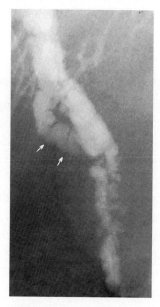

Figure 24-6 Severe extrahepatic duct stricture. Transhepatic cholangiogram shows severe narrowing of intrahepatic ducts, the ductal confluence, and common hepatic and common bile ducts. Skip lesions are present in the common bile duct.

Figure 24-7 Ductal dilatation with mural nodularity. The extrahepatic ducts are diffusely dilated. Coarse mural nodules are present. (Reproduced with permission from Kadir S, Diagnostic Angiography, WB Saunders, Philadelphia, 1986.)

Figure 24-8 Sacculations and annular strictures of the common duct. There is also dilatation of the cystic duct, and fine mural serrations are present (arrows).

PANCREATIC DUCT (FIG. 24-1)

Pancreatic duct abnormalities are seen in ~8% of patients (MacCarty et al, 1983). These may be secondary to chronic pancreatitis, which frequently accompanies sclerosing cholangitis, or due to autoimmune pancreatitis (Ichimura et al, 2002). Pancreatic duct abnormalities are nonspecific and include serrations, beading, smooth strictures, and ectasia.

Differential Diagnosis

In most cases, clinical and laboratory data and results of imaging studies provide sufficient information to differentiate PSC from diseases that may mimic it. Difficulty may arise in patients who have either eluded the diagnosis, previously undergone biliary tract surgery, or developed complications. Advanced biliary cirrhosis, cholangiocarcinoma, benign and malignant strictures, secondary cholangitis, and metastases may simulate PSC on cholangiography.

In advanced cirrhosis, only intrahepatic ducts are involved. Cholangiocarcinoma may be difficult to differentiate from PSC because clinical and cholangiographic similarities exist and PSC also predisposes to cholangiocarcinoma. Additionally, carcinoma of the pancreas and gallbladder occur with a higher frequency in patients with PSC. In both cholangiocarcinoma and PSC, the junction of left and right hepatic ducts is most frequently and severely affected and both are associated with ulcerative colitis. Differentiating features include absence of focal strictures, diverticula, and fine serrations in cholangiocarcinoma (MacCarty et al, 1983). Progressive or marked ductal dilatation secondary to a hilar or extrahepatic stricture, progressive narrowing of a stricture, or development of a mass (seen in half the patients) suggest a neoplasm (MacCarty et al, 1985). However, these criteria can only be used if serial cholangiograms are available to demonstrate the changes. Differentiation may not be possible in the presence of the diffuse sclerosing-type cholangiocarcinoma, or coarse or papillary nodularity. Brush cytology (46% sensitivity) and serum tumor markers (CEA and CA19–9) have been used with some success (Siqueira et al, 2002).

Prognosis, Complications, and Management

Untreated, the disease slowly progresses to hepatic cirrhosis, portal hypertension, and hepatic failure. Neoplasms are now the most common cause of death (44%) (Bergquist et al, 2002). The median survival to death or liver transplantation is 18 years (Ponsioen et al, 2002). The prognosis is poorer in severe intrahepatic and diffuse strictures, which are also associated with advanced liver disease (Craig et al, 1991; Ponsioen et al, 2002). Decreased survival is also seen in patients with long confluent strictures and ductal dilatation.

Patients with chronic PSC are at a greater risk than the general population of developing hepatobiliary (cholangiocarcinoma, hepatocellular, and gallbladder carcinoma), colorectal, and pancreatic neoplasms (Bergquist et al, 2002). About 37% of the hepatobiliary neoplasms are detected within 1 year of diagnosis of PSC and the subsequent annual incidence is 1.5% per year. The risk for colorectal neoplasms is increased 10-fold (~7%) and that for carcinoma of the pancreas is 14-fold over the general population (Bergquist et al, 2002; Soetikno et al, 2002). Cholangiocarcinoma develops in up to 13% of patients with PSC (Bergquist et al, 2002; Ponsioen et al, 2002; Siqueira et al, 2002). In these patients, the prognosis is poor, with the median survival <6 months unless the tumor is detected incidentally in an explanted liver.

Other complications of the disease include cholelithiasis, usually pigment calculi, metabolic bone disease, steatorrhea and vitamin deficiency, and bacterial cholangitis. Chronic pancreatitis is observed in almost half the patients.

Treatment of choice in patients without neoplasia is liver transplantation. In some patients balloon dilatation of the dominant strictures has been successful. Transhepatic drainage may be required after failed endoscopic catheterization or complications thereof.

PEARLS AND PITFALLS

- The etiology of primary sclerosing cholangitis appears to be an autoimmune process.
- The diagnosis is based on cholangiography and histological findings.
- The most common abnormality is multifocal strictures of intra- and extrahepatic ducts.
- The affected extrahepatic ducts are thickened and cordlike, and extensive, nonspecific fibrosis is seen on microscopy.
- Untreated, the disease progresses to hepatic cirrhosis, portal hypertension, and hepatic failure.
- Patients with chronic PSC are at a greater risk of developing hepatobiliary, colorectal, and pancreatic neoplasms, which are the most common cause of death.

Further Reading

Angulo P, Maor-Kendler Y, Lindor KD. Small-duct primary sclerosing cholangitis: a long-term follow-up study. Hepatology 2002;35:1494–1500

Bergquist A, Ekbom A, Olsson R, et al. Hepatic and extrahepatic malignancies in primary sclerosing cholangitis. J Hepatol 2002;36:321–327

Broome U, Glaumann H, Lindstom E, et al. Natural history and outcome in 32 Swedish patients with small duct primary sclerosing cholangitis (PSC). J Hepatol 2002;36:586–589

Cameron JL, Gayler BW, Sanfey H, et al. Sclerosing cholangitis: anatomical distribution of obstructive lesions. Ann Surg 1984;200:54–60

Campbell WL, Ferris JV, Holbert BL, et al. Biliary tract carcinoma complicating primary sclerosing cholangitis: evaluation with CT, cholangiography, US, and MR imaging. Radiology 1998;207:41–50

Craig DA, MacCarty RL, Wiesner RH, et al. Primary sclerosing cholangitis: value of cholangiography in determining the prognosis. AJR Am J Roentgenol 1991;157:959–964

Ichimura T, Kondo S, Ambo Y, et al. Primary sclerosing cholangitis associated with autoimmune pancreatitis. Hepatogastroenterology 2002;49:1221–1224

Lee YM, Kaplan MM. Management of primary sclerosing cholangitis. Am J Gastroenterol 2002; 97:528–534

Li-Yeng C, Goldberg HI. Sclerosing cholangitis: broad spectrum of radiographic features. Gastrointest Radiol 1984;9:39–47

MacCarty RL, LaRusso NF, May GR, et al. Cholangiocarcinoma complicating primary sclerosing cholangitis: cholangiographic appearances. Radiology 1985;156:43–46

MacCarty RL, LaRusso NF, Wiesner RH, et al. Primary sclerosing cholangitis: findings on cholangiography and pancreatography. Radiology 1983;149:39–44

Majoie CB, Reeders JW, Sanders JB, et al. Primary sclerosing cholangitis: a modified classification of cholangiographic findings. AJR Am J Roentgenol 1991;157:495–497

May GR, Bender CE, LaRusso NF, et al. Nonoperative dilatation of dominant strictures in primary sclerosing cholangitis. AJR Am J Roentgenol 1985;145:1061–1064

Olsson R, Danielsson A, Jarnerot G, et al. Prevalence of primary sclerosing cholangitis in patients with ulcerative colitis. Gastroenterology 1991;100:1319–1323

Ponsioen CY, Vrouenraets SME, Prawirodirdjo W, et al. Natural history of primary sclerosing cholangitis and prognostic value of cholangiography in a Dutch population. Gut 2002;51:562–566

Siqueira E, Schoen RE, Silverman W, et al. Detecting cholangiocarcinoma in patients with sclerosing cholangitis. Gastrointest Endosc 2002;56:40–47

Soetikno RM, Lin OS, Heidenreich PA, et al. Increased risk of colorectal neoplasia in patients with primary sclerosing cholangitis and ulcerative colitis: a meta-analysis. Gastrointest Endosc 2002;56:48–54

Xu B, Broome U, Ericzon BG, et al. High frequency of autoantibodies in patients with primary sclerosing cholangitis that bind biliary epithelial cells and induce expression of CD44 and production of interleukin 6. Gut 2002;51:120–127

CHAPTER 25 AIDS-Related Cholangiopathy

Saadoon Kadir

Clinical Presentation

A 20-year-old male with acquired immunodeficiency syndrome (AIDS) presented with abdominal pain, fever, diarrhea, and right upper quadrant tenderness.

Radiological Studies

Computed tomography (CT) of the abdomen showed dilatation of intra- and extrahepatic bile ducts, duct wall thickening, and dilatation of the pancreatic duct (**Fig. 25-1**). There was also gallbladder distention and thickening of the wall (**Fig. 25-2**).

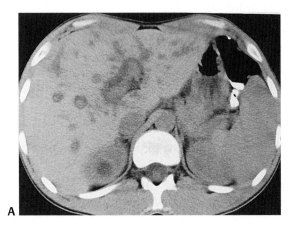
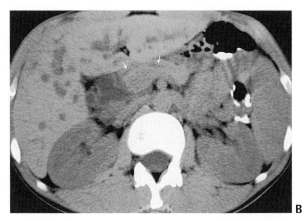

Figure 25-1 (**A**) Noncontrast computed tomography of the abdomen shows dilated intra- and extrahepatic bile ducts and periportal edema. (**B**) There is also dilatation of the pancreatic duct (arrows) and thickening of the distal common bile duct wall.

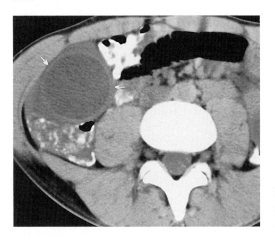

Figure 25-2 A lower section from the same study shows distention of the gallbladder (arrows), thickening of the wall, and pericholecystic fluid.

Differential Diagnosis

Dilatation of both the bile and the pancreatic ducts indicates a juxta-ampullary obstruction, which could be due to several causes such as a calculus, stricture, lymphadenopathy, or neoplasm. Tumors that occur in AIDS patients are Kaposi's sarcoma and non-Hodgkin's lymphoma, and adenopathy may be secondary to tumor or an opportunistic infection. However, neither a tumor mass nor adenopathy was present in this patient. On the other hand, edema with stenosis at the papilla of Vater is a common complication of AIDS-related cholangiopathy (ARC). In addition, stenoses of the adjacent pancreatic duct segment are also common in these patients. Gallbladder wall thickening by itself is a nonspecific finding and can have multiple causes other than ARC. These include cholecystitis, hypoalbuminemia, ascites, congestive cardiac failure, hepatitis, and renal diseases. With the exception of cholecystitis, in most of these cases the gallbladder is not distended. Thickening of the wall with distention of the gallbladder and right upper quadrant tenderness are suspicious for acalculous cholecystitis (also see Chapter 30).

Although the abnormalities seen on the images are not specific because they can be caused by several diseases, in the context of the underlying disease process (i.e., AIDS) they provide the diagnosis of ARC.

Diagnosis

AIDS-related cholangiopathy

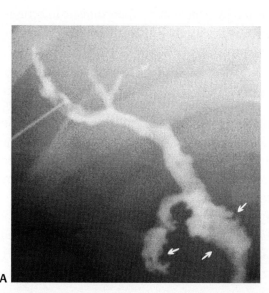
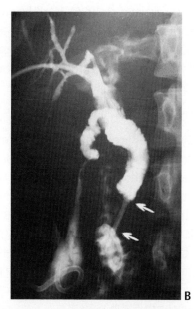

A   B

Figure 25-3 (**A**) Image from the percutaneous transhepatic cholangiogram shows dilated ducts and a nodular appearance in the common bile and cystic ducts (arrows). (**B**) Cholangiogram following drainage catheter placement shows a long segment of severe stenosis in the distal common bile duct (arrows). The common duct is dilated and several intrahepatic ducts show stenoses. The contour of several ducts is shaggy/nodular. A cholecystostomy catheter is in place and there is thickening of the duodenal mucosal folds. Note: There is incomplete opacification of the intrahepatic ducts because of free flow of contrast into the duodenum via the drainage catheter. This incomplete opacification could be misinterpreted as pruning and diminished arborization.

Treatment

Initially, acalculous cholecystitis was suspected to be the cause of the patient's symptoms and percutaneous cholecystostomy was performed. As this provided only some symptomatic relief, transhepatic cholangiography and biliary drainage were undertaken. On the cholangiograms, the intra- and extrahepatic ducts were dilated, and an irregular, shaggy contour was present in the common duct with a long segment of distal stenosis (**Fig. 25-3**). A drainage catheter was placed in the duodenum for internal drainage. Following biliary drainage, the abdominal pain subsided. Bile samples were positive for *Cryptosporidium parvum.*

Discussion

There is a high incidence of hepatobiliary infections in AIDS patients with CD4 counts below 100 per mm^3 (Keaveny and Karasik, 1998). ARC is the most common infectious biliary complication in human immunodeficiency virus (HIV)-positive/AIDS patients and can be caused by several opportunistic agents affecting one or more segments or the entire biliary system. In one study of HIV-positive patients evaluated for biliary symptomatology, cholangiographic criteria of ARC were found in 86% (Ducreux et al, 1995). ARC may be a primary hepatobiliary infection or secondary to a process elsewhere in the body. It is usually a late complication of AIDS, but in the rare instance, ARC may be the initial manifestation (Mukhopadhyay et al, 2001).

Gallbladder involvement can be severe, leading to acalculous cholecystitis. An infectious cholangitis of the bile ducts occurs more frequently. Both the intra- and extrahepatic ducts are affected in 67% of cases and isolated involvement of the intrahepatic or extrahepatic bile ducts is seen in 27% and 6%, respectively (Ducreux et al, 1995). In addition, a distal common bile duct (CBD) and ampullary stenosis is common. The pancreas is also frequently affected by pancreatitis, opportunistic infections, or a malignancy (Cappell, 1997). The relevance of pancreatic disease in ARC is often underestimated because biliary disease usually dominates the clinical picture.

Presentation

The most common symptoms are chronic upper abdominal (right upper quadrant and epigastric) pain and tenderness and low-grade fever. Liver function tests are abnormal and indicative of cholestasis. Some patients also have diarrhea and hepatomegaly. Two thirds of HIV-positive patients being investigated for cholestasis or abdominal pain have ARC on endoscopic retrograde cholangiopancreatography (ERCP), although a history of abdominal pain is elicited in up to 90% of patients with ARC (Forbes et al, 1993; Cappell, 1997). The abdominal pain is often severe. Clinical jaundice and pruritus are uncommon (<10% of cases). Elevation of the cholestatic liver enzymes (alkaline phosphatase and gamma-glutamyl transferase) is seen in over half the patients (Forbes et al, 1993; Ducreux et al, 1995). Regardless of the type of infection, the disease course is similar. Hepatobiliary disease unrelated to the AIDS may also occur in these patients.

Etiology

ARC is an infection of the biliary epithelium (a secondary cholangitis) in an immunodeficient host, which can be caused by any of several agents including viral, bacterial, fungal, and other opportunistic organisms. A causative agent is identified in 75% of patients (Farman et al, 1994; Nash and Cohen, 1997; Keaveny and Karasik, 1998). Pathogens that have been linked to ARC are listed in **Table 25-1**. The responsible pathogens can usually be isolated from bile and stool samples. On occasion, they are

Table 25-1   Agents Responsible for Opportunistic Hepatobiliary Infections in AIDS Patients[a]

Bacteria	Protozoa	Fungi	Viruses
Mycobacterium avium intracellulare	Cryptosporidium parvum	Candida albicans	Cytomegalovirus
Mycobacterium kansasii	Microsporidia	Histoplasma capsulatum	Hepatitis
Mycobacterium tuberculosis	Pneumocystis carinii	Cryptococcus neoformans	Herpes
Campylobacter spp	Toxoplasma gondii	Coccidioides immitis	
Salmonella spp	Giardia lamblia	Isospora belli	
Enterobacter			

[a]Farman et al, 1994; Nash and Cohen, 1997; Keaveny and Karasik, 1998; Sheikh et al, 2000; Chen and LaRusso, 2002.

identified only in tissue biopsy specimens using special staining and culture techniques (Keaveny and Karasik, 1998; Sheikh et al, 2000).

Cryptosporidium parvum is the most commonly isolated pathogen (Chen and LaRusso, 2002). It is an intracellular parasite that infects mucosal epithelial cells. In experimental cryptosporidiosis, it was observed to induce rapid cell death by apoptosis in cultured human biliary epithelial cells (Chen et al, 1999). In addition, it stimulates peribiliary ductal inflammation, which may explain the cholangiographic findings in ARC.

Microsporidia species responsible for opportunistic infection in AIDS patients are *Encephalitozoon intestinalis*, which causes cholangitis, and *Enterocytozoon bieneusi*, which causes diarrhea (Sheikh et al, 2000). The effects of systemic viruses on the biliary system depend upon the host immune status. Hepatitis viruses can cause a lymphocytic cholangitis in which the ductal abnormality is reversible and has no adverse effect on the disease course (Burgart, 1998). The hepatitis C, and to a lesser degree, the hepatitis B virus is frequently associated with cholangitis. Hepatitis A and E virus cholangitis appears to be mild. Cytomegaly virus infections are more common in liver transplant patients than those with AIDS immunosupression.

Imaging Findings

Imaging modalities used for evaluation are ultrasound, CT, and ERCP. Transhepatic cholangiography is useful in some cases. Ultrasound, which is frequently the initial imaging modality, shows gallbladder and bile duct abnormalities. Although the findings on sonography and CT are nonspecific, together with the clinical picture, they may suggest the diagnosis of cholangitis in a significant number of the cases.

GALLBLADDER

A gallbladder abnormality is seen in virtually all patients with ARC but may not be relevant clinically (i.e., it is not a source of symptoms). Thickening of the wall without gallbladder distention, pericholecystic fluid, and, occasionally, sludge are present in the lumen. Calculi, if present, are incidental and unrelated to the ARC disease process. Wall thickness of up to 15 mm has been reported and may change between examinations, probably as a result of fluid/edema shifts (Romano et al, 1988). The thickened wall enhances on CT after intravenous contrast administration. Distention of the gallbladder and other sonographic features of acalculous cholecystitis may be present.

EXTRAHEPATIC BILE DUCTS

There is a variable degree of bile duct dilatation and thickening of the duct wall. An extrahepatic duct wall diameter of up to 15 mm has been reported (Romano et al, 1988). Ductal dilatation is relatively uniform without proximal duct strictures. The duct wall may be shaggy or nodular. The dilated common duct tapers to a narrowing in the ampullary region (papillary stenosis). On ultrasound, an echogenic nodule is seen in distal common bile duct in two thirds of patients and is believed to be from edema at the papilla (Da Silva et al, 1993). This corresponds to the abnormality seen on ERCP, and biopsy of this area has shown inflammation. A papillary stenosis may be present in up to 80% of patients and is usually associated with cholangiographic manifestations of intra- and extrahepatic cholangitis. In some patients, papillary stenosis may be an isolated abnormality.

Small polyp-like structures (with or without stalks) consisting of granulation tissue may be seen on cholangiography in the CBD and larger intrahepatic ducts in around 26% of patients (Collins et al, 1993). Their presence does not correlate with the prognosis or type of infection. In descending order of frequency, a diffuse cholangitis is most common (two thirds of patients), followed by isolated intrahepatic duct and extrahepatic duct abnormalities (Ducreux et al, 1995).

INTRAHEPATIC BILE DUCTS

In the presence of extrahepatic ductal dilatation, the intrahepatic ducts are usually dilated but may also demonstrate focal narrowing or occasionally severe strictures. The duct wall is often shaggy in appearance. Pruning and diminished arborization of peripheral intrahepatic ducts have also been reported (Teixidor et al, 1991). The shaggy contour and shallow narrowing are supposedly due to the sclerosing/fibrosing inflammatory process (Miller et al, 1996). However, a more likely explanation is the presence of the often extensive periductal edema that is demonstrated on CT examinations in these patients (see **Fig. 25-1**). Observed changes in duct (and gallbladder) wall thickness that do not correlate with the disease course are also in keeping with this impression. The edema is lymphatic in origin.

CHOLANGIOGRAPHIC DIFFERENTIAL DIAGNOSIS

Cholangiography in ARC is reported to show some features similar to those of primary sclerosing cholangitis (Teixidor et al, 1991; Farman et al, 1994; Nash and Cohen, 1997; Sheikh et al, 2000). Bile duct strictures, focal or diffuse dilatation, and beading of bile ducts have been reported. A closer look at the published images reveals few consistent similarities. For example, incomplete opacification of intrahepatic ducts simulates pruning and diminished arborization, and also, these ducts may occasionally appear strictured. Beading in larger or proximal ducts is a nonspecific finding and is frequently seen in chronic obstructions (**Fig. 25-4**). Absence of proximal extrahepatic duct strictures, diverticula/sacculations, long segmental strictures and skipped lesions of intrahepatic ducts, and the clinical picture readily differentiate the two diseases. (Also see Chapter 24.)

PANCREAS

CT may demonstrate abnormalities involving the pancreas, and CT-guided pancreatic aspiration biopsy may be necessary for establishing a diagnosis. Pancreatitis, pseudocysts, retroperitoneal adenopathy, or a neoplasm may be seen (**Fig. 25-5**). A higher incidence of pancreatic neoplasms is reported to occur in AIDS patients (Bonacini, 1991; Cappell, 1997). In papillary stenosis, a stricture of the juxta-ampullary pancreatic duct is seen in about half the patients and dilatation of the more peripheral pancreatic ducts, often combined with features of chronic pancreatitis (Farman et al, 1994; Cappell, 1997).

Treatment

Medical therapy focuses on the causative agent and demonstrates a variable effectiveness. Distal CBD obstruction is usually managed endoscopically by sphincterotomy and stents in some patients (Cordero et al, 2001). This relieves abdominal pain in some patients with papillary stenosis but does not appear to alter the clinical disease course or the cholangiographic appearance (Ducreux et al, 1995; Nash and Cohen, 1997).

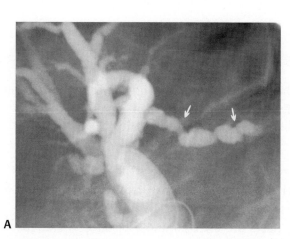
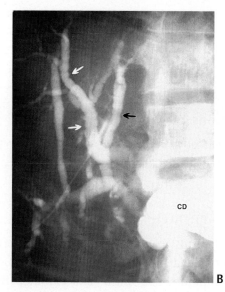

A   B

Figure 25-4 Beading of ducts as a nonspecific cholangiographic sign. (**A**) Cholangiogram from an 80-year-old woman with an ampullary tumor and slowly progressive jaundice. There is beading of an intrahepatic duct (arrows). (**B**) Cholangiogram from a patient with metastatic breast carcinoma. There is beading of several intrahepatic ducts (arrows). The obstructed common duct (CD) is markedly dilated. In neither of these patients was there a history of AIDS, hepatic cirrhosis or other hepatic parenchymal disease, inflammatory bowel disease, or sclerosing cholangitis.

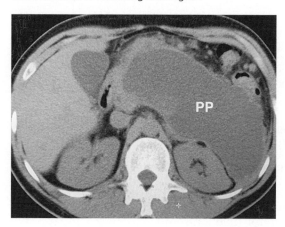

Figure 25-5 Abdominal computed tomography from a different AIDS patient with chronic abdominal pain. A large pancreatic pseudocyst (PP) is present. This was subsequently drained, with alleviation of symptoms.

Abdominal pain refractory to endoscopic sphincterotomy may be pancreatic in origin. CT-guided celiac plexus blockade with absolute alcohol and bupivacaine has provided relief in a small number of patients with refractory right upper quadrant and epigastric pain due to ARC (Collazos et al, 1996). Recurrent stenosis may occur after endoscopic sphincterotomy necessitating repeat intervention. An occasional patient with a longer stricture may be best treated by a metallic stent. The role of balloon dilatation has not been determined.

Acute acalculous cholecystitis requires prompt recognition and gallbladder decompression. Cholecystectomy has provided durable relief of symptoms in such patients. The role of decompressive percutaneous cholecystostomy without subsequent cholecystectomy as the only management of acalculous cholecystitis in this setting is undetermined.

Prognosis

The bile duct injury appears to be progressive with little or no improvement in the cholangiographic picture despite successful management of the infection. Prognosis depends upon the stage of HIV infection, and late-stage and older AIDS patients are at a higher risk for developing ARC (Ducreux et al, 1995; Burgart, 1998). The prognosis is generally poorer in younger individuals affected by ARC and survival is short (Forbes et al, 1993). The 1-year survival is 41% (Ducreux et al, 1995).

Complications

Procedure-related complications are essentially the same as in patients undergoing transhepatic biliary drainage or percutaneous cholecystostomy for other indications. (See Chapters 22 and 30.)

PEARLS AND PITFALLS_____

- ARC is the most common infectious biliary complication in HIV-positive/AIDS patients. It is a secondary cholangitis, which can be caused by several opportunistic organisms.
- Most commonly, both intra- and extrahepatic ducts are affected and a distal CBD/ampullary stenosis is present.
- Abdominal pain is frequently relieved by treatment of the distal CBD obstruction. The cholangiographic abnormalities may persist or worsen even after successful management of the infection.

Further Reading

Bonacini M. Pancreatic involvement in human immunodeficiency virus infection. J Clin Gastroenterol 1991;13:58–64

Burgart LJ. Cholangitis in viral disease. Mayo Clin Proc 1998;73:479–482

Cappell MS. The pancreas in AIDS. Gastroenterol Clin North Am 1997;26:337–365

Chen XM, Gores GJ, Paya CV, et al. *Cryptosporidium parvum* induces apoptosis in biliary epithelia by a Fas/Fas ligand-dependent mechanism. Am J Physiol 1999;277:G599–G608

Chen XM, LaRusso NF. Cryptosporidiosis and the pathogenesis of AIDS-cholangiopathy. Semin Liver Dis 2002;22:277–289

Collazos J, Mayo J, Martinez E, et al. Celiac plexus block as treatment for refractory pain related to sclerosing cholangitis in AIDS patients. J Clin Gastroenterol 1996;23:47–49

Collins CD, Forbes A, Harcourt-Webster JN, et al. Radiological and pathological features of AIDS-related polypoid cholangitis. Clin Radiol 1993;48:307–310

Cordero E, Lopez-Cortes LF, Belda O, et al. Acquired immunodeficiency syndrome-related cryptosporidial cholangitis: resolution with endobiliary prosthesis insertion. Gastrointest Endosc 2001;53:534–535

Da Silva F, Boudghene F, Lecomte I, et al. Sonography in AIDS-related cholangitis: prevalence and cause of an echogenic nodule in the distal end of the common bile duct. AJR Am J Roentgenol 1993;160:1205–1207

Ducreux M, Buffet C, Lamy P, et al. Diagnosis and prognosis of AIDS-related cholangitis. AIDS 1995;9:875–880

Farman J, Brunetti J, Baer JW, et al. AIDS-related cholangiopancreatographic changes. Abdom Imaging 1994;19:417–422

Forbes A, Blanshard C, Gazzard B. Natural history of AIDS-related sclerosing cholangitis: a study of 20 cases. Gut 1993;34:116–121

Keaveny AP, Karasik MS. Hepatobiliary and pancreatic infections in AIDS, I: AIDS Patient Care STDS 1998;12:347–357

Miller FH, Gore RM, Nemcek AA Jr, et al. Pancreatobiliary manifestations of AIDS. AJR Am J Roentgenol 1996;166:1269–1274

Mukhopadhyay S, Monga A, Rana SS, et al. AIDS cholangiopathy as initial presentation of HIV infection. Trop Gastroenterol 2001;22:29–30

Nash JA, Cohen SA. Gallbladder and biliary tract disease in AIDS. Gastroenterol Clin North Am 1997;26:323–335

Romano AJ, vanSonnenberg E, Casola G, et al. Gallbladder and bile duct abnormalities in AIDS: sonographic findings in eight patients. AJR Am J Roentgenol 1988;150:123–127

Sheikh RA, Prindiville TP, Yenamandra S, et al. Microsporidial AIDS cholangiopathy due to *Encephalitozoon intestinalis*: case report and review. Am J Gastroenterol 2000;95:2364–2371

Teixidor HS, Godwin TA, Ramirez EA. Cryptosporidiosis of the biliary tract in AIDS. Radiology 1991;180:51–56

CHAPTER 26 Removal of Bile Duct Calculi

Saadoon Kadir

Clinical Presentation

A 34-year-old white woman sought medical attention because of pruritus and jaundice. She had previously undergone a cholecystectomy and hepaticojejunostomy for cholelithiasis. Laboratory studies indicated obstructive jaundice.

Radiological Studies

A percutaneous transhepatic cholangiogram (PTC) was obtained. This showed dilated ducts with castlike intraductal material suggesting the presence of either intraductal thrombus or calculi (**Fig. 26-1**). The hepaticojejunostomy was stenosed. The aspirated bile was clear.

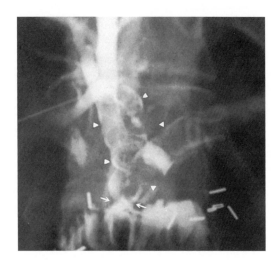

Figure 26-1 Image from the percutaneous transhepatic cholangiogram in a slight oblique projection shows a castlike filling defect in the intrahepatic ducts (arrowheads). A stricture is present at the hepaticojejunstomy (arrows).

Diagnosis

Obstructive jaundice and recurrent intrahepatic biliary calculi due to stenosis of the hepaticoje-junostomy.

Treatment Options and Treatment

In the presence of a hepaticojejunostomy, there are very few endoscopic options. A transgastric endoscopic approach has been described but was not considered. Similarly, surgery was not considered because both the calculi and stricture were amenable to the lesser invasive percutaneous management via the transhepatic route.

Following the PTC, an 8F percutaneous biliary drainage (PBD) catheter was inserted. The jaundice persisted after PBD with only some decrease in the serum bilirubin. The calculi were obstructing both the left and right hepatic ducts and their removal was necessary for relief of the obstructive jaundice. The drainage catheter was exchanged for an 8F vascular sheath. An 8 mm angioplasty balloon was

146

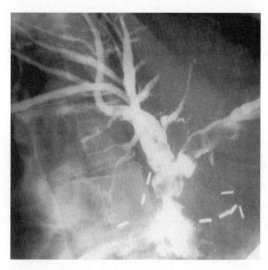

Figure 26-2 Interim cholangiogram shows decompression of the ducts after retrieval of some of the calculi. The stricture is again seen at the hepaticojejunstomy.

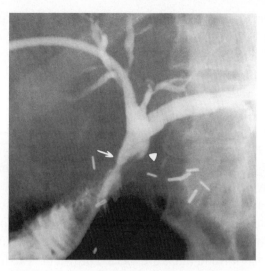

Figure 26-3 Cholangiogram after removal of all calculi. There is a posterior pouchlike dilatation of the duct (arrowhead) proximal to the anastomosis (arrow). Such areas predispose to bile stagnation and calculus formation. The anastomosis was dilated with a 12 mm angioplasty balloon.

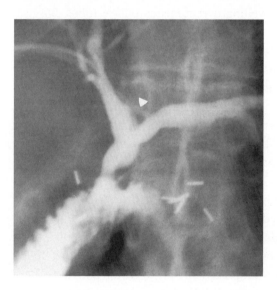

Figure 26-4 Cholangiogram via catheter in the left duct (arrowhead) after a trial of internal drainage. The drainage catheter was subsequently removed.

inserted and the anastomosis was dilated. The soft calculi were crushed with the angioplasty balloon and fragments were flushed into the jejunum or retrieved with a basket (**Fig. 26-2**). Several sessions were needed to clear the system of residual calculi and satisfactorily balloon dilate the anastomosis (**Figs. 26-3** and **26-4**). After a trial of internal drainage, the catheter was removed.

Discussion

Up to 16% of individuals with gallbladder calculi also have common duct calculi. The majority of common duct calculi originate in the gallbladder and ~22% form in the common duct (Bernhoft, 1984). In a large series of patients coming for percutaneous retrieval, intrahepatic calculi were present in 15% (Burhenne, 1980). Intrahepatic calculi are often multiple and occur as a result of hepatobiliary disease (recurrent cholangitis, cirrhosis, ductal ectasia, Caroli's disease, oriental cholangiohepatitis) or secondary to a long-standing obstruction (strictures—benign or malignant, in ducts obstructed by long-term drainage catheters and proximal to a surgical anastomosis). In the absence of intrinsic hepatobiliary disease, these concretions are usually the result of bile precipitation (stasis stones) and are relatively soft and easily crushed. Treatment is directed toward the underlying bile duct obstruction (i.e., the stricture) as well as the calculi.

From their gross appearance, gallstones are classified as either cholesterol, pigment, or mixed type. About 60 to 80% of biliary calculi contain significant amounts of cholesterol. These are typically whitish or yellow colored. Pigment stones account for ~20% of gallstones and are black or dark brown and contain a significant proportion of unconjugated bilirubin (Schwesinger et al, 1985; Bowen et al, 1992). The mixed type are tan or brown in color. Analysis of biliary calculi shows that only ~10% are mainly composed of either cholesterol or calcium bilirubinate and are considered "pure stones," whereas another 10% are "combined stones" consisting of a nucleus and an outer shell, each of a different composition (either pure or mixed). The remainder are of a mixed composition. Calcium is present in sufficient quantity to permit radiographic detection in ~15%. Calculi that form in ducts are usually brown or "earthlike" in color, soft, and easily crushed (Saharia et al, 1977).

Preoperative endoscopic sphincterotomy and calculus removal and intraoperative choledocoscopy have contributed to a decrease in the incidence of retained common duct calculi. Despite these efforts, some calculi escape detection and require an additional procedure for removal.

Most patients with biliary calculi are now managed by endoscopic techniques. This includes the removal of retained biliary calculi in patients with indwelling percutaneous biliary tubes. Surgical patients with cholelithiasis are subjected to endoscopic sphincterotomy or balloon sphincteroplasty for removal of common duct calculi while the gallbladder is subsequently removed laparoscopically (Snow et al, 1999; Cuschieri, 2000). The added cost, longer patient recovery time, and morbidity associated with the endoscopic procedures may be factors that have contributed toward a more selective rather than routine use of preoperative endoscopy. Depending upon the availability and involvement of local interventional radiological expertise, in the presence of a choledochal or transcystic duct catheter, percutaneous methods should be more appealing because of the lower cost, lower periprocedure morbidity, and patient comfort (Navarrete et al, 1998; Stein et al, 1998; Mahmud et al, 2001).

Endoscopy requires deep sedoanalgesia, and a sphincterotomy is necessary prior to calculus removal, although balloon dilatation of the sphincter can also be used. Endoscopic sphincterotomy is associated with a complication rate as high as 9.1% (Halme et al, 1999). Although uncommon, there is a definite risk of developing papillary stenosis after endoscopic sphincterotomy (Prat et al, 1996). Severe complications necessitating a second procedure may occur in up to 4% of patients. These include pancreatitis, hemorrhage, and abscess formation (**Fig. 26-5**). Thus, in the patient with an indwelling biliary drainage catheter, cystic duct, or common duct tube, there is little reason to subject the patient to an endoscopic sphincterotomy when available interventional radiological expertise and established percutaneous techniques offer successful management of retained bile duct calculi.

In the postoperative patient with a T-tube or cystic duct catheter, the cholangiogram remains the method of choice for detecting retained calculi. However, there are reports that indicate a significant failure rate for tube cholangiography to detect retained calculi that were then seen during a subsequent cholangioscopy (Weickert et al, 2003). This is not surprising because the intraoperative or postendoscopy cholangiogram is often obtained in only a single projection utilizing undiluted contrast. Radiological experience shows that the cholangiogram must be of optimal quality to facilitate detection of calculi. An initial image prior to injection of contrast is necessary for the detection of calcified calculi. The cholangiogram is then performed with diluted contrast (20–30% concentration). After obtaining the necessary images (frontal and both oblique projections), the contrast is drained. A second cholangiogram is then obtained with undiluted contrast. Small and

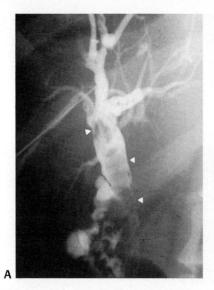 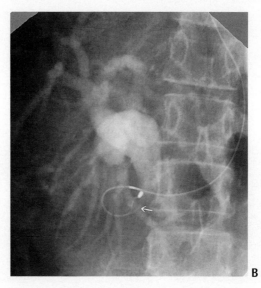

Figure 26-5 Complications of attempted endoscopic removal of calculi. (**A**) Percutaneous transhepatic cholangiogram in a patient with postendoscopic sphincterotomy hemorrhage and biliary obstruction shows dilatation and obstruction of the intrahepatic ducts by thrombus in the common bile duct (CBD) (arrowheads). The patient had undergone endoscopic retrograde cholangiopancreatography for removal of a retained CBD calculus. (**B**) Image from a different patient taken prior to percutaneous transhepatic biliary drainage shows biliary obstruction with a transendoscopic retrieval basket around a large calculus (arrow). The calculus could not be removed and the basket could not be disengaged.

partially calcified calculi are best detected with dilute contrast and are obscured by dense contrast (**Fig. 26-6**). Smaller radiolucent calculi may not be seen if only dilute contrast is used.

Interventional radiological methods for the removal of biliary calculi utilize the standard four- and eight-wire stone-retrieval baskets, balloon catheters, forceps, intracorporal lithotripsy, and lasers. The procedure may be guided by cholangioscopy or fluoroscopy. Guiding catheters or modified angiographic catheters are used to guide placement of the stone-retrieval baskets. Balloon catheters (usually a Fogarty or a Swan) are used primarily to dislodge calculi from inaccessible locations such as the intrahepatic ducts. Angioplasty and occlusion balloons have been used to push distal common duct calculi into the duodenum. Glucagon-induced sphincter relaxation or balloon dilatation of the sphincter usually precedes. In addition, soft, straight catheters (red rubber or silicone) can be useful for suction retrieval of smaller calculi.

Technique

Percutaneous retrieval of retained calculi is usually an outpatient procedure. The patients are instructed to remain on clear liquids after midnight of the day before the procedure. Venous access is obtained in the left arm. Sedation with Valium or Versed and analgesia (fentanyl or Demerol) is given intravenously before beginning the procedure, and additional doses are administered as the need arises. An intravenous dose of a broad spectrum antibiotic is given preprocedure to patients with cholangitis or suspected infection. Antibiotic coverage may also be prudent in patients requiring prolonged instrumentation. The patient is monitored in the usual fashion (visual assessment, vitals, oxygen saturation, and electrocardiogram). The procedure is performed using sterile operating conditions. The skin around the percutaneous access site is prepped with Betadine or other antiseptic and then sterile draped. As most T-tubes and transcystic duct catheters are brought out anteriorly, the image intensifier is angled to minimize radiation exposure to the operator's hands.

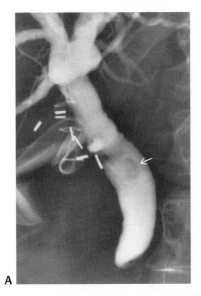
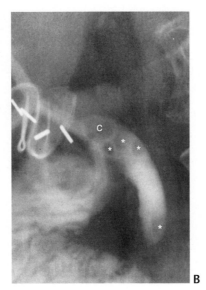

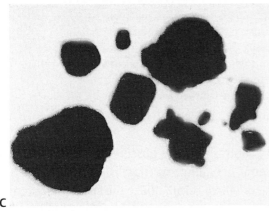

Figure 26-6 Importance of proper contrast concentration for cholangiographic detection of calculi. (**A**) Cholangiogram with undiluted contrast shows a single calculus (arrow). (**B**) Repeat cholangiogram with 20% concentration contrast reveals several additional calculi (*). In addition, the calculus (c) is actually larger than it appeared in (**A**). (**C**) Photograph of the retrieved calculi.

REMOVAL OF CALCULI VIA THE CHOLEDOCHAL CATHETER TRACT

The tract is allowed 4 to 6 weeks for maturation. In some cases, coaxial tubes inserted during surgery facilitate earlier calculus extraction (Stein et al, 1998). If a small size catheter (or T-tube) has been used, the mature tract can be dilated to 10F with coaxial fascial dilators. However, calculi can usually be managed through an 8F tract. Depending upon size, the calculus can also be removed with a T-tube in place.

A cholangiogram is obtained before removal of the choledochal catheter (or T-tube). This serves to identify the calculi, common duct anatomy, and course of the tract. An occasional small calculus may have passed spontaneously or be relocated to another segment of the duct. The T-tube is removed in an atraumatic fashion by application of constant, gentle traction. Forceful removal may traumatize the duct and predispose to stricture formation. If small calculi are present, a syringe is attached to the catheter/T-tube and suction is applied as the tube is removed. This frequently removes one or more smaller calculi.

A "safety" wire should be inserted prior to catheter/T-tube removal if the tract is small (≤10F), ≤4 weeks old, or a traumatic removal is anticipated. A 0.035 in. or 0.038 in. J guide wire is advanced into the intrahepatic or the common bile duct. The T-tube assumes a Y-shape when traction is applied, permitting the guide wire to be directed into the liver or common bile duct (CBD). Following removal of the T-tube, proximally located calculi frequently migrate into the distal CBD and distally located calculi might shift into the intrahepatic ducts. This may also occur during cholangiography. After completing the calculus retrieval, a straight catheter (sterile red rubber, pediatric feeding tube) is inserted into the common duct. Cholangiograms are obtained in different projections to assess the intra- and extrahepatic ducts for residual calculi and complications.

REMOVAL OF CALCULI VIA A CYSTIC DUCT ACCESS

The cystic duct is used as access for choledocoscopy during laparoscopic surgery. Patients requiring direct common duct exploration may receive a cystic duct drainage catheter. This access can be used for cholangiography and removal of retained common duct calculi (Snow et al, 1999; Mahmud et al, 2001). Such access is also available in patients with a surgical or percutaneous cholecystostomy. Catheter manipulation through a redundant cystic duct can be frustrating for the operator and the spasm severely painful for the patient. Sublingual nitroglycerine has provided relief of spasm. The cystic duct can also be balloon dilated after administration of analgesics to permit placement of a larger catheter. The calculus retrieval technique is similar to that for the choledochal catheter/T-tube tract. (Also see Chapter 31).

TRANSHEPATIC RETRIEVAL OF CALCULI

This approach is used for common or intrahepatic duct calculi in patients without an available direct choledochal (T-tube or transduodenal endoscopic) access or failed endoscopic retrograde cholangiopancreatography (ERCP). Ultrasound-guided PTC enables selection of a suitable duct for PBD catheter placement. From this approach, calculi in the common duct and also in the ipsi- and contralateral intrahepatic branches are accessible for removal. The calculi can be removed in the same sitting (i.e., immediately after PBD insertion) or after tract maturation. An 8 or 9F sheath placed in the hepatic or proximal common duct is used for passage of the instruments.

BASKET METHOD

Selection of the retrieval basket is determined by the duct diameter and calculus size. In general, the basket diameter should equal that of the duct in which the calculus is located. It may be difficult to engage and secure a calculus with an inappropriate-diameter basket. For example, if a 6 or 8 mm diameter basket is used for a 6 mm calculus in a common duct that measures 1 cm, the calculus may slip out as it is being engaged or as the basket is withdrawn or closed. However, this occurs less frequently with eight-wire baskets (Cook Incorp., Bloomington, IN). The retrieval basket is introduced via a large lumen (8–9F) angiographic catheter. The wire basket may also be removed from its catheter and the latter is positioned over a guide wire. The basket is then reinserted for engaging and removing the calculus.

After removal of the surgical tube, the tract may be opacified with contrast to facilitate catheterization. The angiographic/guiding catheter is inserted into the duct (over a guide wire or the contrast opacified mature tract is negotiated without a leading guide wire) and the tip is positioned beyond the calculus. The retrieval basket is inserted and the angiographic/guiding catheter is then withdrawn to expose the unopened basket (**Fig. 26-7**). The basket is then opened by withdrawing the basket catheter and is brought alongside the calculus. A gentle, short back and forth excursion will engage the calculus. Occasionally a slight rotation of the basket may be necessary. If the calculus moves with the basket, this usually indicates that it is in the basket. The whole assembly is then removed in one continuous motion.

The basket can be left open if the calculus is large and if the tract is relatively straight (i.e., without acute bends). The calculus may fall out when going around a bend or if the assembly removal is jerky. The basket may be closed by advancing the catheter over it. A tight closure may fragment the calculus. The eight-wire baskets can usually remain open because calculus dislodgment is infrequent.

The procedure is repeated for additional calculi. A cholangiogram is obtained upon completion and a multiple-hole catheter is inserted. For common duct calculi, I place the catheter in an intrahepatic duct and into the common duct if intrahepatic calculi have been removed. A sterile red rubber catheter or pediatric feeding tube (with two to three side holes made close to the tip) can

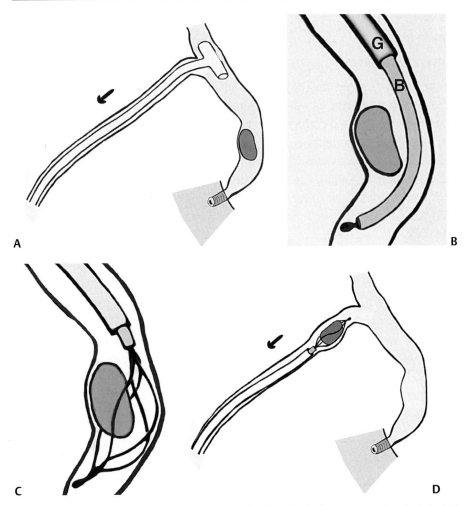

Figure 26-7 Technique for calculus removal. (**A**) After the cholangiogram, the choledochal tube/catheter is removed. (**B**) The basket (B) and guiding (G) catheter are inserted past the calculus. The guiding catheter is withdrawn, leaving the basket catheter along side the calculus. (**C**) The basket catheter is pulled back to unsheath the basket. (**D**) The calculus is engaged and removed.

also be used for this purpose. The catheter is capped with a "Christmas tree" adapter to permit internal bile drainage. If there was extensive manipulation at the papilla and edema is observed, the catheter is left to external drainage for 24 hours and subsequently converted to internal drainage. Reevaluation for ductal patency, residual calculi, and eventual catheter removal is scheduled after 2 to 3 days.

OTHER METHODS

Other percutaneous methods for the removal of biliary calculi include suction; irrigation; electrohydraulic; laser and mechanical lithotripsy; dissolution; and transampullary expulsion following balloon dilatation of the papilla or glucagon-aided relaxation, balloon-aided fragmentation, and extraction (Gil et al, 2000; Bonnel et al, 2001; Mahmud et al, 2001; Ilgit et al, 2002; Ozcan et al, 2003). These procedures can be guided by fluoroscopy or cholangioscopy.

REMOVAL OF INTRAHEPATIC CALCULI

Calculi lodged in smaller intrahepatic ducts may not be accessible for removal by the standard wire basket retrieval methods. These must be brought into a major duct for basket retrieval or adjunctive techniques must be used to insert baskets into remote locations (see Chapter 27). Intrahepatic calculi can be approached from a transductal (choledochal, cystic duct) or transhepatic route (Kadir and Gadacz, 1987; Neuhaus, 1999).

Outcome

Approximately 20% of calculi either pass spontaneously or disappear as a result of fragmentation. These are usually <6 mm in diameter. Calculi can be removed by percutaneous techniques in over 95% of cases. Multiple and intrahepatic calculi often necessitate several sessions.

Complications

The overall complication rate is between 4 and 6% (Burhenne, 1980). Serious complications from removal of biliary calculi via the T-tube/cystic duct tract are very uncommon. With the transhepatic approach, the incidence is higher and the complications are usually from the PTC and PBD and can be minimized by careful access selection and ultrasound guidance. Complications have included cholangitis, pleural effusion, and bleeding. Other rare complications include tract disruption, loss of calculus in the subcutaneous tissues or peritoneal cavity, and pancreatitis.

Biliary-Enteric Stricture Management

An anastomotic stricture after hepaticojejunostomy for benign disease is uncommon (McDonald et al, 1995). Such strictures are inaccessible to endoscopy unless a transjejunal or transgastric approach is used. Treatment is usually surgical revision or percutaneous transhepatic management. A percutaneous transjejunal approach can also be used via an attached or an unattached jejunal loop (see Chapter 29).

The short- to midterm results of percutaneous dilatation of anastomotic strictures are good with no recurrence in 73% at 30 months (Vos et al, 2000). Most benign anastomotic strictures are treated by balloon angioplasty alone. Success of balloon dilatation is usually determined by a clinical trial of internal drainage with the drainage catheter placed above the treated anastomosis and the hub capped. Alternatively, biliary manometry can be used and provides comparable predictive value (Savader et al, 1994).

Metallic stents are used only occasionally in benign disease. If calculi have been removed or crushed, the presence of a stent also facilitates passage of calculus fragments. Overlooked or residual fragments could not only reobstruct but also provide a nidus for development of larger calculi (Weickert et al, 2003).

PEARLS AND PITFALLS_____

- Percutaneous biliary calculus retrieval should be considered the first option in patients with a percutaneous access such as a choledochal, cystic duct, or transhepatic catheter.
- The calculus retrieval procedure is highly successful and can be performed on an outpatient basis with a low rate of serious complications.

Further Reading

Bernhoft RA, Pellegrini CA, Motson RW, et al. Common duct stones: primary or secondary? Am J Surg 1984;148:77–85

Bonnel D, Liguory C, Lefebvre JF, et al. Traitement percutané de la lithiase intra-hépatique. Gastroenterol Clin Biol 2001;25:581–588

Bowen JC, Brenner HI, Ferrante WA, et al. Gallstone disease: pathophysiology, epidemiology, natural history, and treatment options. Med Clin North Am 1992;76:1143–1157

Burhenne HJ. Percutaneous extraction of retained biliary tract stones: 661 patients. AJR Am J Roentgenol 1980;134:888–898

Cuschieri A. Ductal stones: pathology, clinical manifestations, laparoscopic extraction techniques, and complications. Semin Laparosc Surg 2000;7:246–261

Gil S, de la Iglesia P, Verdu JF, et al. Effectiveness and safety of balloon dilation of the papilla and the use of an occlusion balloon for clearance of bile duct calculi. AJR Am J Roentgenol 2000;174:1455–1460

Halme L, Doepel M, von Numers H, et al. Complications of diagnostic and therapeutic ERCP. Ann Chir Gynaecol 1999;88:127–131

Ilgit ET, Gurel K, Onal B. Percutaneous management of bile duct stones. Eur J Radiol 2002;43:237–245

Kadir S, Gadacz TR. Adjuncts and modifications to basket retrieval of retained biliary calculi. Cardiovasc Intervent Radiol 1987;10:295–300

Mahmud S, McGlinchey I, Kasem H, et al. Radiological treatment of retained bile duct stones following recent surgery using glucagons. Surg Endosc 2001;15:1359–1360

McDonald ML, Farnell MB, Nagorney DM, et al. Benign biliary strictures: repair and outcome with a contemporary approach. Surgery 1995;118:582–590

Navarrete CG, Castillo CT, Castillo PY. Choledocholithiasis: percutaneous treatment. World J Surg 1998;22:1151–1154

Neuhaus H. Intrahepatic stones: the percutaneous approach. Can J Gastroenterol 1999;13:467–472

Ozcan N, Erdogan N, Baskol M. Common bile duct stones detected after cholecystectomy: advancement into the duodenum via the percutaneous route. Cardiovasc Intervent Radiol 2003;26:150–153

Prat F, Malak NA, Pelletier G, et al. Biliary symptoms and complications more than 8 years after endoscopic sphincterotomy for choledocholithiasis. Gastroenterology 1996;110:894–899

Saharia P, Zuidema GD, Cameron JL. Primary common duct stones. Ann Surg 1977;185:598–604

Savader SJ, Cameron JL, Pitt HA, et al. Biliary manometry versus clinical trial: value as predictors of success after treatment of biliary tract strictures. J Vasc Interv Radiol 1994;5:757–763

Schwesinger WH, Kurtin WE, Levine BA, et al. Cirrhosis and alcoholism as pathogentic factors in pigment gallstone formation. Ann Surg 1985;201:319–322

Snow LL, Weinstein LS, Hannon JK, et al. Management of bile duct stones in 1572 patients undergoing laparoscopic cholecystectomy. Am Surg 1999;65:530–545

Stein DE, Sclafani SJ, Kral JG. Management of T tubes for common bile duct stones: a new technique. Dig Surg 1998;15:279–282

Vos PM, van Beek EJR, Smits NJ, et al. Percutaneous balloon dilatation for benign hepaticojejunostomy strictures. Abdom Imaging 2000;25:134–138

Weickert U, Jakobs R, Hahne M, et al. Cholangioskopie nach erfolgreicher Therapie einer komplizierten Choledocholithiasis: ist Steinfrei wirklich Steinfrei? Dtsch Med Wochenschr 2003;128:481–484

CHAPTER 27 Intrahepatic Calculi and Monolobar Caroli's Disease

Saadoon Kadir

Clinical Presentation

A 30-year-old woman with a history of upper abdominal pain underwent cholecystectomy and choledocotomy for cholelithiasis. A postoperative cholangiogram showed abnormal bile ducts and intrahepatic calculi. There was no history of portal hypertension, sclerosing cholangitis, or inflammatory bowel disease.

Radiological Studies

Cholangiogram obtained through a surgically placed choledochal catheter showed multiple small calculi in the peripheral left hepatic ducts (**Fig. 27-1**). Several stenoses as well as fusiform and saccular ductal dilatations were also present.

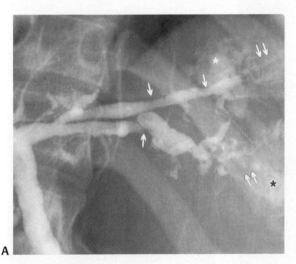
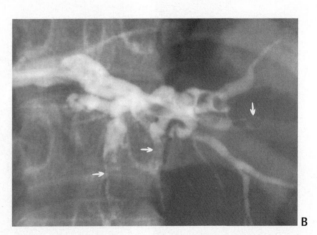

Figure 27-1 (**A**) Cholangiogram of the left hepatic ducts through a common duct catheter shows numerous small calculi in peripheral ducts (double arrows). Other ducts packed with calculi are not opacified. Abnormal duct caliber is present with strictures (single arrows) and dilatation. Contrast is present in the stomach (*). (**B**) Cholangiogram through a catheter in the left hepatic duct shows additional ducts filled with calculi (arrows).

Diagnosis

Intrahepatic bile duct calculi and Caroli's disease

Treatment Options and Treatment

Calculi in the larger intrahepatic ducts are accessible to endoscopic intervention. Those in remote locations, as in this patient, are not easily reached by transduodenal endoscopy. The surgical treatment option for multiple intrahepatic calculi is hepatic resection and hepaticojejunostomy. The presence of percutaneous access allowed direct access to the calculi. Cholangioscopic or fluoroscopy guidance could be used. The anatomy of the calculi-bearing peripheral left hepatic duct appeared to be more easily negotiated with angiographic catheters using fluoroscopy. Therefore, the latter was chosen.

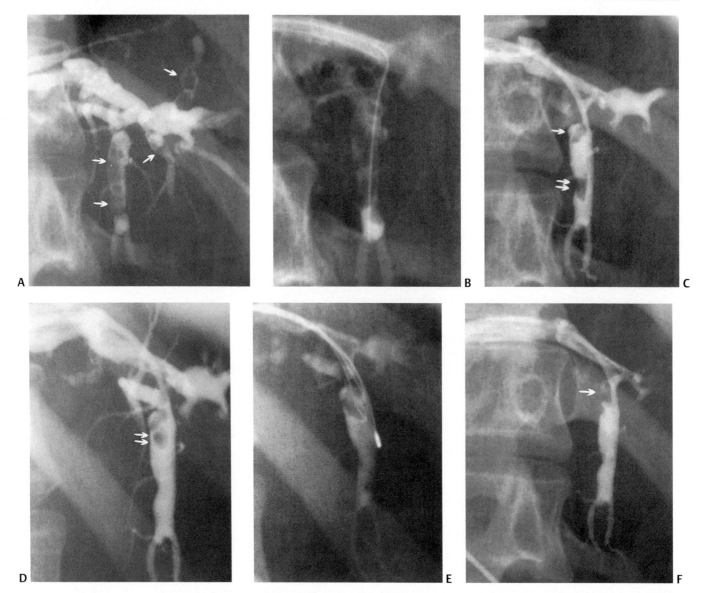

Figure 27-2 (**A**) After retrieval of some of the calculi, additional ducts with calculi are better opacified (arrows). (**B**) Fogarty balloon embolectomy catheter is used to relocate calculi from the distal duct. (**C**) Irrigation/flushing method for relocating a distal calculus (double arrows) into (**D**) the proximal duct for (**E**) basket retrieval. Single arrow in (**C**) points to a second calculus. (**F**) Cholangiogram after retrieval shows fusiform duct dilatation. A proximal stricture is present (arrow).

An 8F guiding catheter (nontapered angiographic catheter) was advanced into the left hepatic duct, and accessible calculi were removed using a retrieval basket. Those in inaccessible locations (side branches or the peripheral duct) were relocated into a larger or more central duct and subsequently removed with a basket. Calculi deep inside the side branches or small ducts were dislodged with a Fogarty embolectomy catheter or by irrigation/flushing (**Fig. 27-2**). For the latter, the tip of an angiographic catheter was positioned peripheral to the calculus, and dilute contrast (~10% concentration) was slowly injected. This dislodged the calculi. Once in a larger duct, the calculi were retrieved using standard basket techniques. Several sessions were necessary to remove all calculi. Images obtained during and after the procedures showed abnormal-caliber ducts with fusiform and saccular dilatation (**Figs. 27-2** and **27-3**).

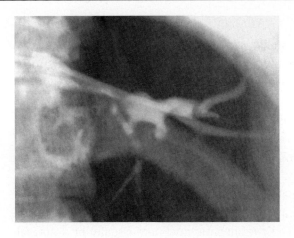

Figure 27-3 Cholangiogram after retrieval of all calculi. There is saccular ductal dilatation.

Discussion

Intrahepatic Calculi

Intrahepatic calculi (hepatolithiasis) were found in 20% of postcholecystectomy patients referred for removal of retained calculi (Burhenne, 1980). One fourth of these patients also had extrahepatic duct calculi. The actual incidence of intrahepatic calculi is much lower at ~1% of patients with cholelithiasis (Guma et al, 1999). They are seen more commonly in East Asian populations and occur in about equal frequency in men and women. Not all patients with intrahepatic calculi are symptomatic. In one series, over one third of patients were asymptomatic at the time of diagnosis and only 11.5% of these patients developed related symptomatology over a mean follow-up period of 10 years (Kusano et al, 2001). The most common presenting symptoms are abdominal pain, cholangitis, pancreatitis in ~6% of patients, and manifestations of hepatic cirrhosis (Guma et al, 1999). The onset of symptoms frequently correlates with the migration of a calculus (or several calculi) into the common duct, resulting in obstruction or colic.

Intrahepatic calculi are usually multiple and both lobes are affected. In approximately one third of patients, there is monolobar disease of the left lobe. Lobar atrophy may be present and occurs more commonly in patients with symptomatic hepatolithiasis (Kusano et al, 2001). Associated common duct calculi are found in 28% and gallbladder calculi occur in about one third of cases (Guma et al, 1999; di Carlo et al, 2000). Most intrahepatic calculi are composed predominantly of bile pigment. Pure intrahepatic cholesterol calculi have been observed in ~3% of cases (Kim et al, 2001). In the majority of patients, there is an underlying anatomical or physiochemical abnormality that is responsible for the formation of calculi in the intrahepatic ducts. In descending order of frequency, these include: a benign stricture (usually postoperative), ductal dilatation (due to Caroli's disease or syndrome), cholangiocarcinoma, parasites (*Ascaris lumbricoides*), sickle cell anemia, and thallasemia (Pridgen et al, 1977; Lee et al, 2001).

The diagnosis is most accurately made by cholangiography. For the determination of the extent of involvement, magnetic resonance cholangiopancreatography (MRCP) is the preferred diagnostic modality, with an accuracy that surpasses that of endoscopic retrograde cholangiopancreatography (ERCP) (Kim et al, 2002). Cholangioscopy has also been used for diagnosis and management of these patients. Despite the diligent use of different nonsurgical retrieval methods, residual calculi are left behind in a significant number of patients. Calculi may be particularly difficult to remove in patients with ductal strictures.

Caroli's Disease and Caroli's Syndrome

There are two forms of this entity. Caroli's *disease* is characterized by congenital dilatation of the intrahepatic ducts without associated hepatic parenchymal or cystic renal abnormalities. In Caroli's *syndrome*, there is presence of periportal (congenital hepatic) fibrosis and cystic kidney disease. The mode of inheritance remains uncertain, although it is believed that Caroli's syndrome may be transmitted as an autosomal recessive abnormality, whereas Caroli's disease may not be inherited (Desmet, 1998).

Clinical manifestation may be observed during infancy and childhood or later in life (Pinto et al, 1998). It is characterized by saccular and, frequently, fusiform dilatation of segmental and subsegmental bile ducts. The disease may involve all hepatic segments or be localized to one or more segments or a lobe. In addition, the degree of dilatation may vary. The left lobe is affected most commonly in localized disease (Gillet et al, 1999). The extrahepatic ducts are usually of a normal caliber but may also be dilated. An unusual number of extrahepatic ductal abnormalities were reported in one review (Levy et al, 2002).

Caroli's syndrome occurs more commonly (Caroli, 1973; Dagli et al, 1998). Symptoms common to both forms include upper abdominal or right upper quadrant pain, recurrent bouts of cholangitis, which may lead to sepsis and abscesses, and formation of calculi or concretion of sludge (or both) in the dilated bile ducts. Common duct calculi are reported to be present in the majority of cases (Gillet et al, 1999). Reports of the presence of cholecystolithiasis vary from complete absence to almost all adult patients (Dagli et al, 1998; Gillet et al, 1999). In Caroli's syndrome, symptoms of hepatic cirrhosis and its complications may be present. Particularly in children with congenital hepatic fibrosis, symptoms of advanced liver disease are seen more commonly (Pinto et al, 1998). Renal tubular ectasia and renal cysts are found in association with Caroli's syndrome, although their presence may not be clinically manifested in all cases. Renal abnormalities may be responsible for hypertension, recurrent pyelonephritis, and calculi (Reilly and Neuhauser, 1960).

The diagnosis may be established by MRCP or contrast cholangiography (retrograde or percutaneous). Cross-sectional imaging findings include ductal dilatation, calculi, and manifestations of cirrhosis and portal hypertension. Characteristic features include the intraductal bridging seen on ultrasound, which represents intraductal septae and the "dot sign" on computed tomography (CT), which is produced by contrast enhancement of a portal vein branch surrounded by dilated bile ducts (Marchal et al, 1986; Choi et al, 1990). Corresponding to the severity and extent of disease, there is a wide range of abnormalities from a mild segmental ductal abnormality (see **Fig. 27-3**) to diffuse saccular and sometime fusiform ductal dilatation affecting the entire liver (**Fig. 27-4**).

Differential Diagnosis

Diseases that may simulate Caroli's disease include recurrent pyogenic cholangitis, sclerosing cholangitis, liver abscesses, long-standing biliary obstruction, and polycystic liver disease (on CT or ultrasound). Sclerosing cholangitis may occasionally demonstrate diffuse ductal dilatation with a shaggy contour and has been mistaken for Caroli's disease. Clinical symptoms may be similar, and calculi and cirrhosis may also be present.

Prognosis

Untreated, the prognosis is poor in diffuse disease because the course may be complicated by the sequelae of recurrent cholangitis, hepatic cirrhosis, and portal hypertension. In addition, cholangio-carcinoma has been reported to occur with some frequency (Nagasue, 1984; Abdalla et al, 1999; Kusano et al, 2001; Ammori et al, 2002). Calculi have been managed by endoscopic or percutaneous

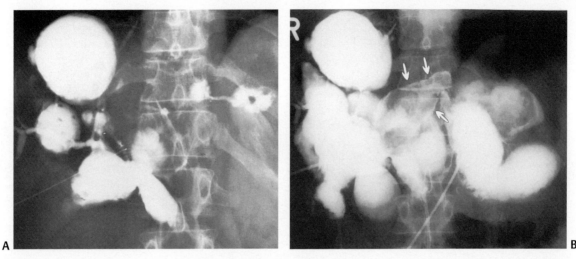

Figure 27-4 Cholangiogram in a patient with extensive involvement of both hepatic lobes by Caroli's disease. (**A**) Early image from a percutaneous transhepatic cholangiogram shows large, saccular ducts. Several of the communicating ducts are either mildly dilated or of a normal caliber. (**B**) Image obtained after insertion of drainage catheters shows the diffuse abnormality. Arrows point to a cast of claylike concretions in a dilated duct. (Figure 27-4B reproduced with permission from Kadir S, Diagnostic Angiography, WB Saunders, 1986.)

techniques, especially in localized disease. However, the treatment of choice is surgical. In monolobar disease, hepatic resection has been recommended, whereas diffuse disease is treated by liver transplantation (Nagasue, 1984; Gillet et al, 1999; Ammori et al, 2002).

Technique for Removal of Intrahepatic Calculi (Figs. 27-5 to 27-7)

An available access such as a choledochal catheter, cystic duct catheter, or transhepatic catheter can be used for cholangioscopic or fluoroscopic guidance, whereas in other cases, a percutaneous access may be planned for this purpose (Kadir and Gadacz, 1987; Neuhaus, 1999). The cystic duct may be used for access to intrahepatic calculi, depending upon the anatomy of the cystic–common duct junction. Most of intrahepatic duct calculi are small and soft (high pigment content) and are easily

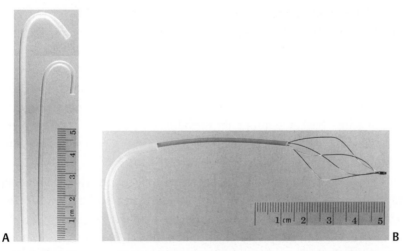

Figure 27-5 Catheters used for retrieval of calculi from the peripheral branches. (**A**) Left: thin-walled, nontapered angiographic catheter (8–9 French) with steam-shaped curve. A large diameter Sidewinder can also be used after modification. Right: modified 7F Sidewinder I catheter with the distal limb shortened. (**B**) Four-wire retrieval basket inserted through a nontapered angiographic catheter.

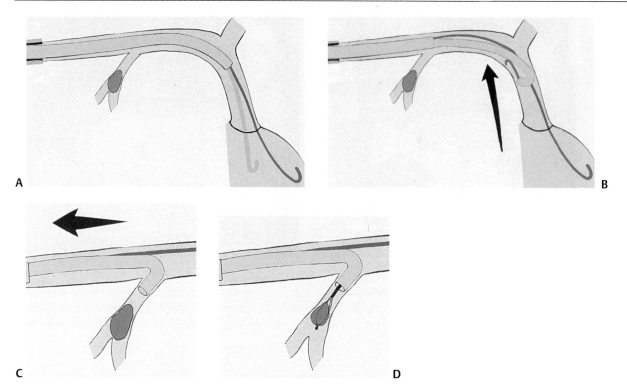

Figure 27-6 Drawings illustrating transhepatic catheterization technique for intrahepatic duct calculus retrieval. (**A**) A vascular sheath is placed and two guide wires are inserted. One wire is left in the bowel for reaccess (safety wire), whereas the other is used to insert the modified angiographic catheter. (**B**) The reverse curve of the catheter is reformed in the bowel (or through an anastomosis as illustrated) or in a contralateral duct. With the J-wire leading, the catheter is pulled back to the level of the calculus-bearing duct. Prior to insertion of the modified angiographic catheter, the vascular sheath may either be removed entirely or withdrawn to permit access to the desired branch. (**C**) The desired branch is entered, the guide wire is removed, and the retrieval basket is inserted. (**D**) The calculus is engaged and removed.

removed with baskets, and, therefore, do not require dissolution or electrohydraulic or laser fragmentation.

Calculi lodged in smaller or peripheral intrahepatic ducts are usually not accessible for removal by the standard basket retrieval methods and either they must be brought into a major duct for basket retrieval or adjunctive techniques must be used to insert baskets into remote locations. Modified angiographic catheters are used for catheterizing such peripheral ducts (**Fig. 27-5**). For branches in the ipsilateral lobe that arise at an acute angle, a modified sidewinder catheter is used (7F, Simmons I catheter with distal limb cut off with a sharp blade). The lumen is large enough to permit insertion of a 2F Fogarty or stone basket without its introducer catheter. A stem-shaped, nontapered, thin-walled 8 or 9F angiographic catheter permits insertion of the retrieval basket with its introducer catheter (**Fig. 27-5B**).

A calculus that is wedged in a small duct can often be dislodged with a J guide wire. Depending upon the diameter and location of the duct, a 5F balloon-tipped catheter can also be used for this purpose. A multiple-hole angiographic or a wedge Swan-Ganz or Berman catheter is passed peripheral to the calculus. Diluted contrast (or saline) is injected to flush out the calculus and the balloon is partially inflated and pulled back. **Figs. 27-6** and **27-7** demonstrate the technique for retrieving calculi from an ipsilateral side branch via the transhepatic approach.

As intrahepatic calculi are usually multiple, several sessions may be required to clear the ducts. In some cases, residual calculi remain despite a diligent effort. Procedure-related complications are uncommon. Potential risks include duct perforation from an overinflated balloon or use of the

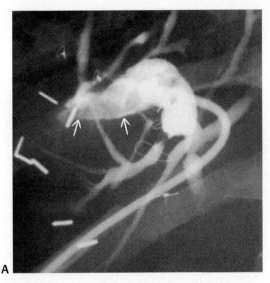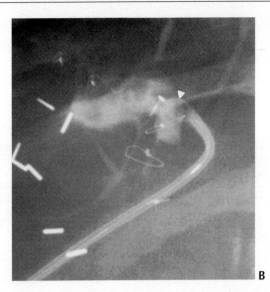

Figure 27-7 (**A**) Cholangiogram through a modified 7F Sidewinder I catheter shows multiple calculi in the duct (arrows). (**B**) A calculus is trapped in a four-wire basket (arrowhead). The basket, which was inserted without its own catheter, is closed because the calculus was to be removed around a bend. A reaccess or safety guide wire is not present because the tract was mature.

guide wire or basket in the smaller ducts. The injury is usually self-limited and can be avoided if the instruments are used cautiously.

PEARLS AND PITFALLS

- Intrahepatic calculi are found in ~1% of patients with cholelithiasis. They are usually multiple, and both lobes are affected, although in about one third of patients there is monolobar disease of the left lobe.
- Conditions associated with hepatolithiasis include benign strictures (usually postoperative), ductal dilatation (Caroli's disease or syndrome), tumor, parasites, sickle cell anemia, and thallasemia.
- In Caroli's *disease* there is dilatation of the intrahepatic ducts without hepatic parenchymal or cystic renal abnormalities. Caroli's *syndrome* is associated with periportal (congenital hepatic) fibrosis and cystic disease of the kidney.
- Caroli's disease may involve all hepatic segments or be localized to one or more segments or a lobe. The left lobe is affected most commonly in localized disease. The extrahepatic ducts are usually of a normal caliber but may also be dilated.

Further Reading

Abdalla EK, Forsmark CE, Lauwers GY, et al. Monolobar Caroli's disease and cholangiocarcinoma. HPB Surg 1999;11:271–276

Ammori BJ, Jenkins BL, Lim PCM, et al. Surgical strategy for cystic diseases of the liver in a Western hepatobiliary center. World J Surg 2002;26:462–469

Burhenne HJ. Percutaneous extraction of retained biliary tract stones: 661 patients. Garland lecture. AJR Am J Roentgenol 1980;134:889–898

Caroli J. Diseases of the intrahepatic biliary tree. Clin Gastroenterol 1973;2:147–161

Caroli J, Soupault R, Kossakowski J, et al. Congenital polycystic dilation of the intrahepatic bile ducts: attempt at classification [in French]. Sem Hop 1958;34:488–495

Choi BI, Yoen KM, Kim SH, et al. Caroli disease: central dot sign in CT. Radiology 1990;174:161–163

Dagli U, Atalay F, Sasmaz N, et al. Caroli's disease: 1977–1995 experiences. Eur J Gastroenterol Hepatol 1998;10:109–112

Desmet VJ. Pathogenesis of ductal plate abnormalities. Mayo Clin Proc 1998;73:80–89

di Carlo I, Sauvanet A, Belghiti J. Intrahepatic lithiasis: a Western experience. Surg Today 2000; 30:319–322

Gillet M, Favre S, Fontolliet C, et al. Maladie de Caroli monolobaire: a propos de 12 cas. Chirurgie 1999;124:13–18

Guma C, Viola C, Apestegui M, et al. Hepatolithiasis and Caroli's disease in Argentina: results of a multicenter study [in Spanish]. Acta Gastroenterol Latinoam 1999;29:9–15

Kadir S, Gadacz TR. Adjuncts and modifications to basket retrieval of retained biliary calculi. Cardiovasc Intervent Radiol 1987;10:295–300

Kim TK, Kim BS, Kim JH, et al. Diagnosis of intrahepatic stones: superiority of MR cholangiopancreatography over endoscopic retrograde cholangiopancreatography. AJR Am J Roentgenol 2002; 179:429–434

Kim HJ, Kim MH, Lee SK, et al. Characterization of primary pure cholesterol hepatolithiasis: cholangioscopic and selective cholangiographic findings. Gastrointest Endosc 2001;53:324–328

Kusano T, Isa T, Ohtsubo M, et al. Natural progression of untreated hepatolithiasis that shows no clinical signs at its initial presentation. J Clin Gastroenterol 2001;33:114–117

Lee SK, Seo DW, Myung SJ, et al. Percutaneous transhepatic cholangioscopic treatment for hepatolithiasis: an evaluation of long-term results and risk factors for recurrence. Gastrointest Endosc 2001;53:318–323

Levy AD, Rohrmann CA Jr, Murakata LA, et al. Caroli's disease: radiologic spectrum with pathologic correlation. AJR Am J Roentgenol 2002;179:1053–1057

Marchal GJ, Desmet VJ, Proesmans WC, et al. Caroli disease: high frequency US and pathologic findings. Radiology 1986;158:507–511

Nagasue N. Successful treatment of Caroli's disease by hepatic resection: report of six patients. Ann Surg 1984;200:718–723

Neuhaus H. Intrahepatic stones: the percutaneous approach. Can J Gastroenterol 1999;13:467–472

Pinto RB, Lima JP, da Silveira TR, et al. Caroli's disease: report of 10 cases in children and adolescents in southern Brazil. J Pediatr Surg 1998;33:1531–1535

Pridgen JE, Aust JB, McInnis WD. Primary intrahepatic gallstones. Arch Surg 1977;112:1037–1044

Reilly BJ, Neuhauser EBD. Renal tubular ectasia in cystic disease of the kidneys and liver. Am J Roentgenol Radium Ther Nucl Med 1960;84:546–554

CHAPTER 28 Giant Common Duct Calculi

Saadoon Kadir

Clinical Presentation

A 70-year-old man with multiple medical problems presented with jaundice. He had previously undergone cholecystectomy. Endoscopic retrograde cholangiography (ERC) was attempted but was unsuccessful because of an obstruction at the papilla.

Radiological Studies

Computed tomography (CT) of the liver (not shown) demonstrated dilated intra- and extrahepatic ducts. The percutaneous transhepatic cholangiogram (PTC) showed obstruction of the distal common bile duct by a 16 × 21 mm, relatively low density lesion with smooth margins (**Fig. 28-1**). A transhepatic biliary drainage catheter was inserted for the relief of obstructive jaundice.

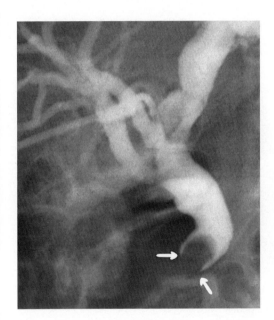

Figure 28-1 Cholangiogram after transhepatic drainage catheter placement shows a large obstructing lesion in the distal common bile duct (arrows). There is contrast surrounding the smooth upper margins and no contrast passage is seen into the duodenum.

Differential Diagnosis

Causes of distal common duct obstruction in patients of this age that may have a similar cholangiographic appearance include neoplasms (carcinoma of the pancreas, cholangiocarcinoma, tumors arising at or adjacent to the papilla, duodenal tumors, and intraductal metastases), calculi, and rare nonmalignant conditions (arterial aneurysms, pancreatic pseudocysts, and hydatid cysts). As no tumor or mass effect was seen on CT or endoscopy and the patient had undergone cholecystectomy for cholecystolithiasis, a wedged calculus was the most likely diagnosis.

High cholesterol content and lower radiographic density, when present, can be useful for differentiating a calculus from a tumor. However, most common duct calculi contain pigment and are thus difficult to differentiate from tumors on the basis of radiographic density alone

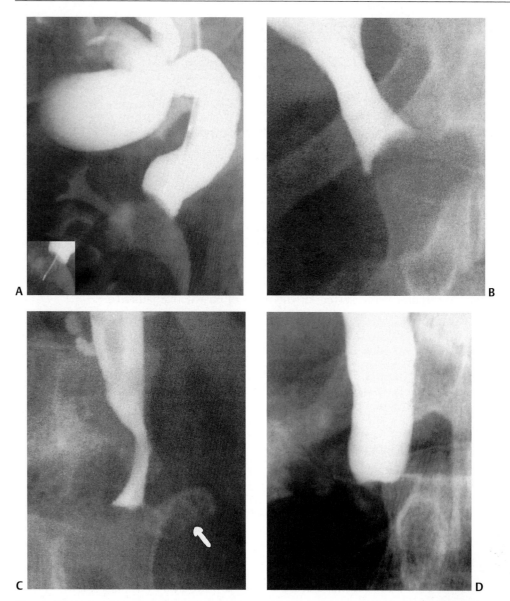

Figure 28-2 Opacity and margins of a mass in the distal common bile duct are inaccurate for differentiating between tumor and calculus. Also see **Fig. 28-1**. (**A**) Cholangiogram in a patient with carcinoma of the pancreas. The obstructing tumor shows a superior meniscus. Inset shows a guide wire passing through the center of the lesion. (**B**) Obstructing distal common duct calculus. (**C**) Distal common duct obstruction by a calculus and small pancreatic carcinoma. Incidental pancreatic calculi are seen (arrow). (**D**) Ampullary carcinoma simulating an obstructing calculus.

(**Fig. 28-2**). Occasionally, a calculus and carcinoma may coexist. A feature that may occasionally help is the location of the traversing guide wire. A guide wire that passes through the center indicates a tumor (**Fig. 28-2A** inset). A calculus displaces the guide wire to the side. An occasional tumor with eccentric growth may also displace the guide wire to the side.

Diagnosis

Obstructing giant common bile duct calculus

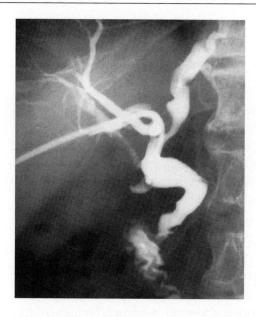

Figure 28-3 Cholangiogram obtained prior to catheter removal (after fragmentation and removal of the giant common duct calculus) shows no residual calculus or obstruction at the papilla. (Same patient as in **Fig. 28-1**.)

Treatment Options

Treatment options were endoscopic (sphincterotomy and basket removal or lithotripsy), surgical, or percutaneous. Endoscopic cannulation failed because the calculus was wedged. Surgery was not considered an option because of the patient's medical problems. The different percutaneous treatment options were fluoroscopically or cholangioscopically guided lithotripsy followed by forceps or basket removal or transampullary expulsion of the fragments, fluoroscopically guided fragmentation, and basket removal of the calculus fragments. The presence of obstructive jaundice necessitated biliary drainage catheter placement, which also provided the percutaneous access to the calculus.

Treatment

Following PTC, a biliary drainage catheter was inserted. Two weeks later, transhepatic retrieval of the calculus was undertaken. This delay permitted normalization of the laboratory parameters and tract maturation. The drainage catheter was exchanged for a long 8F sheath. The calculus was dislodged from the distal common duct with a hockey stick–shaped catheter and J guide wire. Following biliary decompression, the calculus was no longer firmly wedged in the distal common bile duct and was easily dislodged. A standard four-wire stone retrieval basket was inserted and the calculus was engaged but could not be crushed. Its large size precluded extraction through the transhepatic sheath or expulsion into the jejunum.

At this point, the treatment options were intracorporal or mechanical lithotripsy.

Mechanical lithotripsy was chosen because it was readily available. The drainage catheter was removed over a guide wire and the transhepatic tract was dilated with fascial dilators, and a 16F sheath was inserted. A reaccess or "safety" guide wire was advanced into the duodenum. The mechanical lithotriptor (Wilson-Cook, Bloomington, IN) was inserted and the calculus was engaged and crushed and the fragments removed. A 14F nephrostomy catheter was inserted into the common duct. It was left to internal drainage because no manipulations had been performed at the papilla and there was no obstruction to contrast passage. A final cholangiogram was performed 1 day later and showed satisfactory drainage (**Fig. 28-3**). The catheter was removed over a guide wire. There was no bleeding, cholangitis, or other complications.

Discussion

A calculus is called "giant" when it is >2 cm in diameter. The density, not the size, determines how easily the calculus can be crushed. Most large calculi are soft and therefore easily crushed. Those with a high cholesterol content are usually hard. Treatment options for large, difficult to fragment calculi are surgical removal, extracorporal shock wave lithotripsy (ESWL) or various endoscopic methods: mechanical, intracorporal electrohydraulic or laser lithotripsy, and dissolution (Classen et al, 1988; Guldutuna et al, 1991; Dorman et al, 1998; Leung et al, 2001). The latter attempts to decrease the size and make the calculus manageable by other endoscopic techniques. Although a relatively safe procedure, electrohydraulic lithotripsy may require multiple endoscopic sessions to clear all calculi (Leung and Chung, 1989). The expense associated with multiple endoscopic procedures is not insignificant and the incidence of complications can be high (Matsumoto et al, 1988). Failure of endoscopic management in some common duct calculi has led to the use of the percutaneous transhepatic approach (Matsumoto et al, 1997).

Percutaneous techniques for managing large or hard to crush calculi include cholangioscopically aided sonic or electrohydraulic lithotripsy and cholangioscopically or fluoroscopically guided laser lithotripsy (Ell et al, 1993; Nadler et al, 2002). In selected cases, transhepatic mechanical lithotripsy can be used. Thus, with the available methods, most large common duct calculi no longer require surgery.

The Soehendra mechanical lithotripsy device consists of a 14F metallic sheath and a high tensile strength wire basket. After the calculus is engaged, the basket is tightened by pulling it against the tip of the sheath. The pressure exerted by the wires cuts into the calculus, causing it to fragment. The fragments can then be retrieved using standard extraction techniques. The device necessitates the insertion of a large diameter (≥16F) transhepatic sheath. This is not associated with any problems if an appropriate peripheral duct is catheterized in preparation for this procedure. Furthermore, 20F transhepatic Silastic tubes have been used routinely by some surgeons to stent hepaticojejunostomies (Crist et al, 1987). Such placement occurs through existing percutaneous biliary drainage (PBD) tracts that may or may not enter a duct peripherally and has not been associated with any significant morbidity.

Indications, Patient Selection, and Preparation

The main indications for percutaneous transhepatic mechanical lithotripsy of a giant common duct calculus are (1) failed endoscopic management and (2) unsuccessful transhepatic fragmentation and removal using standard calculus retrieval methods.

Through a percutaneous transhepatic access, first an attempt should be made to fragment and remove the giant calculus by using standard techniques. If these are unsuccessful, mechanical lithotripsy can be attempted. Cholangioscopically assisted intracorporal lithotripsy is the other alternative. For biliary procedures, it requires expertise that is usually unavailable outside of larger medical centers and is also unavailable at short notice. Percutaneous transhepatic mechanical lithotripsy also requires an interventional radiologist experienced in complex biliary interventions. Advantages of fluoroscopically guided mechanical lithotripsy include the decreases in procedure duration and expense.

The usual precautions for PTC and PBD are observed (i.e., the patients are instructed to remain on clear liquids after midnight before the day of the procedure). Laboratory parameters are checked for clotting and renal function. Venous access is obtained in the left arm. Sedation with Valium or Versed and analgesia (fentanyl or Demerol) is given intravenously before beginning the procedure and additional doses are administered as the need arises. An intravenous dose of a broad spectrum antibiotic is also given preprocedure. The right upper quadrant and lower chest and subxiphoid region are prepped and sterile draped. The patient is monitored in the usual fashion (visual assessment, vitals, oxygen saturation, and electrocardiogram [EKG]).

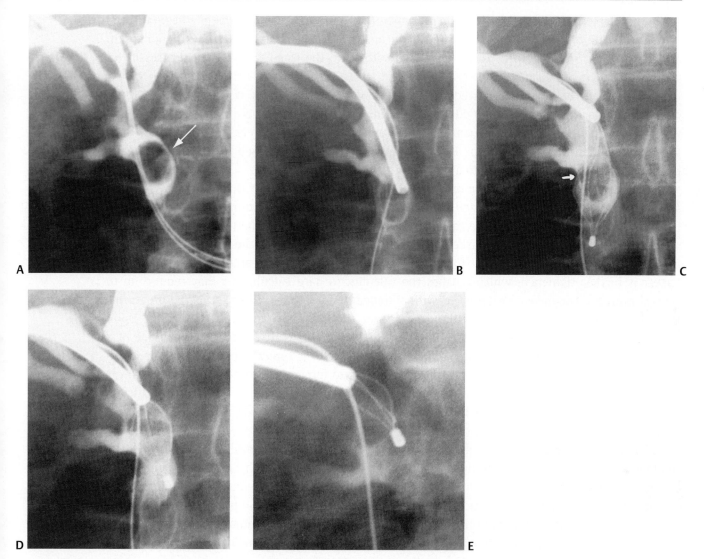

Figure 28-4 Technique for mechanical fragmentation of giant common duct calculus. (**A**) The large calculus (arrow) has been dislodged from the wedged position. Two guide wires have been passed into the duodenum. One of these will remain as a reaccess (safety) wire, while the other is used to insert the sheath used for the calculus fragmentation and retrieval systems. (**B**) The sheath tip is advanced to the calculus. The basket is exposed alongside the calculus by withdrawing the sheath. (**C**) The calculus (arrow) is engaged in the basket. (**D**) The calculus is trapped by advancing the sheath over the basket. (**E**) The basket diameter becomes smaller as the calculus begins to fragment from the pressure applied.

Technique (Fig. 28-4A-E)

PBD is performed via the right transcostal approach. In some instances, a left duct with suitable anatomy may be selected. A peripheral duct is accessed (utilizing ultrasound guidance) and a 10F drainage catheter is inserted and left to external (gravity) drainage. Depending upon the patient's condition and if the drainage catheter tip is in the duodenum (or jejunum through a hepaticoje-junostomy), a cholangiogram is obtained 24 to 48 hours later and the catheter is converted to internal drainage. If the procedure was performed electively, the patient is discharged home if there were no complications. About 2 weeks later, the patient returns for the lithotripsy. This delay permits maturation of the transhepatic tract. In inpatients, the mechanical lithotripsy may be undertaken sooner if the clinical condition permits or, preferably, it is also scheduled for a later date.

The patient returns for mechanical lithotripsy, having been instructed to remain on clear liquids after midnight before the day of the procedure. Venous access is obtained in the left arm and sedation

(Valium or Versed) and analgesia (fentanyl or Demerol) are given intravenously before beginning the procedure. Additional doses are administered as the need arises. The access site and surrounding skin are prepped and sterile draped. The patient is monitored in the usual fashion (visual assessment, vitals, oxygen saturation, and EKG).

The drainage catheter is removed over a guide wire and the tract is dilated to 16F using over-the-wire fascial (nephrostomy) dilators (Cook Incorp., Bloomington, IN). Two 0.035 in. J guide wires are inserted. One of these remains as a reaccess (safety) wire, whereas the other one is used to insert a 16F sheath (Cook Incorp., Bloomington, IN). The sheath is used to bridge the hepatic parenchyma, and the tip extends into a major duct.

There are two ways of using the mechanical lithotripsy device. Either the device is assembled and inserted as a unit or it is inserted in stages (some newer devices are preassembled). For the latter, the basket is inserted and the calculus is engaged. The sheath of the mechanical lithotripsy device is then threaded over the basket cable until it is in contact with the calculus. The cable is attached to a handle, which is used to pull and thus tighten the basket around the calculus. The basket is further tightened, which crushes the calculus. In hard calculi, this may require up to several minutes. Fragments are removed with a standard stone retrieval basket. If the preassembled device is used, it can be difficult to maneuver the basket to engage the calculus. Upon completion of the procedure, a 12 or 14F nephrostomy catheter is inserted. In the absence of a distal stricture or post-procedure edema, the drainage catheter is typically placed in the common duct (or proximal to a bilioenteric anastomosis) and left to internal drainage. A cholangiogram is obtained the following day and if no residual fragments or debris are seen and there is satisfactory contrast passage into the bowel, the catheter is removed over a guide wire (in the presence of a mature tract).

If a stricture is present in the distal bile duct or at a bilioenteric anastomosis, this must be dilated and managed accordingly by balloon dilatation or stenting with large diameter Silastic tubes (Born et al, 1999; Vos et al 2000). Metallic stents are used only occasionally in benign disease, in patients who are not being considered for surgical management, in the presence of significant medical problems that may not permit a repeat intervention, and in inflammatory strictures, which respond poorly to balloon dilatation. A stent also facilitates passage of smaller calculi and residual fragments.

Outcome

Endoscopic techniques are successful in removing >95% of common duct calculi. Larger calculi frequently necessitate multiple sessions, and excessive manipulation is associated with a higher incidence of cholangitis (Matsumoto et al, 1988). In the patients in whom we have used this technique, all fragments were removed in one session and there were no complications related to the PBD or mechanical lithotripsy.

Studies have shown that stone fragments can be overlooked on cholangiography (Weickert et al, 2003). A residual fragment could not only reobstruct but may form a nidus for a subsequent larger calculus. Unsatisfactory cholangiography technique is usually responsible for the inability to detect retained calculi or fragments on postintervention or intraoperative cholangiograms. Contributing factors include technical factors, presence of air or thrombus, and inappropriate contrast medium concentration.

Appropriate concentration of contrast medium avoids one of the major pitfalls in cholangiography for the detection of calculi. The standard undiluted contrast concentration is very dense and may obscure even large calculi (**Fig. 28-5**). The ideal concentration is between 20 and 30%, with the contrast diluted with normal saline. If no calculi are detected with diluted contrast, I repeat the

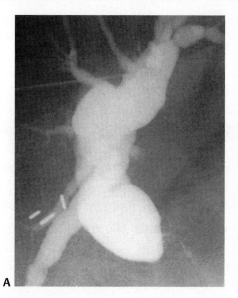 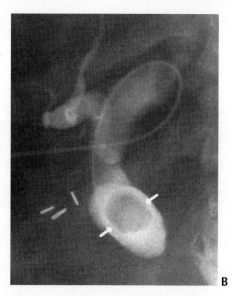

Figure 28-5 Contrast concentration may determine the ability to visualize a calculus on cholangiography. Images from another patient. (**A**) Cholangiogram using undiluted contrast does not shows any calculus. (**B**) Cholangiogram using 20% contrast shows the giant common duct calculus (arrows).

cholangiogram with more concentrated contrast. The latter is better suited for detection of larger radiolucent calculi, whereas dilute contrast visualizes the partially calcified calculi to better advantage. In either case, images should be obtained in several projections.

Complications

Potential complications of the transhepatic procedure include hemobilia, common duct injury, and cholangitis. Following endoscopic sphincterotomy, spontaneous passage of large calculi has been observed with the potential risk of a gallstone ileus (Halter et al, 1981). Other complications that are usually seen after endoscopic sphincterotomy and common duct manipulation include bleeding, pancreatitis, perforation with sepsis, and abscess formation (Halme et al, 1999).

PEARLS AND PITFALLS

- A calculus that is larger than 2 cm in maximal dimension is called a "giant" calculus.
- In cases where endoscopic management is unsuccessful, percutaneous transhepatic mechanical lithotripsy can be used for managing giant calculi.

Further Reading

Born P, Rosch T, Bruhl K, et al. Long-term results of endoscopic and percutaneous transhepatic treatment of benign biliary strictures. Endoscopy 1999;31:725–731

Classen M, Hagenmueller F, Knyrim K, et al. Giant bile duct stones: nonsurgical treatment. Endoscopy 1988;20:21–26

Crist DW, Kadir S, Cameron JL. Proximal biliary tract reconstruction: the value of preoperatively placed percutaneous biliary catheters. Surg Gynecol Obstet 1987;165:421–424

Dorman JP, Franklin ME Jr, Glass JL. Laparoscopic common bile duct exploration by choledochotomy: an effective and efficient method of treatment of choledocholithiasis. Surg Endosc 1998;12:926–928

Ell C, Hochberger J, May A, et al. Laser lithotripsy of difficult bile duct stones by means of a rhodamine-6G laser and an integrated automatic stone-tissue detection system. Gastrointest Endosc 1993;39:755–762

Guldutuna S, Hellstern A, Leuschner M, et al. Endoskopie, Stosswellenlithotripsie und lokale Lyse bei komplizierten Pigmentsteinen der extra- und intrahepatischen Gallengaengen. Dtsch Med Wschr 1991;116:288–293

Halme L, Doepel M, von Numers H, et al. Complications of diagnostic and therapeutic ERCP. Ann Chir Gynaecol 1999;88:127–131

Halter F, Bangerter U, Gigon JP, et al. Gallstone ileus after endoscopic sphincterotomy. Endoscopy 1981;13:88–89

Leung JW, Chung SS. Electrohydraulic lithotripsy with peroral choledocoscopy. BMJ 1989;299:595–598

Leung JW, Neuhaus H, Chopita N. Mechanical lithotripsy in the common bile duct. Endoscopy 2001;33:800–804

Matsumoto S, Ikeda S, Maeshiro K, et al. Management of giant common bile duct stones in high-risk patients using a combined transhepatic and endoscopic approach. Am J Surg 1997;173:115–116

Matsumoto S, Ikeda S, Tanaka M, et al. Nonoperative removal of giant common bile duct calculi. Am J Surg 1988;155:780–782

Nadler RB, Rubenstein JN, Kim SC, et al. Percutaneous hepatolithotomy: the Northwestern University experience. J Endourol 2002;16:293–297

Vos PM, van Beek EJR, Smits NJ, et al. Percutaneous balloon dilatation for benign hepaticojejunostomy strictures. Abdom Imaging 2000;25:134–138

Weickert U, Jakobs R, Hahne M, et al. Cholangioskopie nach erfolgreicher Therapie einer komplizierten Choledocholithiasis: ist steinfrei wirklich steinfrei? Dtsch Med Wochenschr 2003;128:481–484

CHAPTER 29 Transjejunal Biliary Intervention

Robert N. Gibson

Clinical Presentation

A 51-year-old woman was referred for surgical repair of a high bile duct injury sustained at the time of cholecystectomy. Hepatojejunostomy was performed with anastomosis to the confluence of the right and left hepatic ducts and surgical fixation of the efferent limb of the Roux-en-Y jejunal loop to the parietal peritoneum of the anterior abdominal wall. She was lost to follow-up but returned 2 years later with cholangitis and jaundice. On abdominal computed tomography (CT, not shown) the intrahepatic bile ducts were dilated. Percutaneous transjejunal cholangiography showed a stricture at the hepatojejunostomy effectively separating the right posterior and anterior hepatic ducts and the left hepatic duct (**Fig. 29-1**). Calculi were present above the strictures in the left and to a lesser extent in the right hepatic ducts.

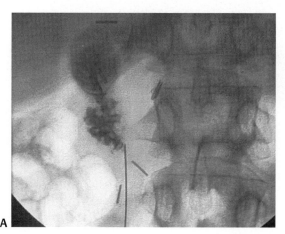
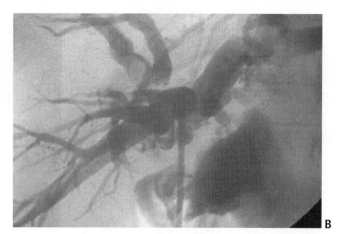

Figure 29-1 (**A**) The jejunal loop is punctured with a 22 gauge Chiba needle at site of surgical fixation, which is marked by clips. Contrast injected via the needle opacifies the jejunum. (**B**) A catheter has been used to negotiate the jejunal loop and cross the biliary-enteric anastomosis. Strictures are seen affecting the right anterior and right posterior hepatic ducts and the left hepatic duct.

Diagnosis

Benign anastomotic biliary stricture

Treatment

Percutaneous transjejunal biliary stricture dilatation and stone removal were performed immediately following the transjejunal cholangiography. Transjejunal access was gained by puncturing the Roux-en-Y loop under fluoroscopy using the surgical marking clips for guidance. Small amounts of contrast were injected via a 22 gauge Chiba needle until the needle tip was positioned in the

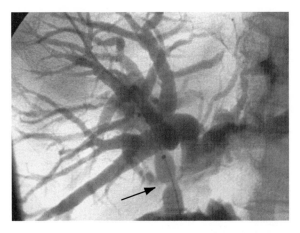

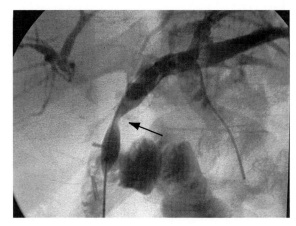

Figure 29-2 A waist is seen on the angioplasty balloon inflated across the right anterior hepatic duct stricture (arrow).

Figure 29-3 The left hepatic duct stricture (arrow) is dilated.

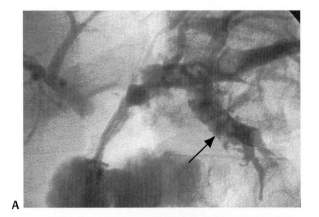

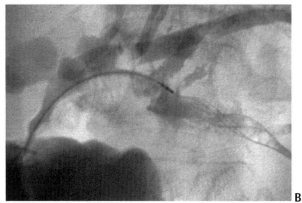

A

B

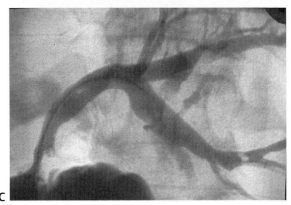

C

Figure 29-4 (**A**) Multiple calculi are present in the left hepatic duct, in particular, in segment 3 (arrow). (**B**) A stone retrieval basket has been advanced into the duct. The calculi were removed with the basket and saline flushing. (**C**) Left hepatic duct cholangiogram following stone removal.

lumen. A Neff introduction set was then used to insert a 0.035 in. J-shaped guide wire (Cook, Brisbane, Australia). A catheter with a very short distal bend and high torque (Gibson Biliary Manipulation Catheter, Cook, Brisbane, Australia) was then used with the guide wire to negotiate the bowel lumen. Once the anastomosis was reached, the J guide wire was replaced by an Amplatz wire (Cook, Brisbane, Australia), which was used to cross the anastomosis and strictures, controlling direction with the catheter. The strictures were dilated with a 6 mm angioplasty balloon catheter (Cook, Brisbane, Australia) (**Figs. 29-2** and **29-3**). The intrahepatic calculi were cleared with a biliary stone retrieval basket combined with flushing with normal saline through a catheter placed peripheral to the calculi (**Fig. 29-4**). A good cholangiographic result was achieved

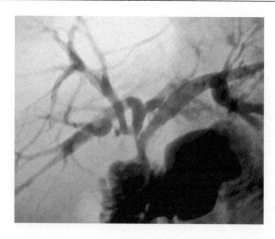

Figure 29-5 Follow-up transjejunal cholangiogram shows no residual stricture or calculi.

(**Fig. 29-5**) and the patient has been managed since with periodic transjejunal cholangiography and dilatation of the strictures and removal of accumulated calculi, with only occasional episodes of cholangitis.

Discussion

Bile duct injury, most often a result of cholecystectomy, is best managed by surgical repair. However, even with the best surgical care, there is a moderately high incidence of stricture recurrence (20–30%), with some occurring years after the initial repair. Furthermore, any associated intrahepatic strictures or calculi are difficult to treat surgically.

Without adequate treatment, the clinical pattern of biliary strictures is that of recurrent episodes of cholangitis, secondary biliary fibrosis and cirrhosis, and portal hypertension. When surgical repair is either unsuccessful or not possible, one option is to treat the strictures by transhepatic dilatation, which often necessitates placement of indwelling catheters for longer periods. Nevertheless, recurrence of the strictures and/or calculi occurs in at least 30% of patients.

Percutaneous transjejunal intervention provides an attractive adjunct to surgery in managing this difficult group of patients and is most easily performed if there is deliberate surgical fixation of the jejunal anastomotic Roux-en-Y loop at the time of surgical repair, as in the patient described.

Transjejunal intervention offers several advantages over the transhepatic approach:

1. It allows access to all segments of the intrahepatic biliary tree from a single percutaneous puncture. Strictures involving both the right and left hepatic ducts cannot be readily dilated or stented via a single transhepatic approach. Similarly, calculi in multiple intrahepatic ducts and intrahepatic strictures require multiple accesses if a transhepatic approach is used. The latter is associated with increased patient discomfort and morbidity.
2. The transjejunal approach provides long-term access for cholangiography and repeat dilatations, and removal of calculi, without the need for multiple transhepatic catheterizations or long-term indwelling tubes, the latter having often been used in the past to maintain biliary access.
3. The transjejunal approach is exceptionally well tolerated and can be performed with a short hospitalization. The major and minor complication rates are very low (2% each), which compare very favorably with transhepatic procedures. Major complications have included venous hemorrhage from abdominal wall varices, detachment of the jejunal loop from the anterior abdominal wall, and superficial abscess at the puncture site. Episodes of clinical septicemia are rare compared with percutaneous transhepatic procedures. In the latter, communications between the intrahepatic bile ducts and vessels created by the transparenchymal tract predispose to septic complications.

The technical success rate for gaining percutaneous loop access is at least 95%. Distension of the jejunal loop by injection of saline or air is often helpful. Most loops can be negotiated, even in the presence of some tortuosity, by using a combination of a guide wire and torqueable catheter. In difficult cases, the insertion of a sheath of up to 12 to 14F can be helpful to reduce the tortuosity and provide a more stable access to the anastomosis. This can be very useful as a "working channel," especially for the removal of multiple intrahepatic calculi.

The important principles for surgical fixation are to have the loop as short and as straight as possible and to have the fixation site secure and well marked for fluoroscopically guided puncture. Our center prefers to fix the efferent limb to the parietal peritoneum in a right anterior location, approximately midway between the costal margin and the right iliac fossa. This fixation site allows the radiologist's hands to remain outside the primary x-ray beam and usually gives good access to both the right- and left-sided ducts. Occasionally, I make use of the afferent limb fixed in the epigastrium, which sometimes allows a more direct approach to inferior right hepatic ducts. Regardless of the site of fixation, the surgeon should attempt to make the access loop straight and short.

Some reports have described successful transjejunal access of a conventional, unfixed Roux-en-Y loop used for biliary-enteric anastomosis. This approach is generally more difficult than puncturing deliberately fixed loops and most centers secure the access loop at the time of surgery with some form of marking to allow subsequent access. Even if the jejunal loop has not been fixed and marked in this way at the time of the original biliary-enteric bypass, it is relatively simple to reoperate at a later date with the sole purpose of fixing the loop, which then becomes a permanent access loop.

If percutaneous puncture of an unfixed loop is performed, it is important to first obtain a CT with bowel opacification and, if necessary, a percutaneous transhepatic cholangiogram immediately prior to the loop puncture. This will allow identification of the segment of the jejunal loop, which is anteriorly placed and close to the biliary-enteric anastomosis, to provide a safe puncture as well as a short pathway to the anastomosis.

Although the main use of transjejunal intervention is in the treatment of benign biliary strictures and intrahepatic calculi, it can also be used to improve palliation in patients undergoing surgery for malignant hilar biliary strictures. Biliary stents can be deployed and brachytherapy can be delivered via a transjejunal approach. The major appeal of this technique is that it provides safe long-term percutaneous access to the entire biliary tree without the need for repeated transhepatic catheterization or long-term indwelling catheters.

PEARLS AND PITFALLS

- Benign biliary strictures are usually the result of injury at cholecystectomy. Following surgical repair or transhepatic dilatation, there is a significant rate of recurrence often associated with intrahepatic calculi.
- The percutaneous transjejunal approach allows long-term percutaneous access to the entire biliary tree for radiological treatment of benign strictures and intrahepatic duct calculi, management of malignant strictures by stent insertion, and delivery of brachytherapy.
- The procedure is performed preferably via a jejunal loop that has been securely attached to the anterior abdominal wall during surgery, and the fixation site is well marked for fluoroscopically guided puncture.
- This approach has a very low complication rate, is exceptionally well tolerated, and does not require long-term indwelling catheters.

Further Reading

Gibson RN. Transjejunal biliary intervention. Intervention 1999;3:35–41

Gibson RN, Adam A, Yeung E, et al. Percutaneous techniques in benign hilar and intrahepatic benign biliary strictures. Journal of Interventional Radiology 1988;3:125–130

Hutson DG, Russell E, Schiff E, et al. Balloon dilatation of biliary strictures through a choledochojejuno-cutaneous fistula. Ann Surg 1984;199:637–647

Krige JE, Beningfield SJ. Surgery and interventional radiology for benign bile duct strictures. HPB Surg 1993;7:94–97

Matthews JB, Blumgart LH. In: Blumgart LH, ed. Surgery of the Liver and Biliary Tract. 2nd ed. Edinburgh: Churchill Livingstone; 1994:865–894

McPherson SJ, Gibson RN, Collier NA, et al. Percutaneous transjejunal biliary intervention: 10-year experience with access via Roux-en-Y loops. Radiology 1998;206:665–672

Mueller PR, van Sonnenberg E, Ferrucci JT, et al. Biliary stricture dilatation: multicenter review of clinical management of 73 patients. Radiology 1986;160:17–22

Pitt HA, Miyamoto T, Parapatis SK, et al. Factors influencing outcome in patients with postoperative biliary stricture. Am J Surg 1982;144:14–21

Russell E, Yrizzary JM, Huber JS, et al. Percutaneous transjejunal biliary dilatation: alternate management for benign strictures. Radiology 1986;159:209–214

CHAPTER 30 Acute Cholecystitis

Saadoon Kadir

Clinical Presentation

A 78-year-old patient presented with a several-day history of right upper quadrant and epigastric pain. On examination, there was right upper quadrant tenderness and fever. Laboratory tests showed an elevated white blood count (WBC).

Radiological Studies

Ultrasound of the abdomen showed wall thickening and distension of the gallbladder with echogenic material in the lumen (**Fig. 30-1**).

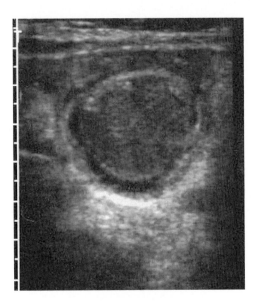

Figure 30-1 Sonogram shows thickened, edematous gallbladder wall, small pericholecystic fluid collection, and nonshadowing intraluminal echoes.

Diagnosis

Acute cholecystitis

Treatment Options

The treatment options were either percutaneous or surgical decompression of the gallbladder. Endoscopic placement of a drainage catheter is also possible via the cystic duct. However, this is rarely necessary because direct percutaneous and surgical methods for decompression are available and less cumbersome. In this setting, surgical mortality for a cholecystectomy is high, making percutaneous drainage the initial treatment of choice.

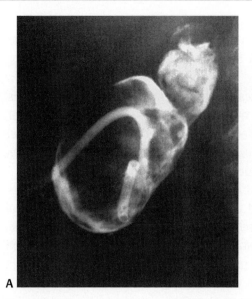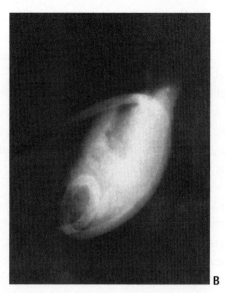

Figure 30-2 (**A**) Contrast injection through the drainage catheter shows an asymmetrical lumen contour due to an edematous gallbladder wall and intraluminal thrombus. (**B**) Cholecystogram after acute symptoms had subsided. There is normalization of the lumen contour.

Treatment

Ultrasound guidance was used to place a sheath needle into the gallbladder. Approximately 5 mL bile was aspirated and sent for Gram stain and culture. The aspirated bile was nonpurulent, thick, and hemorrhagic. Contrast (2–3 mL) was injected to opacify the gallbladder lumen. A guide wire (Rosen, Cook Incorp., Bloomington, IN) was inserted and carefully coiled in the gallbladder. The sheath needle was removed and an 8F pigtail drainage catheter was inserted. A small volume of contrast was then injected to assess catheter position and to look for contrast leakage or perforation (**Fig. 30-2**). The pain and fever subsided after gallbladder decompression. Antibiotics that had been started at the time of admission were continued for several days after the procedure.

Discussion

In acute cholecystitis, calculi may or may not be present in the gallbladder. Clinically, both forms (calculous and acalculous cholecystitis) are indistinguishable and their initial treatment is the same (i.e., decompression of the gallbladder). Although patients with acalculous cholecystitis may not necessitate a second procedure, those with calculous cholecystitis or manifested complications of the disease usually undergo cholecystectomy. In some patients, percutaneous decompression followed by percutaneous removal of calculi may also provide durable relief.

Although acute cholecystitis may occur in the otherwise healthy individual, it is most frequently seen in severely ill patients with serious comorbid conditions: patients in intensive care, respiratory failure, after major surgery or severe trauma, and burn victims. It may also occur in immunosupressed patients with acquired immunodeficiency syndrome (AIDS) and viral and fungal infection, those on parenteral nutrition, and in association with parasitic infestation. Acute cholecystitis is also seen in some patients with unexplained sepsis (Eggermont et al, 1985; Boland et al, 1994). It remains unclear whether the gallbladder is the source or is affected as a complication.

Patient age is usually over 30 years in acute *calculous* cholecystitis and the past history is often indicative of gallbladder disease (i.e., the person has experienced symptoms in the preceding weeks or months). Acute *acalculous* cholecystitis can occur in individuals of all ages, including young children (Roca et al, 1988).

Symptoms and signs may be nonspecific and are occasionally absent. Fever with leucocytosis, elevated bilirubin and liver enzymes, sepsis, right upper quadrant or epigastric pain, and a tender, palpable right upper quadrant mass may be present. The latter is due to a severely distended gallbladder and is seen in ~30 to 40% of patients. Similar symptomatology may occur in the absence of gallbladder disease, in pancreatitis, peptic ulcer, liver abscess, right-sided pyelonephritis, or gastroenteritis.

Bile cultures are positive in over 80% of patients, and frequently, there are multiple organisms. Gram-negative organisms are most common (~70%) and anaerobes are found in less than 10% of cases. The most commonly encountered organisms are *Escherichia coli,* enterococcus, and *Klebsiella.* Other cultured organisms include proteus, streptococcus, staphylococcus, *Pseudomonas, Candida,* and salmonella (Vauthey et al, 1993; Tseng et al, 2000). The presence of organisms in the bile may in itself be unreliable for the diagnosis of acute cholecystitis because bacteria have been found in bile samples in the absence of clinical biliary tract disease (Dye et al, 1978).

The aspirated bile may be of a normal consistency or thickened, purulent in empyema, blood tinged, or even grossly bloody depending upon severity of the disease. It is usually hemorrhagic in pregangrenous or gangrenous gallbladders, coagulopathy, trauma, or tumor and in patients on anticoagulation.

Complications of the disease include gallbladder empyema, focal or diffuse gallbladder wall necrosis (gangrene), and perforation. Gangrene of the gallbladder occurs in ~2% of patients with acute cholecystitis (Morfin et al, 1968). Gangrene predisposes to perforation and may be associated with sepsis. Gallbladder perforation is reported in ~3% of patients (Smith, 1981). In most cases, this leads to a localized pericholecystic or hepatic abscess. Less frequently, there is perforation with free spillage into the peritoneal cavity resulting in peritonitis. Occasionally, a cholecystoenteric fistula may develop. Though the incidence of complications generally increases with duration of symptoms, gallbladder perforation can also occur acutely, early in the disease (Warshauer et al, 1987).

Imaging

Sonography is the diagnostic imaging modality of choice for evaluation of patients suspected of having acute cholecystitis. Sonographic findings include distended gallbladder (transverse diameter >5 cm), thickened gallbladder wall (>3 mm), transducer-elicited focal tenderness over the gallbladder (positive sonographic Murphy's sign, which has >90% positive predictive value), gallbladder calculi, nonshadowing echoes (sludge, blood, pus, or gas), and pericholecystic fluid (Ralls et al, 1985). Gallbladder calculi are present in the majority of patients (>80%) and a significant number also have common duct calculi.

In *acalculous* cholecystitis, there is absence of calculi but sludge may be present in a distended gallbladder with thickened wall. Pericholecystic fluid, when present, may be indicative of gangrene (Harshfield et al, 1991). Other sonographic findings in gangrene are asymmetrical wall thickening, mural irregularity simulating masses, and intraluminal debris (Jeffery et al, 1983). Sloughed mucosa may be seen as a thin, echogenic, intraluminal membrane. Contrast cholecystography shows an irregular lumen with mural indentations secondary to edema or hemorrhage. Although no histological proof is available, the patient described probably had a pregangrenous gallbladder.

In the appropriate clinical setting, the presence of wall thickening, a positive sonographic Murphy's sign, and calculi allows the diagnosis of acute cholecystitis in ~94% of patients (Ralls et al, 1985). Sonography has several pitfalls: (1) the gallbladder wall thickening may also occur in other diseases as well as some normal gallbladders (Sanders, 1980); (2) calculi are found in individuals without gallbladder symptoms; (3) the patient's status (e.g., severely ill, comatose) may not elicit a response to pain stimuli (negative sonographic Murphy's sign); and (4) the sonographic Murphy's sign is frequently absent in gallbladder gangrene (Simeone et al, 1989).

Etiology

Several factors have been implicated in the etiology:

Cystic duct obstruction by a calculus leading to gallbladder distention and bacterial invasion of the wall

Infection (hematogenous or regional lymphatic spread)

Ischemia. This may play a major role in acalculous cholecystitis. Further, hypoperfusion secondary to one or more factors such as visceral atherosclerosis, low cardiac output, and cardiopulmonary bypass have been implicated.

Chemical inflammation secondary to reflux of pancreatic secretions

Rare causes are due to volvulus of the gallbladder, polyarteritis nodosa (LiVolsi and Perzin, 1973), sclerosing cholangitis, and embolic cystic artery occlusion.

Emphysematous Cholecystitis

Emphysematous cholecystitis is an uncommon manifestation of acute cholecystitis. It is characterized by the presence of gas in one or more of the following: gallbladder wall, lumen, biliary radicles, and pericholecystic spaces (**Fig. 30-3**). It occurs more commonly in men (76%), in association with acalculous cholecystitis, and ~35% of the patients are diabetics (Keller et al, 1971). Bile cultures are positive in the majority of patients, with frequent occurrence of *Clostridium welchii*. There is a higher incidence of gallbladder perforation and associated mortality than in other forms of acute cholecystitis. Ischemia and necrosis of the gallbladder with secondary invasion by gas-forming bacteria are believed to be responsible.

Treatment

The initial treatment of acute cholecystitis is decompression of the gallbladder. This is accomplished by one of two methods: (1) placement of a drainage catheter or (2) simple aspiration of the gallbladder via an 18 gauge needle, without drainage catheter insertion. The latter is an attractive method for

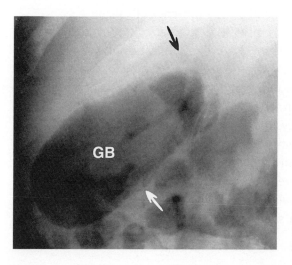

Figure 30-3 Emphysematous cholecystitis. Radiograph of the abdomen from a different patient shows gas in the gallbladder lumen (GB) and wall (arrows).

diagnosing and treating patients suspected of having acalculous cholecystitis. Relief of symptoms following gallbladder aspiration not only establishes the diagnosis but also provides the treatment. Thus several patients with acalculous cholecystitis may be satisfactorily treated by simple gallbladder aspiration and not require cholecystostomy or cholecystectomy (Chopra et al, 2001). Patients with gallbladder calculi usually undergo elective cholecystectomy, although there are reports suggesting that the drainage catheter may be removed while leaving the calculi in situ because these were not symptomatic prior to onset of the acute cholecystitis. Patients with empyema or those developing complications (gangrene, perforation, peritonitis, emphysematous cholecystitis) require cholecystectomy.

The gallbladder may be drained through a transhepatic or direct transperitoneal approach. In acute cholecystitis, the distended gallbladder often extends below the liver margin, making it available for direct puncture. Either the Seldinger technique or a one-step trocar technique is used. A 22 gauge needle may also be used to opacify the gallbladder for subsequent insertion of a preloaded catheter.

The advantages of a transhepatic approach include (1) a lower risk of accidental colon or duodenal puncture, (2) a lower risk of accidental loss of access as the gallbladder is decompressed, (3) a lower risk of bile spillage into the peritoneal cavity, and (4) the possibility for mechanical tract occlusion at the time of catheter removal, if the tract is immature.

The section of liver that is traversed is usually peripheral and without significant-diameter vasculature. Theoretical considerations of the risk of hepatic parenchymal injury with bleeding have not materialized in my experience even with the use of large-caliber sheaths.

I use ultrasound to guide the initial access with fluoroscopy for subsequent maneuvers. A drainage catheter can also be inserted at the bedside using only ultrasound guidance. This may be the preferred method for patients deemed too sick to be moved. I use a direct transperitoneal approach whenever the gallbladder is readily accessible. In most cases, I prefer the transhepatic approach and the Seldinger technique for catheter placement.

After access is obtained with an 18 gauge needle, ~5 mL bile is removed to partially decompress the gallbladder and provide a sample for Gram stain and culture. Contrast (2–3 mL) is slowly injected to opacify the lumen, determine needle tip position, and detect bile leakage or perforation. This practice also provides a target for repeat needle puncture, should there be accidental loss of access. An 8 or 10F pigtail-shaped drainage catheter (e.g., nephrostomy) is inserted over a stiff-shaft J guide wire. After the catheter has been secured, the gallbladder is partially emptied or, preferably, the catheter is left to drain via gravity. Rapid evacuation of the gallbladder is avoided because it may trigger a vasovagal reaction.

A cholecystogram may be obtained upon completion of the procedure but is usually omitted because the gallbladder wall may be necrotic and friable and predisposed to rupture. Instead, a cholecystogram is obtained a few days later, after the acute symptoms have subsided. This is used to assess patency of the cystic and common bile ducts and for the presence of calculi.

Following percutaneous decompression, there is usually a dramatic improvement in the symptoms in up to 90% of cases (Hultmann et al, 1996). Failure of clinical improvement within 24 to 48 hours is indicative of some other etiology or signals the presence of complications. The latter are associated with an increased mortality. Gangrene of the gallbladder should be suspected if there is persistence of symptoms following decompression (Lo et al, 1995).

In patients with uncomplicated acalculous cholecystitis, a second procedure (i.e., cholecystectomy) may not be necessary. Therefore, the catheter is removed after cholangiographic determination of the absence of calculi or other outflow obstruction (e.g., stricture, tumor). Follow-up studies in patients treated by catheter cholecystostomy indicate a low incidence of recurrent symptoms after catheter removal (Hamy et al, 1997). In calculous cholecystitis, the catheter usually remains in place because most patients undergo cholecystectomy. In some, the calculi can be retrieved through the percutaneous access (see Chapter 31).

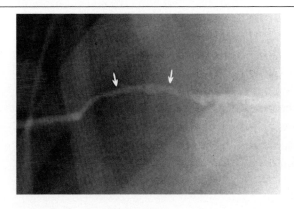

Figure 30-4 Assessment of transhepatic tract maturity. Sinogram shows a mature tract without extravasation of contrast into the surrounding tissues (arrows).

Catheter Removal

The drainage catheter should be removed only after the tract has matured. The transhepatic tract usually matures in 2 to 3 weeks and after 3 or more weeks if a transperitoneal access was used (Hatjidakis et al, 1998). Thus the drainage catheter can be removed safely after ~3 or more weeks, provided there is no outflow obstruction. However, in some individuals, tract maturation make take longer depending upon several factors such as impaired healing secondary to malnutrition, steroids, infection, diabetes, coagulopathy, ascites, and others. Catheter removal in the presence of an immature tract may be associated with pain, fever, peritonitis, and sepsis (D'Agostino et al, 1991; Picus et al, 1992). Therefore, if such conditions exist or there is concern about tract maturity for any reason, a sinogram should be obtained prior to catheter removal.

To accomplish this, the drainage catheter is removed over a guide wire and a 15 cm long vascular sheath with side arm is inserted. The guide wire is left in place and contrast is injected through the side arm while the sheath is withdrawn. An image is obtained or the last image hold on the monitor is stored and used to assess the tract. In mature tracts, there is a continuous column of contrast from the gallbladder to the skin (**Fig. 30-4**). In immature tracts, there is peritoneal, pericholecystic, subcapsular, or hepatic parenchymal extravasation of contrast. The guide wire then permits the reinsertion of a drainage catheter.

Management of the Immature Tract

The presence of an immature tract requires reinsertion of a drainage catheter to avoid complications (pain, fever, peritonitis, sepsis). The immature tract can be managed in the following fashion:

1. A drainage catheter can be left in place for an additional period of time and tract maturity is reassessed prior to removal.
2. If the transperitoneal approach was used initially, a second transhepatic catheter is inserted and the original transperitoneal catheter is removed. Tract maturity for the new access is evaluated after 2 to 3 weeks. If the tract is mature, the catheter is removed or if the tract has not matured, it is occluded by embolization.
3. The transhepatic tract is embolized.
4. A Foley-type catheter is inserted through a peel-away sheath and left in place for ~2 to 3 weeks. This is used for transperitoneal catheter placements. Latex induces a stronger tissue reaction, which may contribute to tract maturation. This option cannot be used in patients with a latex allergy.

Technique for Tract Embolization

The technique for embolization of the transhepatic tract is identical to that used for embolization of the postbiopsy or transhepatic portal vein access tracts. Either coils or Gelfoam (or both) are used.

Coils (3 or 4 mm diameter, Cook Incorp., Bloomington, IN) are deployed close to the gallbladder through a short angiographic catheter or vascular sheath obturator. Gelfoam is cut into 4 × 5 mm plugs. These are inserted through a vascular sheath with a detachable hub. The Gelfoam is pushed to the desired location with the vascular sheath obturator. Frequently, I will place a second coil or Gelfoam plug in the hepatic parenchyma ~15–20 mm from the hepatic capsule.

Complications

Procedure-related complications vary with the severity of the disease (and comorbid conditions) and choice of access (transhepatic or transperitoneal). Overall, minor complications (leakage of small amounts of bile, hemorrhage, or catheter dislodgment) are reported in up to 26%. Bile leakage may occur during catheter placement using the Seldinger technique. This is minimized by aspiration of some bile after needle placement. Serious complications such as gallbladder perforation (usually in gangrenous gallbladders), colonic and duodenal puncture, vasovagal reactions, and death are uncommon.

PEARLS AND PITFALLS_____

- The diagnosis of acute cholecystitis may be difficult despite laboratory tests and imaging studies. In the appropriate setting, there must be a high index of suspicion.
- When clinical suspicion is high and test results are equivocal, needle aspiration of the gallbladder or trial placement of a cholecystostomy may provide both the diagnosis and the therapy.
- Relief of acute symptoms can be expected in up to 90% treated by aspiration or cholecystostomy.
- Persistence of symptoms following decompression is indicative of either a different etiology or signals onset of complications (i.e., gallbladder gangrene).

Further Reading

Boland GW, Lee MJ, Leung J, et al. Percutaneous cholecystostomy in critically ill patients: early response and final outcome in 82 patients. AJR Am J Roentgenol 1994;163:339–342

Chopra S, Dodd GD III, Mumbower AL, et al. Treatment of acute cholecystitis in non–critically ill patients at high surgical risk: comparison of clinical outcomes after gallbladder aspiration and after percutaneous cholecystostomy. AJR Am J Roentgenol 2001;176:1025–1031

D'Agostino HB, van Sonnenberg E, Sanchez RB, et al. Imaging of the percutaneous cholecystostomy tract: observations and utility. Radiology 1991;181:675–678

Dye M, MacDonald A, Smith G. The bacterial flora of the biliary tract and liver in man. Br J Surg 1978;65:285–287

Eggermont AM, Lameris JS, Jeekel J. Ultrasound guided percutaneous transhepatic cholecystostomy for acute acalculous cholecystitis. Arch Surg 1985;120:1354–1356

Hamy A, Visset J, Likholatnikov D, et al. Percutaneous cholecystostomy for acute cholecystitis in critically ill patients. Surgery 1997;121:398–401

Harshfield DL, McGahan J, Teefey S, et al. Pericholecystic fluid collections in acute cholecystitis: diagnostic and therapeutic implications. JVIR 1991;2:31

Hatjidakis AA, Karampekios S, Prassopoulus P, et al. Maturation of the tract after percutaneous cholecystostomy with regard to the access route. Cardiovasc Intervent Radiol 1998;20:36–40

Hultman CS, Herbst CA, McCall JM, et al. The efficacy of percutaneous cholecystostomy in critically ill patients. Am Surg 1996;62:263–269

Jeffrey RB, Laing FC, Wong W, et al. Gangrenous cholecystitis: diagnosis by ultrasound. Radiology 1983;148:219–221

Keller HL, Ferstl M, Rupp N. Roentgenologic and general aspects of emphysematous cholecystitis [in German]. Fortschr Geb Rontgenstr Nuklearmed 1971;115:475–482

LiVolsi VA, Perzin. Polyarteritis nodosa of the gallbladder presenting as acute cholecystitis. Gastroenterology 1973;65:115–123

Lo LD, Vogelsang RL, Braun MA, et al. Percutaneous cholecystostomy for the diagnosis and treatment of acute calculous and acalculous cholecystitis. J Vasc Interv Radiol 1995;6:629–634

Morfin E, Ponka JL, Brush BE. Gangrenous cholecystitis. Arch Surg 1968;96:567–573

Picus D, Hicks ME, Darcy MD, et al. Percutaneous cholecystolithotomy: analysis of results and complications in 58 consecutive patients. Radiology 1992;183:779–784

Ralls PW, Colletti PM, Lapin SA, et al. Realtime sonography in suspected acute cholecystitis: prospective evaluation of primary and secondary signs. Radiology 1985;155:767–771

Roca M, Sellier N, Mensire A, et al. Acute acalculous cholecystitis in salmonella infection. Pediatr Radiol 1988;18:421–423

Sanders RC. The significance of sonographic gallbladder wall thickening. J Clin Ultrasound 1980;8:143–146

Simeone JF, Brink JA, Mueller PR, et al. The sonographic diagnosis of acute gangrenous cholecystitis: importance of Murphy's sign. AJR Am J Roentgenol 1989;152:289–290

Smith EB. Perforation of the gallbladder: a clinical study. J Natl Med Assoc 1981;73:333–335

Tseng LJ, Tsai CC, Mo LR, et al. Palliative percutaneous transhepatic gallbladder drainage of gallbladder empyema before laparoscopic cholecystectomy. Hepatogastroenterology 2000;47:932–936

Vauthey JN, Lerut J, Martini M, et al. Indications and limitations of percutaneous cholecystostomy for acute cholecystitis. Surg Gynecol Obstet 1993;176:49–54

Warshauer D, Scott G, Gottschalk A. Focal acute acalculous cholecystitis. AJR Am J Roentgenol 1987;149:505–506

CHAPTER 31 Cholecystolithiasis

Saadoon Kadir

Clinical Presentation

A 77-year-old patient with multiple cardiovascular problems was evaluated for colicky right upper quadrant pain. On physical examination, there was right subcostal and epigastric tenderness. The gallbladder was not palpable. Laboratory tests were unrevealing.

Radiological Studies

Abdominal ultrasound (not shown) and computed tomography (CT) demonstrated multiple gallbladder calculi (**Fig. 31-1**).

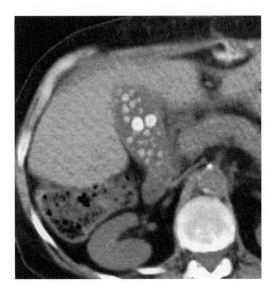

Figure 31-1 Image from an abdominal computed tomographic scan shows multiple gallbladder calculi, many of which are densely calcified. A narrow liver segment is interposed between the gallbladder and anterior abdominal wall.

Diagnosis

Cholecystolithiasis with biliary colic

Treatment Options

The treatment options were surgical cholecystostomy or cholecystectomy or percutaneous cholecystostomy and subsequent removal of calculi. Endoscopic catheterization of the gallbladder via the cystic duct may provide temporary drainage but does not address the calculi. The percutaneous method was chosen because of the high operative risk associated with the multiple comorbid conditions.

Treatment

The presence of multiple calcified calculi provided a target for CT-guided gallbladder catheterization. An 18 gauge sheath needle was inserted into the gallbladder via a transhepatic approach. A 1.5 mm J stiff-shaft guide wire (Cook, Bloomington, IN) was inserted, the tract was dilated with vascular

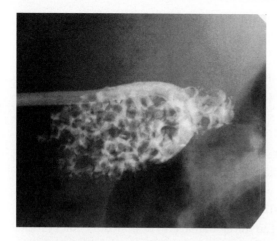

Figure 31-2 Contrast injection after drainage catheter insertion reveals numerous calculi.

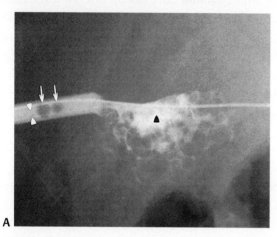

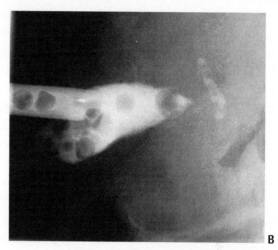

Figure 31-3 (**A**) An Amplatz sheath is in place and a reaccess (safety) guide wire has been inserted. Smaller calculi (arrows) are flushed out by irrigating the gallbladder with an 8F red rubber catheter (arrowheads). (**B**) Larger calculi are retrieved with a basket.

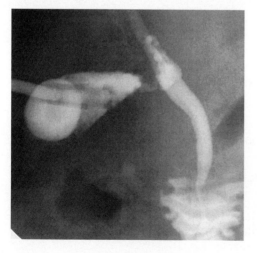

Figure 31-4 Post procedure cholecystogram through a Foley balloon catheter opacifies normal-appearing cystic and common bile ducts. Residual contrast defects seen on the gallbladder wall are a common finding on post-procedure cholecystograms and are probably due to edema. These resolve spontaneously within a few days.

dilators, and a 14F self-retaining pigtail nephrostomy catheter was inserted and left to gravity drainage (**Fig. 31-2**). Ten days later, the patient was brought back for retrieval of the calculi.

The tract was dilated with fascial dilators and an 18F sheath (trimmed to 15 cm length) was inserted (Amplatz, Cook Incorp., Bloomington, IN). The calculi were retrieved using several techniques. Smaller calculi were easily suctioned or flushed out of the gallbladder (**Fig. 31-3A**). Larger calculi were retrieved with stone retrieval baskets (Wittich nitinol basket, Cook eight-wire basket) (**Fig. 31-3B**). At the termination of the session, an 18F Foley catheter was inserted and left to external drainage. After ~24 hours, the catheter was clamped. A cholecystogram was obtained 3 days later and demonstrated unhindered flow and no residual calculi (**Fig. 31-4**). The catheter was removed.

Discussion

Percutaneous cholecystolithotomy (gallbladder calculus removal) should be offered as a primary treatment option for individuals with cholecystolithiasis and significant comorbid conditions. It should also be the primary approach in patients with common duct calculi and indwelling cholecystostomy tubes or surgically inserted transcystic duct catheters. Percutaneous diagnostic gallbladder aspiration and drainage play a major role in the initial management of acute cholecystitis. However, patients with an indwelling cholecystostomy and common duct calculi are often referred for endoscopic intervention. The endoscopic procedure is performed under conscious sedation and requires a sphincterotomy. The latter has been associated with significant complications, including pancreatitis in 6.4% and hemorrhage in 1.7% of patients (Rabenstein et al, 2002). Both can be severe and hemorrhage may necessitate arteriography and embolization (Saeed et al, 1989). Other complications of endoscopic sphincterotomy include ductal injury and development of a stricture, basket entrapment, perforation, and abscess formation (Sugiyama and Atomi, 2002). As the procedure is transoral, bacteria are introduced into the bile ducts.

The advantage of the percutaneous approach to the gallbladder is that the procedure is applicable to a wide range of patients, including those with severe comorbid conditions that preclude surgery and general anesthesia. In the absence of acute cholecystitis, it can be performed as a single-stage procedure, similar to percutaneous nephrolithotomy or more commonly in two stages: cholecystostomy and removal of calculi 10 to 14 days later, after formation of a soft tissue tract. In the short term, percutaneous cholecystolithotomy provides relief of symptoms without surgery. The major disadvantage is that the gallbladder, which is invariably diseased, remains in situ. There is a high incidence of recurrent symptoms and the potential risk of overlooking or the subsequent development of a gallbladder carcinoma (So et al, 1990).

Indications

- Any patient with an indwelling cholecystostomy catheter with gallbladder and/or common duct calculi or a surgically placed transcystic duct catheter and common duct calculi should be offered percutaneous calculus extraction.
- Patients with cholelithiasis and multiple medical problems, high risk, or contraindications for surgery or general anesthesia

Contraindications

- Absence of a safe access route to the gallbladder for the percutaneous cholecystostomy
- Contracted, thick-walled gallbladder
- Abnormal clotting parameters (prolonged international normalized ratio [INR], prothrombin time, activated partial thromboplastin time, or platelet count <60,000). The procedure can be undertaken after correction of the coagulopathy. Heparin and Coumadin must be discontinued.

- Ascites, because a large amount of intraperitoneal fluid displaces the liver margin away from the anterior abdominal wall. This results in an increased length of catheter that is extraparenchymal (i.e., unsupported) and is predisposed to dislodgment as a result of respiratory motion and patient ambulation
- A malignancy in the anticipated path of the catheter, because the tissue may be necrotic, friable, and prone to excessive bleeding and is also less likely to provide adequate substance to assure catheter positioning and retention

Patient Preparation

A broad spectrum cephalosporin is given intravenously ~1 hour before cholecystostomy placement. In the emergency setting, the dose is administered immediately before the procedure. If given for prophylaxis, the antibiotic is continued for 1 to 2 days after the procedure.

Biliary calculus extraction procedures can be painful so sufficient analgesia and sedation are administered before and during the procedure. Fentanyl or Demerol is used together with either Versed or Valium to provide patient comfort. In addition, liberal use of local anesthesia and, if applicable, an intercostal nerve block may be of additional benefit. As with all interventional procedures, a large-bore intravenous line is inserted for giving fluids and medication and vitals are monitored together with electrocardiogram (EKG) and pulse oximetry.

For the cholecystostomy, imaging methods for guidance are ultrasound and CT. Ultrasound can be performed in the interventional suite, obviating the need to move the patient. The entire procedure could also be completed using CT-fluoroscopy.

The percutaneous approach to the gallbladder may be direct transperitoneal (if a free surface is available without interposition of bowel, liver, or rib) or transhepatic. In ~17% of individuals, only a transperitoneal approach is possible because there is no liver parenchyma between the gallbladder and the anterior abdominal wall (Warren et al, 1988). Maturation of the transperitoneal tract requires longer than the transhepatic tract, which may delay calculi retrieval or catheter removal or both. Once it is decompressed, the gallbladder may retract away from the surface, causing bile leakage and loss of access. The transhepatic approach decreases the risk of catheter dislodgment and loss of access during catheter insertion or after gallbladder decompression. Bile leakage, if any, is tamponaded by the liver. There are usually no large blood vessels in the liver periphery, and the risk of major bleeding is low even if the tract is dilated to 18F or larger. Furthermore, the potentially fatal complication of traversing the colon is eliminated.

In the acutely sick patient (e.g., acute cholecystitis), the gallbladder should only be drained (percutaneous cholecystostomy) and no manipulations performed until there is stabilization. A significant number of these patients have calculous cholecystitis. Frequently, the calculi are detected on a subsequent cholecystogram because an initial cholecystogram may have been omitted or the calculi were obscured by the presence of thick bile, blood clots, and sludge in the gallbladder. If calculi are detected in the gallbladder or common duct, these can be removed electively. Depending upon the patient's clinical status, the retrieval of calculi can also be performed as an outpatient procedure.

There are usually two stages to the procedure: (1) placement of a cholecystostomy and (2) retrieval of calculi. In most patients, tract maturation can be expected in 2 to 3 weeks and the catheter can be removed without any problem. (For track maturity assessment, see Post-Procedure Care and Chapter 30.)

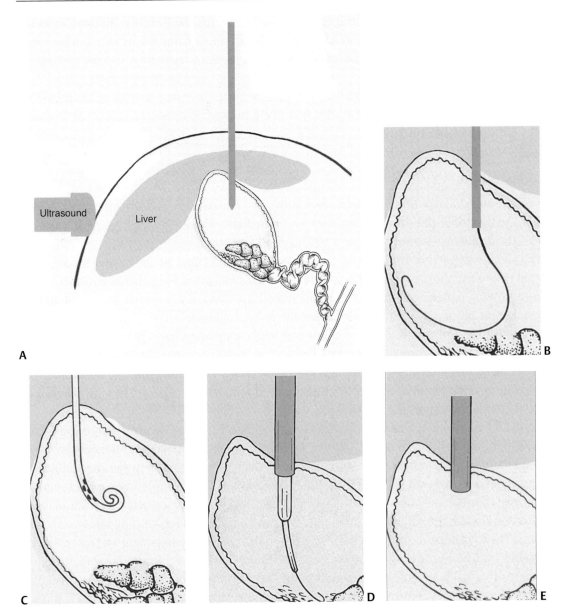

Figure 31-5 Drawings illustrating the techniques for ultrasound-guided percutaneous cholecystostomy and sheath insertion for calculus retrieval. (**A**) With the patient in a supine, ~15 degree right anterior oblique position, the gallbladder is entered from a transhepatic approach with an 18 gauge needle. (**B**) A guide wire is inserted, followed by (**C**) the placement of a pigtail-type drainage catheter, after dilatation of the tract. (**D**) In preparation for calculus retrieval, the drainage catheter is removed over a guide wire and (**E**) a large-diameter sheath (shortened to 15 cm) is inserted over a fascial dilator with coaxially inserted Teflon catheter.

Percutaneous Cholecystostomy (Figs. 31-5A-C)

The patient is placed in the supine or a slight right anterior oblique position. The gallbladder is localized by ultrasound (or CT) and a perpendicular transhepatic (or transperitoneal) path is chosen for catheter placement. An 18 gauge sheath needle is passed into the gallbladder via a single (anterior) wall puncture. Following the aspiration of 2 to 3 mL bile, a similar volume of undiluted contrast is injected to opacify the lumen and confirm the needle tip position. A 0.038 in. J-shaped, stiff mandril guide wire (e.g., Rosen wire, Cook Incorp.) is inserted followed by the placement of a self-retaining nephrostomy catheter (8–14F). A preloaded trocar-catheter can also be used.

In elective procedures, I usually perform a limited cholangiogram to assess cystic duct patency. The catheter is placed to external (gravity) drainage. It is not flushed. An increase in the intracholecystic pressure during flushing may induce a colic or sepsis. Bile cultures from the initial gallbladder aspirate may be positive for organisms in 50% of cases (Picus et al, 1992). If the bile is clear, a cholangiogram is obtained the following day. If there is unobstructed flow, the catheter hub is capped for internal drainage. If the bile is blood tinged or clots are present in the drainage bag, external drainage is maintained for a longer period. The patient is then scheduled to return for retrieval of calculi after 2 to 3 weeks, as an outpatient procedure.

RETRIEVAL OF GALLBLADDER CALCULI (FIGS. 31-5D,E)

Antibiotic coverage is usually not necessary unless excessive manipulation and common duct cannulation are anticipated. A cholecystogram is obtained by gravity infusion or careful injection of diluted contrast (20–30% concentration). Diluted contrast medium allows for better visualization of calculi. The drainage catheter is removed over a guide wire and the tract is dilated with fascial dilators and a Teflon sheath (18–24F, Amplatz, Cook Incorp.) is inserted into the gallbladder. For small calculi, a 16 or 18F sheath may suffice.

Smaller calculi are simply lavaged or suctioned out of the gallbladder (See **Fig. 31-3**). For flushing out the calculi, an 8F red rubber catheter is inserted and the gallbladder is irrigated with saline or diluted contrast (to permit fluoroscopic observation). For suction removal, a 14 to 18F modified red rubber catheter is used. The catheter tip is cut perpendicular to the long axis proximal to the side holes. The proximal end is shortened to permit insertion of a cone-shaped adapter. A 50 mL syringe containing diluted contrast is attached to the adapter and the catheter is inserted into the gallbladder. The diluted contrast is injected to localize and move the calculi by partially distending the gallbladder. As suction is applied, the calculus is caught at the catheter tip and removed. The catheter tip may need to be directed toward a calculus with the help of a guide wire to provide more effective suction. Larger calculi are retrieved with forceps or baskets. Because biliary calculi are frequently soft, they may be crushed with the basket or forceps and the smaller fragments lavaged or suctioned. Occasionally, larger, hard calculi may necessitate adjunctive measures for size reduction prior to extraction (e.g., lithotripsy).

Calculi impacted in the gallbladder neck frequently dislodge spontaneously after the gallbladder is decompressed. Failure to dislodge can be managed as follows: the calculus is dislodged with either a multipurpose or hook-shaped catheter and J guide wire, by flushing with an end-hole catheter, a Fogarty embolectomy catheter, or a short angioplasty balloon.

COMMON DUCT CALCULI (FIGS. 31-6 AND 31-7)

A cholangiogram via the cholecystostomy catheter using continuous gravity infusion usually opacifies the common bile and frequently the intrahepatic ducts. Although individual anatomical peculiarities determine the degree of difficulty, both common hepatic and common bile duct calculi can usually be removed from this approach.

In a dilated system, a guide wire can be advanced into the common bile duct with little difficulty. The natural tortuosity of the cystic duct and valves of Heister may provide some difficulty in nondilated systems. The cystic duct is catheterized using a 4 to 5F straight, hydrophilic catheter and an angled hydrophilic guide wire (Terumo, Boston Scientific, Watertown, MA). This is successful in most cases. A multipurpose hockey-stick–shaped catheter can also be used without a guide wire. Diluted contrast is carefully injected to distend the cystic duct, and the catheter is torqued through it.

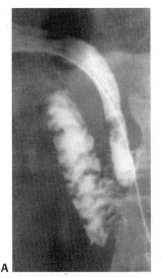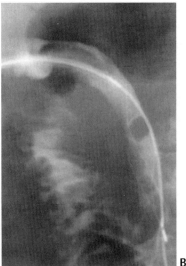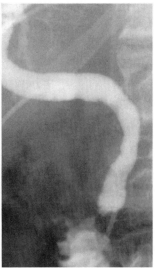

Figure 31-6 (A) Cholangiogram through the 8F sheath in the common duct shows the calculi. A safety wire has been advanced into the duodenum. The wire lies outside the working sheath. **(B)** The calculi have been engaged by the retrieval basket.

Figure 31-7 Cholangiogram after retrieval shows no residual calculi.

Alternatively, an 0.018 in. coronary wire is used. The coronary wire is back loaded into a 4F catheter. Once the catheter is in the common duct, a heavy-duty guide wire is inserted. The tract is dilated to 9F with vascular dilators and an 8F sheath is inserted with its tip well into the common bile duct. Contrast is injected to locate the calculi and a basket is inserted for retrieval. Some smaller calculi can be pushed into the duodenum with either an occlusion balloon or an angioplasty balloon catheter, using glucagon sphincter relaxation (0.5–1.0 mg IV glucagon) or after balloon sphincteroplasty.

Post-Procedure Care

Gallbladder calculi: Following the removal of gallbladder calculi, a 10 or 12F self-retaining catheter (e.g., nephrostomy, Foley, or Malecot) is inserted and left to external drainage. A cholecystogram is obtained 2 or 3 days later to look for residual calculi. If no residual calculi are found and there is free contrast flow through the cystic and common ducts, the catheter is removed. Assessment of tract maturity prior to catheter removal may be required in some hospitalized patients those on steroids or with medical conditions predisposing to poor wound healing, or when track maturity is in question for any reason. To evaluate the tract, a sinogram is obtained through a vascular sheath. (See Chapter 30 for assessment of tract maturity.)

Common duct calculi: Following the removal of common duct calculi, an 8 or 10F biliary drainage catheter is inserted with its tip in the duodenum. It is placed on external drainage for 2 to 3 days, at which time a cholangiogram is obtained. This evaluates patency of the ducts and successful removal of all calculi and fragments and clearing of intraluminal debris and blood clots. The biliary drainage catheter is then exchanged for a self-retaining nephrostomy catheter, which is inserted into the gallbladder and placed on internal drainage. After 24 hours, if there are no problems and the cholangiogram shows free contrast flow into the duodenum, the catheter is removed over a guide wire.

Outcome and Complications

Gallbladder and transcholecystic common duct calculi can be removed in over 90% of patients. Recurrent symptoms and cholecystolithiasis are observed in a significant number of patients (up to 40%) and may necessitate a repeat procedure or cholecystectomy (Courtois et al, 1996). Complications are uncommon in patients undergoing elective retrieval of calculi. Complications may be anticipated in severely ill patients with cholecystitis and comorbid conditions and may be severe in as many as 9% in this setting (Picus et al, 1992). Complications include vasovagal reaction, gallbladder perforation, cholangitis, loss of access, bile leakage, and peritonitis (Picus et al, 1992; Gillams et al, 1992).

Bile leakage after percutaneous cholecystostomy can usually be avoided if a transhepatic approach is used. This approach also avoids accidental colonic injury. Common bile duct injury is avoided by careful use of catheters and wires. Should ductal perforation or bile extravasation occur, external drainage is instituted to prevent bile peritonitis. Pancreatitis is a potential but rare complication of common duct calculus manipulation. This may occur as the result of an obstructing calculus or be related to excessive manipulation at the sphincter (post-instrumentation edema) or transampullary expulsion of large calculi.

PEARLS AND PITFALLS

- Increased use of preoperative retrograde endoscopic cholangiography, intraoperative cholangiography, and choledocoscopy has resulted in a significant reduction in the number of retained common duct calculi.
- Percutaneous transcholecystic retrieval of common duct calculi is an underutilized alternative to the more invasive surgical and endoscopic approaches in such patients.
- Percutaneous cholecystolithotomy can be performed as a semi-elective procedure where the general medical condition of the patient precludes operative intervention or where other methods have been unsuccessful.

Further Reading

Courtois CS, Picus DD, Hicks ME, et al. Percutaneous gallstone removal: long-term follow-up. J Vasc Interv Radiol 1996;7:229–234

Gillams A, Curtis SC, Donald J, et al. Technical considerations in 113 percutaneous cholecystolithotomies. Radiology 1992;183:163–166

Picus D, Hicks ME, Darcy MD, et al. Percutaneous cholecystolithotomy: analysis of results and complications in 58 consecutive patients. Radiology 1992;183:779–784

Rabenstein T, Roggenbuck S, Framke B, et al. Complications of endoscopic sphincterotomy: can heparin prevent acute pancreatitis after ERCP? Gastrointest Endosc 2002;55:476–483

Saeed M, Kadir S, Kaufman SL, et al. Bleeding following endoscopic sphincterotomy: angiographic management by transcatheter embolization. Gastrointest Endosc 1989;35:300–303

So CB, Gibney RG, Scudamore CH. Carcinoma of the gallbladder: a risk associated with gallbladder-preserving treatments for cholelithiasis. Radiology 1990;174:127–130

Sugiyama M, Atomi Y. Risk factors predictive of late complications after endoscopic sphincterotomy for bile duct stones: long-term (more than 10 years) follow-up study. Am J Gastroenterol 2002;97:2763–2767

Warren LP, Kadir S, Dunnick NR. Percutaneous cholecystostomy: anatomic considerations. Radiology 1988;168:615–616

CHAPTER 32 Pancreatic Abscess Drainage

Gerhard R. Wittich

Clinical Presentation

A 46-year-old man presented in the emergency department with an 8-hour history of severe epigastric pain accompanied by episodes of nausea and vomiting. His past history was remarkable for long-term abuse of alcohol and intravenous drugs. On examination, there was mide-pigastric tenderness with an otherwise soft abdomen. Laboratory values revealed an elevated white blood count (WBC 32,500) as well as significantly elevated levels of serum amylase and lipase. He was admitted to the intensive care unit (ICU).

Radiological Studies

Abdominal radiographs (not shown) showed no free intraperitoneal gas. Abdominal computed tomography (CT) was performed on the second hospitalization day. The scout image showed a colon cutoff sign (**Fig. 32-1A**) and the contrast-enhanced images showed extensive pancreatic necrosis (**Fig. 32-1B**).

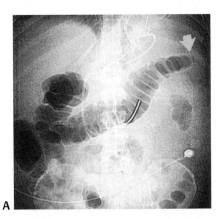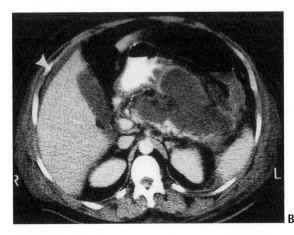

Figure 32-1 Coomputed tomographic scan of the abdomen obtained at the time of admission. (**A**) The scout image shows a colon cutoff sign (arrow). (**B**) Image from the contrast-enhanced scan shows replacement of most of the pancreatic parenchyma by a nonenhancing mass that extends into the lesser sac. This represents pancreatic necrosis with associated acute peripancreatic fluid collection. A small amount of ascites is also present (arrowhead).

Diagnosis

Severe acute pancreatitis

Treatment

Following the diagnostic CT study, the pancreatic fluid was aspirated under CT guidance. Gram stains revealed no bacteria and cultures were negative. The patient's early clinical course was complicated by the onset of pulmonary problems (acute respiratory distress syndrome and *Serratia* pneumonia) from

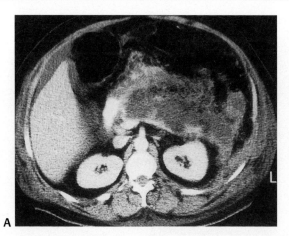
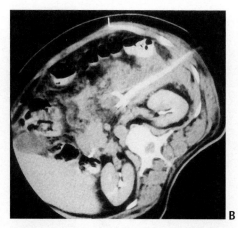

Figure 32-2 Computed tomography (CT) guided pancreatic abscess drainage. (**A**) Contrast-enhanced abdominal CT obtained 6 weeks after admission demonstrates a pancreatic abscess. CT-guided needle aspiration yielded pus and the cultures grew *Klebsiella pneumoniae*. (**B**) A 14F pigtail drainage catheter was placed into the abscess via the left anterior pararenal space.

Table 32-1 Hospital Course and Radiological Management

		Clinical Aspects	**Radiological Procedures**
First hospital admission	Day 1	ICU admission for acute pancreatitis	Abdominal radiographs: negative
	Day 2		CT shows necrotizing pancreatitis (**Fig. 32-1**) CT-guided needle aspiration: negative Gram stain and cultures
	Day 3	ARDS, *Serratia* pneumonia	
	Day 37	Temperature spike, increased WBC	CT-guided abscess drainage (**Fig. 32-2**) Culture grew *Klebsiella pneumoniae*
	Day 50		Additional CT-guided drain placed and catheter changed to 24F
	Day 69	Discharge	
Second hospital admission	Day 89	Readmitted with sepsis	Additional CT-guided abscess drainage
	Day 94	Condition improved	Sinogram shows colon fistula (**Fig. 32-3**)
	Day 96	Discharge	
Third hospital admission	Day 139	Readmitted with sepsis	Repeat CT-guided drainage
	Day 148	Discharge	Sinogram (**Fig. 32-4**)
Follow-up visit	Day 186		Final sinogram, all catheters removed

ARDS, acute respiratory distress syndrome; CT, computed tomography; ICU, intensive care unit; WBC, white blood cell.

which he slowly recovered. On hospitalization day 32, a temperature spike and elevated WBC prompted a repeat CT. A pancreatic abscess was drained under CT guidance (**Fig. 32-2**). A summary of the hospital course, subsequent hospitalizations, and radiological management is shown in **Table 32-1.**

Discussion

Pancreatic abscess is a late complications of acute pancreatitis usually developing >3–4 weeks after the acute episode. The most common etiology is alcoholic, followed by post-traumatic and gallstone pancreatitis. In addition to pus, the abscess usually contains variable amounts of debris from liquefaction

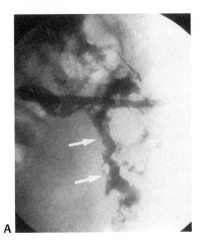
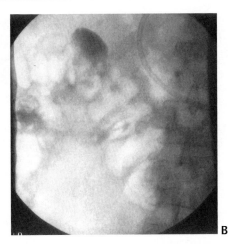

Figure 32-3 Sinogram obtained several days after the second hospital admission for recurrent sepsis. (**A**) An irregular abscess cavity is opacified, extending from the region of the pancreatic tail (catheter) into the left anterior pararenal space, posterior to the descending colon (arrows). (**B**) An image of the hepatic flexure shows contrast within the colon, indicating a pancreaticocolonic fistula.

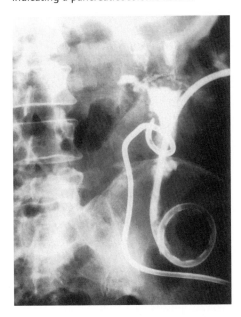

Figure 32-4 Sinogram obtained 7 weeks later shows a small residual cavity with no evidence for a bowel fistula. The initial drainage catheter in the region of the pancreatic body/tail has been removed.

necrosis of the pancreas and peripancreatic tissues. Clinically, it may be difficult to distinguish from a non-infected pseudocyst. Complications of pancreatic abscess include bleeding and fistulization, especially to the gastrointestinal tract. The overall mortality is lower than that for infected pancreas necrosis but can be as high as 20%.

The diagnosis is established by cross-sectional imaging, which demonstrates a fluid collection with or without air. Percutaneous CT-guided aspiration provides a sample for Gram stain and culture. The treatment is drainage. In most patients, percutaneous catheter drainage with antibiotic coverage provides adequate treatment. The method of choice for guiding drainage catheter placement is CT. Careful planning of the access route is important to avoid the colon. The reported success rate for percutaneous management is around 86%.

Other treatment options are surgery and endoscopic drainage. The latter, which has become available more recently, is a relatively invasive procedure that involves endoscopic ultrasound-guided creation of a transmural (transduodenal or transgastric) fistula and balloon dilatation of the created fistula, daily transendoscopic debridement, and lavage. Upon completion of the treatment, the fistula is sealed with tissue glue (cyanoacrylate).

PEARLS AND PITFALLS_____

- Pancreatic abscesses developing after necrotizing pancreatitis are usually more difficult to treat than a well-circumscribed abscess developing after surgery.
- With aggressive, labor intensive management and close clinical monitoring, an 86% cure rate can be expected.
- Percutaneous drainage may be considered as the initial therapy for pancreatic abscesses, with surgery reserved for failures of radiological treatment.

Further Reading

Benziane K. Computed tomography diagnosis of pancreatic abscess and its surgical drainage. J Chir (Paris) 1997;134:301–304

Haaga JR, Nakamoto D. Computed tomography-guided drainage of intra-abdominal infections. Curr Infect Dis Rep 2004;6:105–114

Memis A, Parildar M. Interventional radiological treatment in complications of pancreatitis. Eur J Radiol 2002;43:219–228

Seewald S, Groth S, Omar S, et al. Aggressive endoscopic therapy for pancreatic necrosis and pancreatic abscess: a new safe and effective treatment algorithm. Gastrointest Endosc 2005;62:92–100

van Sonnenberg E, Wittich GR, Goodacre BW, et al. Percutaneous abscess drainage: update. World J Surg 2001;25:362–369

CHAPTER 33 Debridement of Infected Pancreatic Necrosis
Ana Echenique

Clinical Presentation

A 25-year-old female presented to the emergency department with fever and midepigastric pain. Laboratory studies revealed an elevated white blood cell count and elevated alkaline phosphatase. She had a history of gallstones but denied any alcohol ingestion. She was admitted for evaluation and an abdominal computed tomography (CT) scan was obtained.

Radiological Studies

The abdominal CT demonstrated an enlarged pancreas. The anterior portion of the head and body of the pancreas did not enhance after contrast administration (**Fig. 33-1A**). In addition, the mesentery was edematous and fluid was noted along the paracolic gutters and in the retroperitoneum (**Fig. 33-1B**).

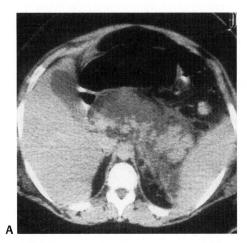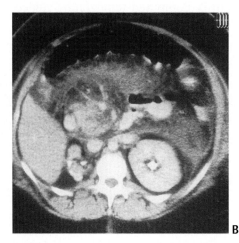

Figure 33-1 Contrast-enhanced abdominal computed tomography shows (**A**) contrast enhancement only of sections of the pancreatic head and body and (**B**) edema and hyperemia of the mesentery and fluid in paracolic gutters.

Diagnosis

Infected pancreatic necrosis

Treatment

A 16F self-retaining drainage catheter was placed into the liquefied pancreatic collection under CT guidance (**Fig. 33-2**). The drainage fluid was tan in color and the culture was positive for *Staphylococcus aureus*. Two days later, the patient was brought back for catheter-directed debridement.

Contrast injected through the drainage catheter revealed an amorphous collection with large contrast defects consistent with pancreatic debris (**Fig. 33-3**). The debris was extracted using a combination of suction debridement and wire basket techniques. Suction debridement was accomplished in the following manner: The existing 16F catheter was removed over a guide wire and a 16F peel-away introducer was inserted. Subsequently, a 14F catheter with enlarged side holes was

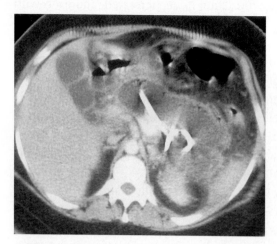

Figure 33-2 Computed tomographic image shows the drainage catheter in the pancreatic fluid collection.

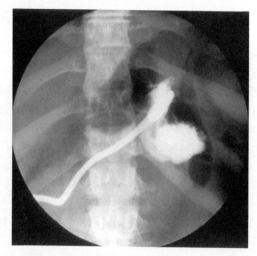

Figure 33-3 Fluoroscopic image obtained after contrast injection through the drainage catheter shows the cavity. The necrotic debris is seen as filling defects.

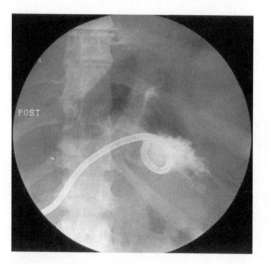

Figure 33-4 Fluoroscopic image shows a small, residual cavity with no debris.

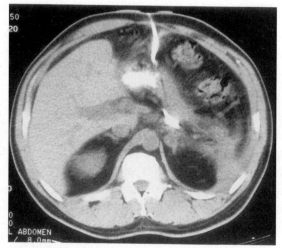

Figure 33-5 Computed tomographic image shows the catheter in the pancreatic bed. There is no residual fluid around the catheter tip.

inserted into the cavity via the introducer. Sixty mL of lavage solution (a mixture of contrast and saline) was rapidly injected into the cavity and suctioned out via the 14F catheter. When the catheter became occluded with debris, it was removed under suction leaving the introducer in place. Stone retrieval baskets were also utilized for debris removal. After a debridement session, a 16F drainage catheter was left in the cavity. The patient returned at 2- to 3-day intervals for a total of 17 sessions. At the final session, contrast injection showed a small, residual cavity with no debris (**Fig. 33-4**). A CT scan confirmed the absence of residual fluid collection and the catheter was removed (**Fig. 33-5**).

Discussion

Infected pancreatic necrosis is one of the most feared complications of acute pancreatitis because of its high morbidity and mortality. It occurs in only 5% of patients with acute pancreatitis but is responsible for 80% of all deaths due to pancreatitis. It is 100% fatal if left untreated, and even with aggressive surgical debridement, there is a high mortality (15–50%).

The standard treatment for infected necrosis is aggressive surgical debridement and open drainage. Recent surgical series have reported improved mortality rates (15%). However, these patients still experience significant morbidity including external pancreatic fistulas (46%), incisional hernias (32%), gastric outlet obstruction (17%), major venous hemorrhage (7%), and intestinal fistulas (7%).

Early attempts at percutaneous therapy for infected pancreas necrosis failed largely because of a lack of means to remove the necrotic tissue. Recent reports have demonstrated effective methods for removal of the necrotic debris, enabling effective management of these patients solely with percutaneous therapy. These results compare very favorably with those of surgical series. In one series of 20 patients with infected pancreatic necrosis who were in hemodynamically stable condition and were treated with catheter drainage and debris removal, there was no procedure-related mortality and very low morbidity. Three patients had self-limited intestinal fistulas and five demonstrated a communication to the pancreatic duct. In all of these patients, the fistulous connections closed spontaneously and no additional therapy was required. No other morbidities, such as seen in surgical series, were noted in these patients. The aggressive percutaneous therapy also resulted in a shorter intensive care unit stay as well as a reduction in the overall hospitalization time because several of the treatment sessions were conducted on an outpatient basis.

Complications

As with any percutaneous drainage of infected material, sepsis remains the predominant postdebridement complication. In fact, it is almost expected after active removal of debris, and therefore, intravenous antibiotic coverage is crucial as well as close patient monitoring during and in the immediate postprocedure period. Early treatment of hypotension and hypoxemia prevents serious consequences.

Often a communication is seen between the abscess cavities and intestinal tract. Drainage via the pancreatic duct into the duodenum is common and of no consequence. Colonic fistulas are not infrequent and may result from involvement of the colonic wall in the inflammatory process. These fistulae limit debridement efforts somewhat and sometimes prolong the duration of drainage.

Erosion into vascular structures (portal and splenic veins or splenic and duodenal arteries) is rarely seen. When this occurs the collection becomes filled with blood and a forceful injection will often opacify the involved vessel. Management is straightforward. The debridement session is terminated; a drainage catheter is reinserted into the collection and capped. This usually stops the bleeding (by tamponading) and the patient remains stable. Serial hematocrits are obtained to rule out continued blood loss. The catheter is again opened in 48 hours, at the next debridement session, and treatment continues. These patients are at a higher risk for sepsis because infected material often enters the vascular system.

PEARLS AND PITFALLS_____

- Infected pancreatic necrosis is uniformly fatal if left untreated and is associated with a high mortality rate of 15 to 50%, even with aggressive surgical debridement.
- Percutaneous catheter–directed debridement is a safe and effective treatment for patients with infected pancreatic necrosis and can be used as the primary means of treatment for the hemodynamically stable patient.
- Open surgical debridement, which carries a higher mortality and morbidity, can be reserved for patients who are hemodynamically unstable and require rapid, large-volume debridement.

Further Reading

Bradley EL III. A fifteen-year experience with open drainage for infected pancreatic necrosis. Surg Gynecol Obstet 1993;177:215–222

Bradley EL III, Allen K. A prospective longitudinal study of observation versus surgical intervention in the management of necrotizing pancreatitis. Am J Surg 1991;161:19–25

Echenique AM, Sleeman D, Yrizarry J, et al. Percutaneous catheter–directed debridement of infected pancreatic necrosis: results in 20 patients. J Vasc Interv Radiol 1998;9:565–571

Frey CF. Management of necrotizing pancreatitis. West J Med 1993;159:675–680

Shonnard KM, McCarter DL, Lyon RD. Percutaneous debridement of infected pancreatic necrosis with nitinol snares. J Vasc Interv Radiol 1997;8:279–282

CHAPTER 34 Pancreatic Biopsy

Khaled K. Toumeh and Kamran Ali

Clinical Presentation

A 65-year-old man was evaluated for abdominal pain. Dilatation of the common bile duct was demonstrated on abdominal computed tomography (CT). He underwent endoscopic retrograde cholangiopancreatography (ERCP), which demonstrated a narrowing of the distal common bile duct. No discrete mass was seen. A brush biopsy was obtained and was interpreted as being negative for malignancy. A common duct stent was placed to decompress the biliary tree. One week later, the patient underwent an inpatient CT-guided biopsy.

Radiological Studies

The three-phase CT of the abdomen showed dilatation of the common bile duct but no mass or liver metastasis was seen (**Fig. 34-1**).

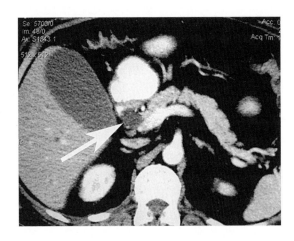

Figure 34-1 Contrast-enhanced computed tomographic scan of the abdomen shows dilatation of the common bile duct (arrow). No mass is seen in the head of the pancreas.

Differential Diagnosis

In the absence of a demonstrable mass, the differential diagnosis would include cholangiocarcinoma, pancreatic head carcinoma, and benign stricture due to chronic pancreatitis. A negative brushing cytology does not exclude a malignancy because it is positive only when the tumor has extended through the mucosa.

Diagnosis

Adenocarcinoma of the pancreas

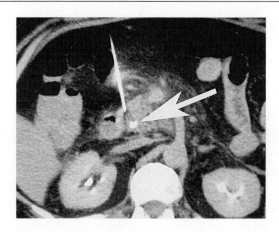

Figure 34-2 Computed tomographic image showing a 20 gauge quick core biopsy needle in the head of the pancreas. Arrow points to the endoscopically placed common duct stent.

Biopsy Procedure

The patient was placed on clear liquids after midnight before the day of the procedure. Prebiopsy coagulation parameters and complete blood count (CBC) were determined and were within normal limits. The procedure was performed under CT guidance, with conscious sedation provided through intravenous Versed and morphine sulfate.

The patient was placed in a supine position and the pancreas was scanned using a biopsy grid. The endoscopically placed common duct stent was to serve as a landmark for biopsy needle placement in the pancreatic head. The skin was prepped with povidone iodine and sterile draped. Lidocaine was injected and a 19 gauge introducer needle was advanced into the pancreatic head. Coaxial fine needle aspiration (FNA) samples were obtained with a 22 gauge, 20 cm length Chiba needle (Meditech, Gainesville, FL). The initial cytological assessment was suspicious for a malignancy. Therefore, two core biopsies were obtained using a quick core biopsy needle (Cook Incorp., Bloomington, IN) (**Fig. 34-2**). The final histology was positive for adenocarcinoma of the pancreas. Post-procedure, the patient was observed on the floor. There were no procedure-related complications.

Discussion

Pancreatic tumors cause nonspecific clinical symptoms such as abdominal pain, weight loss, and jaundice and may rarely manifest with a hypercoagulable state and diarrhea. These tumors are usually detectable by CT, ultrasound (US), or magnetic resonance imaging (MRI). According to Steinberg et al (1998), thin-slice CT with CT angiography (CTA) is probably the best diagnostic test for the evaluation of pancreatic masses. However, even with a negative CT, preoperative laparoscopy has detected metastatic lesions in up to 12% of cases. Most of these represent microimplants on the surface of the liver and peritoneum (Tillou et al, 1996).

Some authors believe that pancreatic biopsy should be performed only in surgically unresectable lesions to confirm the diagnosis, and resectable lesions should not undergo imaging-guided biopsy because in 10 to 20% of cases the biopsy may be falsely negative and there is the risk of malignant seeding of the tract as well as the risk of pancreatitis.

For imaging-guided biopsy, the choice of CT or US guidance is determined by the size and location of the mass, the patient's body habitus, and availability and expertise of the operator. Most gastroenterologists prefer endoscopic US-guided biopsy during the ERCP procedure. There are a few contraindications for pancreatic biopsy, especially when FNA is used. Percutaneous biopsy should not be performed in the presence of a coagulopathy and ascites.

For percutaneous biopsy, CT is preferred to US because it avoids unintended colon and vascular injury. Depending upon the location of the lesion, an anterior or posterior approach may be selected. The direct approach using the shortest distance to the lesion is the preferred method, provided that vascular structures and colon are avoided. Transgastric, transhepatic, and transjejunal approaches are acceptable alternative methods.

There are several types of needles available for FNA of the pancreas. The most commonly used sizes vary between 19 and 22 gauge. Karlson et al (1996) used 18 to 20 gauge core biopsy needles without any increase in the rate of complications. The presence of an experienced cytologist is invaluable for shortening the procedure time and reducing the rate of nondiagnostic samples.

We selected a coaxial system. After placement of a 19 gauge introducer needle, FNA can be performed for immediate cytological assessment. Subsequently, a 20 gauge quick core biopsy needle is used to obtain samples for histology. This type of needle provides a tissue core, which has a better diagnostic yield than the cytological samples obtained by the standard FNA techniques. We make one or two passes with the 22 gauge Chiba needle. The need for additional passes with the core biopsy needle is determined by the results of the immediate reading of the FNA sample.

Outcome and complications

The average sensitivity of image-guided FNA is between 80 and 90% and the specificity is over 90% (Centeno, 1998). A nondiagnostic or negative aspiration due to a sampling error occurs in 10 to 20% of cases and does not exclude the diagnosis of a malignancy. Karlson et al (1996) reported an 87% sensitivity for core biopsy of the pancreas.

Complications occur in 2 to 4% of cases. These include bleeding, infection, and acute pancreatitis. Fistula and pseudocyst formation are less common. The risk of acute pancreatitis and hemorrhage is increased with the use of large bore needles, multiple passes, and biopsy of normal pancreatic tissue.

PEARLS AND PITFALLS_____

- With the coaxial technique, if the FNA cytology is nondiagnostic or inconclusive, a core biopsy can be obtained.
- In the absence of a visible mass, an indwelling biliary stent, a guide wire, or cholangiogram can be used to identify the target for biopsy.
- Biopsy of normal pancreatic tissue increases the risk of acute pancreatitis.

Further Reading

Centeno BA. Fine needle aspiration of the pancreas. Clin Lab Med 1998;18:401–427

David O, Green L, Reddy V, et al. Pancreatic masses: a multi-institutional study of 364 fine-needle aspiration biopsy with histopathologic correlation. Diagn Cytopathol 1998;19:423–427

Dodd LG, Mooney EE, Layfield LJ, et al. Fine-needle aspiration of the liver and pancreas: a cytology primer for radiologists. Radiology 1997;203:1–9

Karlson BM, Forsman CA, Wilander E, et al. Efficiency of percutaneous core biopsy in pancreatic tumor diagnosis. Surgery 1996;120:75–79

Raut CP, Grau AM, Staerkel GA, et al. Diagnostic accuracy of endoscopic ultrasound-guided fine needle aspiration in patients with presumed pancreatic cancer. J Gastrointest Surg 2003;7:118–126

Steinberg WM, Barkin J, Bradley EL III, et al. Controversies in clinical pancreatology. Pancreas 1998;17:24–30

Tillou A, Schwartz MR, Jordan PH Jr. Percutaneous fine needle aspiration of the pancreas. World J Surg 1996;20:283–286

SECTION III
Pelvis

CHAPTER 35 Transgluteal Drainage

Walter M. Romano

Clinical Presentation

A 61-year-old man with T3,N0 rectal carcinoma underwent an uncomplicated low anterior resection with primary anastomosis. Five days after
surgery, he complained of pelvic discomfort. Examination revealed a
temperature of 38°C and the leukocyte count was 28,000. Platelets and
coagulation parameters were within normal limits. He was placed on
intravenous broad spectrum antibiotics.

Radiological Studies

Computed tomography (CT) of the abdomen and pelvis revealed a 4 cm soft mass lying anterior to
the sacrum at the level of the surgical anastomosis (**Fig. 35-1**). The mass showed slightly irregular
margins and there was soft tissue stranding in the adjacent fat.

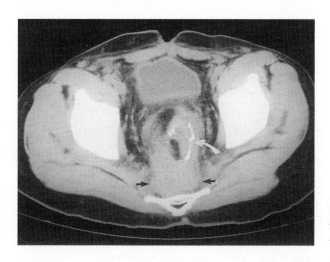

Figure 35-1 Computed tomographic scan of the pelvis demonstrates
the abscess (straight arrows) anterior to the lower sacrum at the level of
the anastomotic staple line (curved white arrow).

Diagnosis

Presacral abscess

Treatment Options

Transrectal drainage was not considered because of the recent surgery and risk of disrupting the
surgical anastomosis. A percutaneous, transabdominal route was prohibited because of overlying
bowel loops and the urinary bladder. Therefore, transgluteal drainage through the left sacrosciatic
foramen was undertaken.

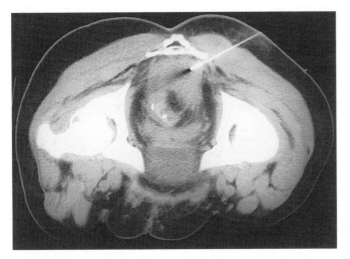

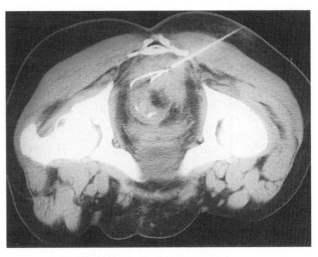

Figure 35-2 Computed tomographic scan of the pelvis with the patient prone. An 18 gauge needle has been advanced into the abscess cavity along a medial trajectory close to the sacrum.

Figure 35-3 A 0.035 in. Amplatz extra-stiff guide wire has been inserted through the needle and is coiled within the abscess cavity.

Treatment

The patient was placed on the CT table in a prone position and rescanned to delineate the relevant anatomy and determine the ideal angle, level, and approach for transgluteal drainage. The optimal entry point was determined and, using the scanner's laser positioning lines, this was marked on the skin with a felt-tipped pen. A radiopaque bead was placed on the mark and a scan obtained at this level to confirm the location of the skin puncture point.

Five milligrams of diazepam and morphine were administered intravenously. The skin was then cleaned with antiseptic solution and the area was sterile draped. Local anesthetic was injected along the intended tract. At the level of the sacrospinous ligament, along a posterolateral course adjacent to the sacrum, an 18 gauge needle was advanced into the collection (**Fig. 35-2**). Purulent fluid was aspirated, a 0.035 in. Amplatz extra-stiff guide wire (Cook Canada, Stouffville, ON) was advanced through the needle and coiled within the abscess cavity (**Fig. 35-3**). The tract was dilated using sequential fascial dilators and a 10F self-retaining drainage catheter (Flexima APDL, Medi-tech, Boston Scientific, Watertown, MA) was inserted over the guide wire (**Fig. 35-4**). The cavity was completely aspirated and then flushed several times with normal saline until the return was nonpurulent. The catheter was left to bag drainage and the patient sent to the ward with instructions to flush the catheter with 20 mL of saline every 6 hours.

Within 24 hours, the patient's fever dropped and leukocyte count returned to normal. Following catheter insertion, the patient experienced moderate pain relating to the tube tract and required parenteral morphine for the first 12 hours. The pain diminished over the course of the next day and was well controlled with oral analgesics thereafter. Over the next 5 days, drainage diminished to 5 mL per 24 hours and the drainage catheter was removed.

Discussion

Deep pelvic abscesses are a well recognized complication of abdominal and pelvic surgery. They are also seen in association with appendicitis, diverticulitis, and Crohn's disease. The efficacy of radiologically guided percutaneous drainage is well known, and it has become the preferred treatment (over open surgical drainage) for most of these collections.

The choice of an appropriate access route is important to optimize drainage and minimize procedural morbidity. In general, the shortest route devoid of solid organs, neurovascular structures,

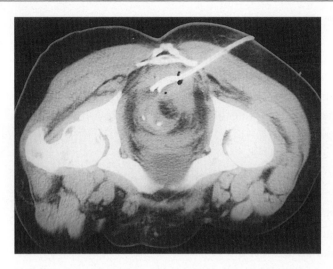

Figure 35-4 A 10F self-retaining drainage catheter has been inserted into the abscess.

bowel, and bladder should be selected. Although an anterior or anterolateral trajectory is suitable for many intra-abdominal collections, the urinary bladder and overlying bowel often preclude such an approach in deep pelvic abscesses. Alternative routes that have been advocated to circumvent these problems include transrectal, transvaginal, and transperineal approaches, all of which have been used with good success. Guidance methods for these procedures include CT, fluoroscopy, and ultrasound. Despite these alternatives, some collections remain inaccessible. High presacral collections that cannot be reached from a transrectal approach or those in patients who have undergone recent anastomosis or surgical removal of the rectum are two examples. CT-guided drainage through the greater sciatic foramen has been shown to be a successful approach for management in these and other select cases.

Use of a transgluteal approach through the greater sciatic foramen requires a thorough knowledge of the anatomical landmarks and excellent pain control during the procedure.

The greater sciatic foramen is an oval space located posterolaterally in the pelvis. It is bounded by the sacrum posteriorly, the sacrospinous ligament inferiorly, the ischium anteriorly, and the ileum superiorly. Several neurovascular structures lie in close proximity to it or transverse the foramen and must be avoided for safe and successful drainage. These include the sacral plexus, which runs on the ventral surface of the piriformis muscle, passing through the center of the foramen. The sacral plexus forms the sciatic nerve, which lies just posterior to the sacrospinous ligament at its insertion anteriorly into the ischial spine. The superior and inferior gluteal arteries and veins cross the foramen in its more cephalad region. Because of the location of these neurovascular structures, safe access to the pelvis through the foramen is best achieved at its inferomedial margin at the level of the sacrospinous ligament. The ideal access site should be as close to the sacrum as possible to avoid injury to the sciatic nerve.

Outcome and Complications

With proper technique, the transgluteal drainage of deep pelvic abscesses has a success rate of over 80%.

Patients often find initial catheter insertion uncomfortable even when the approach is ideal. This is due to the length of the tract and the large amount of muscle and soft tissue that must be traversed. Adequate local anesthesia, parenteral sedation, and analgesia are important in maintaining patient comfort and cooperation during catheter insertion. Occasionally, pain can be pronounced and persistent. This is usually due to the catheter passing through or lying in close proximity to the sacral plexus. In such cases, careful CT evaluation of the access route should be performed. If the discomfort is unrelenting and drainage is needed for an extended period, removal and insertion of a new catheter via a more medial tract may be necessary.

Pelvic hematoma has been described as a complication of transgluteal drainage. This occurs when the tract transects one or more pelvic vessels. Another complication is catheter kinking. This occurs when the patient is supine, causing the catheter to be compressed and kinked at the skin surface. This can be minimized by nursing the patient in a decubitus position and with meticulous post-procedural care on the ward.

PEARLS AND PITFALLS

- For transgluteal abscess drainage through the greater sciatic foramen, the best access route is inferomedial at the level of the sacrospinous ligament. Staying close to the sacrum avoids injury to the sciatic nerve and other neurovascular structures.

- Ample local anesthetic, parenteral sedation, and analgesia are necessary to ensure patient comfort and cooperation during the procedure.

- Persistent catheter-related pain is usually due to close proximity of the tract to the sacral plexus. This can be determined by reevaluation of the access route by CT and may necessitate catheter removal and insertion of a new drainage catheter via a more medial approach.

- Kinking of the catheter at the skin entry site may occur when the patient assumes a supine position. This is avoided by encouraging the patient to lie on the side.

Further Reading

Alexander AA, Eschelman DJ, Nazarian LN, et al. Transrectal sonographically guided drainage of deep pelvic abscess. AJR Am J Roentgenol 1994;162:1227–1230

Butch RJ, Mueller PR, Ferrucci JT, et al. Drainage of pelvic abscesses through the greater sciatic foramen. Radiology 1986;158:487–491

Gazelle GS, Haaga JR, Stellato TA, et al. Pelvic abscesses: CT-guided transrectal drainage. Radiology 1991;181:49–51

Malden ES, Picus D. Hemorrhagic complication of transgluteal pelvic abscess drainage: successful percutaneous treatment. J Vasc Interv Radiol 1992;3:323–328

Michalson AE, Brown BP, Warnock NG, et al. Presacral abscesses: percutaneous transperineal drainage with use of bone landmarks and fluoroscopic guidance. Radiology 1994;190:574–575

Mueller PR, Van Sonnenberg E, Ferrucci JT. Percutaneous drainage of 250 abdominal abscesses and fluid collections, part II: current procedural concepts. Radiology 1984;151:343–347

Sperling DC, Needleman L, Eschelman DJ, et al. Deep pelvic abscesses: transperineal US-guided drainage. Radiology 1998;208:111–115

van Sonnenberg E, D'Agostino HB, Casola G, et al. Percutaneous abscess drainage: current concepts. Radiology 1991;181:617–626

CHAPTER 36 Transrectal Drainage

Roman I. Kozak

Clinical Presentation

A 73-year-old man presented with a 3-week history of pelvic pain, spiking fevers, poor appetite, and diminished energy. He had a past history of unresectable carcinoma of the rectosigmoid colon, which had been managed with a defunctioning colostomy. He had also undergone radiotherapy as well as one cycle of chemotherapy consisting of 5-FU and folinic acid. Physical examination revealed the defunctioning colostomy in the lower abdomen but was otherwise unremarkable. Hemoglobin and leukocyte count were within normal limits.

Radiological Studies

Computed tomography (CT) of the pelvis using oral contrast demonstrated a 6 cm soft tissue mass between the rectum and base of the bladder (**Fig. 36-1**). It had an irregular soft tissue wall with a fluid density center.

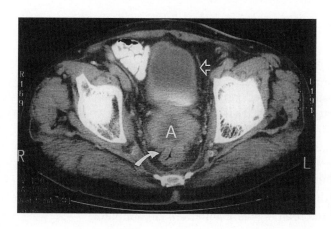

Figure 36-1 Computed tomography of the pelvis using oral contrast demonstrates the abscess (A) between the rectum (curved arrow) and bladder (open arrow).

Diagnosis

Pelvic abscess

Treatment

In preparation for transrectal drainage, the patient was placed on the fluoroscopy table in the left lateral decubitus position. The perineum and anus were cleansed with an antiseptic solution and the area was sterile draped. Topical 2% lidocaine gel was then applied to the perianal region and injected into the rectum using a syringe (Astra Sterile–Pack, Astra Pharma Inc., Mississauga, ON). A modified enema tip (**Fig. 36-2**) was then introduced into the rectum. The enema tip had been preloaded with a 20 cm long 18 gauge needle. The needle tip was positioned proximal to the tip of the tube to prevent needle injury to the anus or rectum during insertion. The rectum was then insufflated with

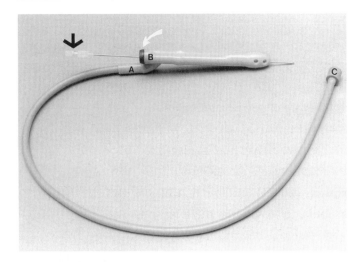

Figure 36-2 Modified enema tip, consisting of a regular plastic enema tube with the barium port (B) cut off close to the side (air) port (A) and then covered with a stopper (curved arrow) to prevent insufflated air from escaping. The 20 cm 18 gauge needle (straight arrow) has been inserted through the stopper. The air insufflation bulb attaches to the end of the side port (C).

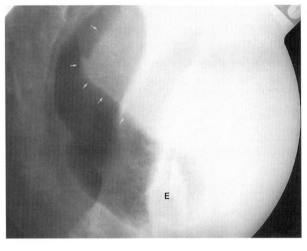

Figure 36-3 Lateral fluoroscopic image following insertion of the modified enema tip (E) with the rectum insufflated clearly demonstrates the abscess bulging the anterior aspect of the rectal air column (arrows).

air, allowing it to be visualized fluoroscopically. The abscess could be clearly seen bulging into the anterior aspect of the air-filled rectum (**Fig. 36-3**). The enema tip was then advanced to the rectal wall in contact with the abscess and the needle advanced through the rectal wall into the abscess. Purulent liquid was aspirated and a sample was sent for microbiological evaluation. An Amplatz extra-stiff guide wire (Cook Canada, Stouffville, ON) was then advanced through the needle and coiled within the abscess. The wire was left in place and the needle and enema tip were removed together. The tract was dilated, following which a 10F self-retaining drainage catheter (Flexima APDL, Medi-tech, Boston Scientific, Watertown, MA) was inserted over the guide wire into the abscess. The cavity was then completely aspirated and flushed with normal saline until the return was nonpurulent. The catheter was placed on bag drainage and taped to the patient's buttock. The patient was sent to the ward with instructions to have the catheter flushed with 20 mL of saline every 6 hours.

Following drainage, the patient's fever rapidly resolved and he became asymptomatic within 24 hours. CT obtained 1 week later showed no residual abscess. Drainage from the catheter tapered off to <10 mL per 24 hours and it was removed after 12 days.

Discussion

Despite diagnostic and therapeutic advances over the past 2 to 3 decades, pelvic abscesses remain an important diagnostic and management challenge. Surgical drainage has long been established as standard therapy for these patients. Antimicrobial drugs, although important, primarily serve in an adjuvant role. With improvements in cross-sectional imaging and advances in catheter technology as well as drainage techniques, the scope of percutaneous treatment of abscesses has expanded such that the majority of infected intra-abdominal fluid collections are now amenable to imaging-guided percutaneous drainage.

Deep pelvic abscesses present specific therapeutic challenges. A conventional transabdominal percutaneous route is often forestalled by intervening structures, such as the bladder or overlying bowel loops. Regardless of the cause, the best drainage approach for pelvic collections depends on the location of the abscess relative to the pelvic organs and rectum. Abscesses posterior or lateral to the rectum can be drained either transrectally or transgluteally. With large pararectal collections, percutaneous transabdominal drainage may occasionally be possible. For collections anterior to the rectum, the transrectal or transvaginal approach may be used. In patients who have had their rectum removed, drainage may still be possible through the rectal stump or, if the collection is low enough, a transperineal approach may be feasible. In most patients, the transrectal approach will reach collections to the level of the sacral promontory. For collections above the level of the true pelvis, transrectal drainage may not be possible.

Transrectal ultrasound and CT guidance have both been suggested for drainage of these collections. We have not found transrectal sonography necessary if the mass effect on the rectum produced by the abscess can be seen fluoroscopically (see **Fig. 36-3**). However, for smaller collections, transrectal ultrasound may be invaluable. Lack of real-time guidance is a significant deficiency of CT for these procedures; however, as experience with CT fluoroscopy grows, this shortcoming may be addressed.

Technique

Prior to drainage, CT of the abdomen and pelvis must be obtained and carefully evaluated to determine the location and number of fluid collections. Oral contrast is given to opacify bowel loops and may be supplemented by contrast administered through a Foley catheter in the rectum. Before undertaking a drainage, the procedure, risks, indications, and alternatives are carefully discussed with the patient and informed consent is obtained. Patients are screened with an International Normalized Ratio (INR) and partial thromboplastin time (PTT), as well as a complete blood count. If necessary, measures may be undertaken to correct any coagulopathy that is detected.

In general, patients should be on appropriate intravenous antibiotics before an infected fluid collection is drained. Intravenous access is established in case fluids, sedation, or analgesia are required.

The procedure is performed with the patient in the left lateral decubitus position on the fluoroscopy table. After the perineum and anus are cleansed with antiseptic solution, 2% lidocaine gel is applied to the anus and injected into the rectum. Other than this, no local anesthesia is generally required. Sedation and intravenous analgesia are given, depending on the patient's anxiety and level of discomfort.

After anesthetizing the rectum, a modified enema tip is introduced. The enema tip consists of a regular plastic enema tip, as used for barium enemas (E-Z-EM Miller Air Tip, Therapex, E-Z-EM, Canada Inc., Montreal, QC). The tube is modified by cutting the barium channel as close to the side port (air channel) as possible. The hole is then covered with an appropriately sized stopper or waterproof tape to prevent insufflated air from escaping (see **Fig. 36-2**). An 18 gauge needle is then preinserted through the stopper to the enema tip (but not past the tip).

The modified enema tip is introduced with the needle inside (to protect the perianal skin and rectal mucosa). The rectum is then distended with air using a bulb attached to the side port. At this point, indentation of the rectal air column by the pelvic collection is usually visualized (see **Fig. 36-3**). With lateral fluoroscopy, reasonably sized anterior and posterior collections are usually evident and puncture of the fluid collection can then be performed appropriately.

Collections lateral to the rectum are more difficult to visualize. Pelvic CT is crucial for correlation and anteroposterior fluoroscopy (using a rotating tube) may demonstrate the abscess indenting the

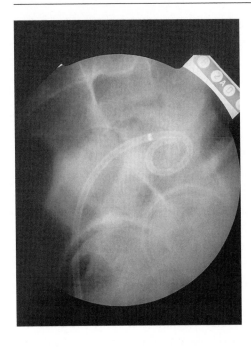

Figure 36-4 Lateral image following transrectal insertion of the abscess drainage catheter.

lateral wall of the rectum. Smaller collections may not produce a discernible indentation on the rectum. In such cases, a transrectal ultrasound probe, covered with a condom, is introduced to visualize the abscess. A guide attached to the probe will direct the needle into the collection once it is demonstrated.

The enema tip is applied to the rectal wall overlying the abscess and the needle is advanced into the fluid collection. The stylet is withdrawn and the lesion aspirated. If the aspirate is purulent, a guide wire (Amplatz extra stiff, Cook Canada, Stouffville, ON) is then advanced through the 18 gauge needle and coiled within the collection. A stiff guide wire is essential because the abscess wall is usually at some distance from the anus and softer wires tend to buckle in the rectum and pull out of the abscess. The needle and the enema tip are then removed together, leaving the guide wire within the abscess. The tract is then dilated with sequential dilators and a 10 or 12F self-retaining catheter (Flexima APDL, Medi-tech, Boston Scientific, Watertown, MA) is advanced into the collection. The guide wire is then removed and the catheter loop is formed within the abscess (**Fig. 36-4**). As much fluid as possible is then aspirated. The cavity is repeatedly flushed with normal saline until the return is nonpurulent. The catheter is left in place and attached to an external drainage bag. The catheter is brought out laterally and taped to the patient's buttocks, which is generally found to be reasonably comfortable. While on the ward, the catheter is managed similar to other abscess drainages (i.e., with instructions to flush the catheter every 6 hours with 20 mL of normal saline).

Ideally, the catheter should remain in place until drainage decreases to 10 mL per day or less. At this point, CT is obtained, and if no residual abscess cavity is demonstrated, the catheter is removed. Often, the catheter will fall out spontaneously, usually after 5 to 7 days, while the patient is having a bowel movement. In general, no attempt is made to reintroduce a drainage catheter as long as the patient's symptoms have improved and there is no persistent evidence of sepsis. If there is continuing high-volume drainage from the catheter, a sinogram is performed to check for possible fistulas.

In patients who have had low colonic resections with primary or secondary reconstructions, it is important to ensure that introduction of a rectal tube will not disrupt the anastomosis.

Outcome

A review of the literature reveals eight recent articles about transrectal drainage of pelvic abscesses. The pooled results are shown in **Table 36-1**, demonstrating a 91% rate of abscess resolution and

Table 36-1   Transrectal Drainage: Combined Results from Eight Studies

Author	# Patients	Success	Complications
Gazelle, et al	10	100%	0%
Alexander, et al	9	100%	0%
Bennett, et al	8	100%—two recurred	0%
Kuligowska, et al	33	84%	0%
Carmody, et al	13	62%	0%
Lomas, et al	5	80%	0%
Chung, et al	7	100%	0%
Kastan, et al	5	100%	0%
TOTAL	90	91%	0%

a 0% complication rate. It should be noted that Kuligowska et al (1995), used aspiration and lavage only and did not place a catheter. With aspiration and lavage only, they achieved an 84% cure rate.

We found transrectal drainage to be both technically easier and better tolerated than the transgluteal approach for deep pelvic abscesses. Very little analgesia is required and sedation is usually only necessary for anxious patients. By topically anesthetizing the anus and rectum, the procedure produces very little discomfort.

PEARLS AND PITFALLS

- The optimal drainage approach for pelvic collections depends upon the location of the abscess relative to the pelvic organs and rectum.
- If the mass effect produced by the abscess cannot be seen on the rectal air column fluoroscopically, transrectal ultrasound may be used for guidance.
- The transrectal approach will reach collections to the level of the sacral promontory in the majority of patients. For collections above the level of the true pelvis, transrectal drainage may not be feasible.
- In patients who have had low colonic resections with primary or secondary reconstruction, it is important to ensure introduction of a rectal tube will not disrupt the anastomosis.
- In patients who have had their rectum removed, drainage may still be possible through the rectal stump.

Further Reading

Alexander AA, Eschelman DJ, Nazarian LN, et al. Transrectal sonographically guided drainage of deep pelvic abscesses. AJR Am J Roentgenol 1994;162:1227–1230

Bennett JD, Kozak RI, Taylor BM, et al. Deep pelvic abscesses: transrectal drainage with radiologic guidance. Radiology 1992;185:825–828

Carmody E, Thurston W, Yeung E, et al. Transrectal drainage of deep pelvic collections under fluoroscopic guidance. Can Assoc Radiol J 1993;44:429–433

Chung T, Hoffer FA, Lund DP. Transrectal drainage of deep pelvic abscesses in children using a combined transrectal sonographic and fluoroscopic guidance. Pediatr Radiol 1996;26:874–878

Finne CO. Transrectal drainage of pelvic abscesses. Dis Colon Rectum 1980;23:293–297

Gazelle GS, Haaga JR, Stellato TA, et al. Pelvic abscesses: CT-guided transrectal drainage. Radiology 1991;181:49–51

Hovsepian DM. Transrectal and transvaginal abscess drainage. J Vasc Interv Radiol 1997;8:501–515

Kastan DJ, Nelson KM, Shetty PC, et al. Combined transrectal sonographic and fluoroscopic guidance for deep pelvic abscess drainage. J Ultrasound Med 1996;15:235–239

Kuligowska E, Keller E, Ferrucci JT. Treatment of pelvic abscesses: value of one-step sonographically guided transrectal needle aspiration and lavage. AJR Am J Roentgenol 1995;164:201–206

Lomas DJ, Dixon AK, Thompson HJ, et al. CT-guided drainage of pelvic abscesses: the peranal transrectal approach. Clin Radiol 1992;45:246–249

Nosher JL, Needell GS, Amorosa JK, et al. Transrectal pelvic abscess drainage with sonographic guidance. AJR Am J Roentgenol 1986;146:1047–1048

van Sonnenberg E, D'Agostino HB, Casola G, et al. US-guided transvaginal drainage of pelvic abscesses and fluid collections. Radiology 1991;181:53–66

CHAPTER 37 Transvaginal Drainage

John P. McGahan

Clinical Presentation

A 44-year-old woman with a prior history of pelvic inflammatory disease presented with fever, elevated white count, and pelvic pain. Bimanual examination of the pelvis elicited excruciating pelvic pain. She had a palpable pelvic mass.

Radiological Studies

A contrast-enhanced computed tomographic (CT) scan of the pelvis (**Fig. 37-1**) demonstrated a well-demarcated fluid collection within the pelvis. An endovaginal ultrasound showed a fluid collection in the cul de sac (**Fig. 37-2**).

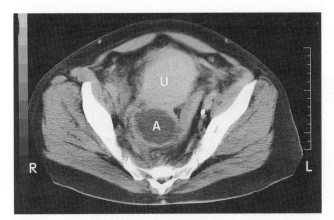

Figure 37-1 Computed tomographic scan shows a well-demarcated fluid collection (A) posterior to the uterus (U). (Used with permission from McGahan et al, 1996.)

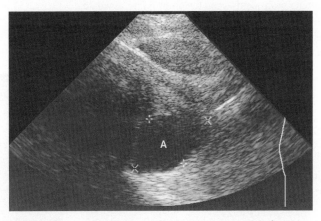

Figure 37-2 Parasagittal endovaginal ultrasound localized the fluid collection (A) in the pelvic cul de sac. (Used with permission from McGahan et al, 1996.)

Diagnosis

Pelvic abscess

Treatment

The preprocedure CT and ultrasound confirmed the clinical suspicion of a pelvic abscess. The patient was consented for transvaginal ultrasound-guided drainage. An anesthesiologist was present and administered intravenous propofol (Diprivan, Stuart Pharmaceuticals, Wilmington, DE) to the patient without intubation but with use of oxygen via nasal cannula. Endovaginal ultrasound was then performed to localize the fluid collection. After the fluid collection was localized, the endoluminal transvaginal probe (Ultramark 9, Advanced Technical Laboratory, Bothel, WA) was modified as follows: there is a groove in the metal biopsy guide attachment, within which a cylindrical plastic needle guide is clipped into place. This plastic guide is closed at both ends, and thus the needle or catheter must be removed when the ultrasound probe is removed. Instead, a 6.7F McGahan drainage

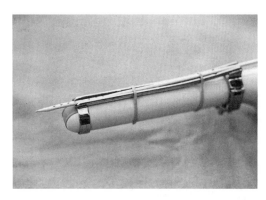

Figure 37-3 Photograph shows a trocar catheter placed into the grooves of the endovaginal probe. The catheter is held in place in the grooves of the metal guide with rubber bands. The distal tip of the catheter protrudes beyond the probe guide, as would occur with the advancement of the trocar into the pelvic fluid collection. (Used with permission from McGahan et al, 1996.)

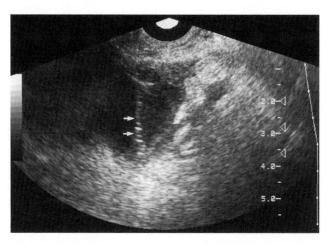

Figure 37-4 Trocar-type catheter is pushed from the endovaginal probe into the pelvic fluid collection. The trocar needle is visualized (arrows) in the fluid collection. (Used with permission from McGahan et al, 1996.)

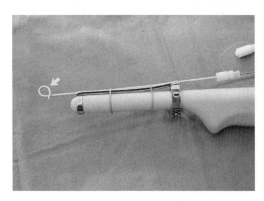

Figure 37-5 Once the trocar catheter is placed into the pelvic abscess and purulent material is aspirated, the stiffening cannula is fixed and the outer catheter pushed from the stiffening cannula. The distal loop is formed (arrow), as shown in the photograph. (Used with permission from McGahan et al, 1996.)

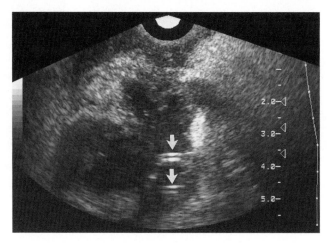

Figure 37-6 Transvaginal ultrasound also shows the distal loop of the catheter (arrows) within the fluid collection. (Used with permission from McGahan et al, 1996.)

catheter (Cook Catheter, Cook Incorp., Bloomington, IN) was placed into the groove where the clips of the needle guide were to be placed (**Fig. 37-3**). The catheter was kept in place by affixing small rubber bands around the catheter and the tranvaginal probe. After the vagina was cleaned with povidon-iodine (Betadine, Purdue Frederick, Norwalk, CT), the probe was placed as firmly as possible against the vaginal vault. The trocar technique was used to place the catheter into the fluid collection under ultrasound guidance (**Fig. 37-4**). Once the trocar catheter was within the fluid collection, the inner cannula was fixed and the catheter pushed from the stiffening cannula into the fluid collection, as illustrated in **Fig. 37-5**. Once within the fluid collection, the string of the distal catheter loop was tightened (**Fig. 37-6**). The probe was then removed, and rubber bands were removed over the catheter. The abscess was completely drained. Irrigation was not immediately performed but was begun 12 hours later. Culture from this fluid revealed bifidobacterium and peptostreptococcus organisms. After 3 days, the catheter was removed, and no further treatment was necessary.

Discussion

Percutaneous image-guided aspiration and drainage of abdominal or pelvic abscesses has been shown to be an effective alternative to surgery. The most common method of draining these abscesses is usually by the transabdominal route for abdomen abscess and by the transgluteal route for pelvic abscesses. Very commonly, CT guidance is used. Transabdominal ultrasound guidance has also been shown to be an effective alternative method to drainage of many of these abscesses. Ultrasound may be utilized for initial needle puncture and catheter placement done via the guide wire exchange technique using either ultrasound or fluoroscopy. Alternatively, in the pelvis, ultrasound has been advocated for drainage of pelvic abscesses by either the transvaginal or the transrectal approach. Kuligowska et al (1995) used a one-step method of sonographically guiding transrectal 16 gauge needle aspiration with lavage to drain pelvic abscesses. This was curative in ~85% of these patients. Van Sonnenburg et al (1991) used ultrasound-guided transvaginal aspiration or drainage to treat pelvic abscesses. There is no difference in clinical outcome of the aspiration or drainage patients. Others, such as Casola et al (1992), reported difficulty inserting the catheter through the vaginal vault using a guide wire exchange technique. In our patient, trocar placement of the catheter was utilized without complications. McGahan et al (1996) demonstrated the feasibility of a trocar method in placement of catheters with an 86% cure rate. This is a one-step method using a trocar-type catheter for drainage of these abscesses.

Hovsepian et al (1999) have compared transvaginal versus transrectal guidance of abscesses. They found in a patient survey that the pain experienced during the insertion procedure was higher for the transvaginal than for the transrectal route. Also, patients felt that the transvaginal catheter limited their activity more than the transrectal catheter. Therefore, they thought that the transrectal route of drainage of abscesses was better tolerated than the transvaginal route.

In our experience, transvaginal abscess drainage is painful for the patient, and, as such, deep conscious sedation or general anesthesia is usually necessary. More commonly, using the transrectal route, conscious sedation rather than general anesthesia may be utilized. We have found that there has been no significant limitation of patient activity using transvaginal drainage.

Thus, it would seem that the transvaginal drainage is best performed using the trocar technique for catheter placement. There is some indication that transrectal catheter drainage may be better tolerated by patients than transvaginal catheter placement. Either route is effective in performance of drainage and is an expedient method for abscess drainage.

PEARLS AND PITFALLS_____

- Transvaginal ultrasound guidance may be utilized for drainage of pelvic abscesses.
- Using the transvaginal route, pain may be experienced by the patient, and, as such, deep conscious sedation or general anesthesia is required.
- When using the transvaginal route, it is recommended that a trocar-type catheter be used instead of performing the drainage by the guide wire exchange technique.

Further Reading

Casola G, van Sonnenberg E, D'Agostino HB, et al. Percutaneous drainage of tubo-ovarian abscesses. Radiology 1992;182:399–402

Feld R, Eschelman DJ, Sagerman JE, et al. Treatment of pelvic abscesses and other fluid collections: efficacy of transvaginal sonographically guided aspiration and drainage. AJR Am J Roentgenol 1994;163:1141–1145

Hovsepian DM, Steele JR, Skinner CS, et al. Transrectal versus transvaginal abscess drainage: survey of patient tolerance and effect of activities of daily living. Radiology 1999;212:159–163

Kuligowska E, Keller E, Ferrucci JT. Treatment of pelvic abscesses: value of one-step sonographically guided transrectal needle aspiration and lavage. AJR Am J Roentgenol 1995;164:201–206

McGahan JP, Brown B, Jones CD, et al. Pelvic abscesses: transvaginal US-guided drainage with the trocar method. Radiology 1996;200:579–581

van Sonnenberg E, D'Agostino HB, Casola G, et al. US-guided transvaginal drainage of pelvic abscesses and fluid collections. Radiology 1991;181:53–56

CHAPTER 38 Female Infertility: An Overview

Noel Peng and Bruce R. Carr

Infertility affects approximately 10 to 15% of couples in the reproductive age group (Gray, 1990; Mosher and Pratt, 1991). Most infertile couples have one or more of three major causes: male factor, ovulatory dysfunction, or tuboperitoneal disease. With the tendency of more couples to practice contraception and delay childbearing until the last 2 decades of reproductive life, an increasing number of women are seeking care for infertility. Several factors account for this: With the epidemic of sexually transmitted diseases such as chlamydia and gonorrhea, pelvic infection may lead to tubal occlusion, pelvic adhesions, and distortion of tubo-ovarian anatomy. Anovulation and spontaneous abortions are also more common in the last decade of reproductive life (James, 1979; Schwartz and Mayaux, 1982; Gindoff and Jewelewicz, 1986). In addition, there may be an increased incidence of endometriosis and uterine pathology such as leiomyomata, intrauterine polyps, and adhesions. Furthermore, fewer infants are available for adoption because of increased use of contraception and abortion.

Infertility evaluation and treatment are often expensive and many major insurance carriers exclude infertility as a reimbursable diagnosis, leaving the financial burden with the infertile couple. This must be considered when counseling patients about available treatment options. Evaluation of fertility issues may be extremely stressful to some couples. Loss of privacy, disruption of spontaneous sexual habits, and a feeling of reproductive failure or inadequacy are frequent causes of depression, anxiety, and grief. Thus the practitioner must be aware of the psychological impact of infertility and be sensitive and understanding to the patient's needs. Referral for counseling or to infertility support groups may be helpful.

The basic investigation of a couple for infertility includes assessment of male factors, evaluation of tubal pathologies, and hormonal testing to evaluate ovulation. The infertility evaluation serves to: (1) determine the etiology(ies) of infertility as expediently as possible; (2) provide recommended treatment protocols; (3) determine expected success rates for recommended therapy; and (4) educate the couple about their specific disorder and available alternatives. Some patients may merely seek a diagnosis and not intend to pursue therapy or cannot afford recommended diagnostic tests or treatment, whereas others proceed with adoption.

Definitions

Infertility is usually defined as the inability of a couple practicing frequent intercourse and not using contraception to conceive a child within 1 year. This definition is based upon investigations on the time required for conception in 1727 planned pregnancies, which was 12 months for 90% conception (Tietze et al, 1950). The chance for conception depends upon the length of exposure, coital frequency, and age of the couple. For fertile couples, there is a 25% chance of conception after 1 month of unprotected intercourse, 70% by 6 months, and 90% by 1 year. Only an additional 5% will conceive after waiting an additional 6 to 12 months. Once fertility therapy is initiated, couples must be counseled that at least 4 to 6 months of therapy are required to test the adequacy for most given treatment regimens.

Primary infertility occurs in couples with no previous history of conception; *secondary infertility* exists when a prior conception has been, at a minimum, documented by a positive β-human chorionic gonadotropin β-hCG) test, histology, or ultrasound. *Fecundability* is the probability of achieving a pregnancy within one menstrual cycle (about 25% in normal couples); *fecundity* is the ability to achieve a live birth within one menstrual cycle.

Evaluation of the infertile couple often reveals one or more causes for failure to conceive. Motivated couples who comply with therapeutic guidelines can expect a 50 to 60% chance of conception. A spontaneous, treatment-independent cumulative pregnancy rate of about 30 to 40% exists in couples in whom no identifiable cause for the infertility can be determined (Collins et al, 1983).

Age Factors

Peak rate of conception in both men and women occurs at age 24 and begins to decline significantly after age 35 so that for every 5 years, the length of time for conception doubles. Thus, in the couple over 30 years of age who meets the definition of either primary or secondary infertility, the workup should be initiated and completed as soon as possible. The rate of conception declines with advancing age in women as well as men (Guzick et al, 1986). With advancing maternal age, the percentage of couples conceiving within 12 months of unprotected intercourse decreases as follows: 86%, 78%, 63%, and 52% in age groups 20 to 24, 25 to 29, 30 to 34, and 35 to 39 years, respectively (Hendershot et al, 1982). The incidence of impaired fertility in women aged less than 25 years was 11.7% compared with 42.1% for women aged 35 years and older (Abma et al, 1997). The results of artificial insemination in 2193 nulliparous women with azoospermic men show that below age 31 years, the pregnancy rate over 1 year was 74%. This decreased to 62% at age 31 to 35 and to 54% in women over 35 years.

As a general rule, couples who have not conceived after 1 year of unprotected intercourse are reasonable candidates for infertility evaluation. Earlier investigation may be recommended based on the woman's age and pertinent history such as oligomenorrhea or amenorrhea, pelvic inflammatory disease (PID), tubal obstruction, endometriosis, intrauterine device (IUD) use, diethylstilbestrol (DES) exposure in utero, ectopic pregnancy, and abdominal surgery. Patients planning chemotherapy should be offered an emergency evaluation.

Causes of Infertility

The incidence of the factors responsible for infertility varies with the population studied. In 15 to 20% of cases, infertility is due to ovulatory dysfunction; in 30 to 40% it is due to pelvic factors such as endometriosis, adhesions, or tubal disease; 30 to 40% are due to male factors such as oligospermia (density <20 million sperm per mL or total count <50 million), azoospermia (absence of sperm), asthenospermia (defects in sperm movement or decreased sperm motility), or teratospermia (defects in morphology); and less than 5% are due to abnormal sperm–cervical mucus penetration or antisperm antibodies. In about 10% of couples, no cause can be found, whereas 20 to 40% may have multiple factors.

The initial workup of the infertile couple consists of a semen analysis, detection and quantification of ovulatory function by various methods, and evaluation of tubal patency by hysterosalpingography (HSG). Further evaluation of pelvic anatomy by either or both laparoscopy and hysteroscopy is considered if there is an abnormality on HSG or if no cause for infertility can be found. Other procedures such as postcoital testing (PCT), antisperm antibodies, or other sperm function tests may be used in certain cases.

Evaluation of the Couple as a Unit

Infertility is a "two-patient disorder." Both the male and the female partner must be thoroughly evaluated, counseled, and included in the therapeutic decision-making processes. A questionnaire is often helpful prior to the first visit and should include questions regarding prior conceptions, contraceptions, coital frequency, and techniques. This serves as a basis for review and in-depth questioning; it does not replace the history.

The most common sexual problems are a misunderstanding of the timing of ovulation and either too frequent or too infrequent intercourse. The optimal time for intercourse is midcycle and the most effective frequency of intercourse is every 48 hours. Both partners should be screened for the use of drugs or alcohol that may affect fertility. Studies in males with heavy marijuana use show reduced testosterone levels, decreased sperm counts, and impotency (Hembree et al, 1976). Alcohol is also known to affect libido and potency. Decreases in gonadotropin levels and ovulation are noted in females with frequent drug or alcohol ingestion. Cigarette smoking has also been implicated in subfertility. Early menopause, reduced spermatogenesis, and decreased steroid production have been noted in individuals who use cigarettes (Hammond et al, 1961). Life table analysis studies demonstrate a longer period of time to conception for smokers when compared with nonsmokers (Baird and Wilcox, 1985; Bolumar et al, 1996). High caffeine intake may also delay conception among fertile women (Bolumar et al, 1997).

Initial Consultation

The basic evaluation consists of a detailed medical history, physical examination, semen evaluation, ovulation, and uterotubal assessment. In women older than 35 years, estradiol and follicle-stimulating hormone (FSH) levels obtained on the third day of the menstrual cycle may be useful (Scott and Hofmann, 1995).

FEMALE

An extensive history and physical examination are conducted. The history includes timing of pubertal development; menarche; menstrual history with cycle length, duration, and amount of bleeding; associated dysmenorrhea; and premenstrual symptoms. In almost all women, spontaneous, regular, cyclic predictable menses is consistent with ovulation, whereas a history of amenorrhea or abnormal or unpredictable bleeding suggests anovulation or uterine pathology. Previous pregnancies, miscarriages, abortions, and birth control history are documented. Dyspareunia and dysmenorrhea may be linked to endometriosis. PID, sexually transmitted disease, ruptured appendix, or other abdominal surgery and past use of an intrauterine device may be associated with tubal disease. Galactorrhea may indicate hyperprolactinemia, and pubertal onset of progressive hirsutism associated with oligomenorrhea may indicate polycystic ovary syndrome or other disorders of hyperandrogenism. Excessive weight loss or gain, stress, and exercise are often associated with ovulatory disorders. Sexual, social, and psychological issues are explored.

MALE

Questions pertaining to prior fertility, impotence, general health, medications, genital surgery, trauma, infection, drug or alcohol abuse, frequent hot tub baths, excessive stress, fatigue, and excessive or infrequent coitus need to be addressed. Medical conditions that may result in infertility include diabetes (lack of emission or retrograde ejaculation), serious debilitating disease (e.g., cystic fibrosis), mumps orchitis (from postpubertal mumps), and pituitary hypofunction, which may all lead to hypogonadism. Herniorrhaphy, varicocele repair, orchiopexy, and bladder neck suspension are potentially associated with infertility.

Review of Records

Most infertile couples have had some prior evaluation and this information is extremely important and should be reviewed. Couples may not understand the complexity of a thorough infertility evaluation. Many times, the infertility evaluation may have been satisfactory by previous standards but inadequate by today's. In addition, the records may suggest a different interpretation: For instance, the woman who is proven to be ovulatory may have a cycle length of 25 days with a biphasic rise of basal body temperature but the temperature elevation lasts only 7 to 11 days, which indicates a short luteal phase. An HSG reported as normal may be of poor quality to adequately rule out uterine filling defects or evaluate tubal patency. In addition, it is not uncommon to see an extensive female partner evaluation and treatment for years without a semen analysis or a reevaluation during that time.

Previous infertility evaluation including HSGs; operative report, photographs, or videotapes; pathological report; and medical therapy should be obtained and reviewed. Hormonal studies including FSH, luteinizing hormone (LH), progesterone (P4), thyrotropin (Thyroid Stimulating Hormone), and prolactin should be evaluated based upon the day in the menstrual cycle the sample was collected. Prior treatment regimens should be evaluated as to efficacy and length of treatment. All medications used by the couple should be reviewed.

Physical Examination

FEMALE

A thorough general physical examination helps define factors that may contribute to infertility, with special attention to signs of endocrine disturbances such as abnormal size or consistency of the thyroid gland, skin hyperpigmentation, or presence of abdominal striae. Acne, oily skin, and hirsutism indicate hyperandrogenism; acanthosis nigricans results from insulin resistance (Conway and Jacobs, 1990); and galactorrhea may be due to hyperprolactinemia. Note is made of surgical scars or significant variation from normal body weight or percent body fat. The degree of estrogenization of the vagina and quality and quantity of cervical mucus should be evaluated in the context of the menstrual cycle phase. Vaginal or cervical infection is evaluated by microscopic examination of a wet prep of a vaginal smear. The cervix is evaluated for anatomical abnormalities due to intrauterine exposure to DES or prior cervical surgery, including cryotherapy, cautery, or laser. Cervical cultures for gonorrhea, chlamydia, and Pap smears may be obtained. The size and contour of the uterus and adnexa and the presence of cervical, uterine, or adnexal tenderness and pelvic masses are assessed on the pelvic examination. The rectovaginal examination is performed to detect uterosacral nodularity found in endometriosis. A sterile plastic catheter is used to measure the length and direction of the uterine cavity and to check for cervical stenosis. This information may be of aid if intrauterine inseminations or embryo transfer is considered.

MALE

A general physical exam is performed with focus on the secondary sexual development, general body habitus, height, arm span, presence of gynecomastia, and abdomen scars from surgical procedures performed during childhood. The examination includes evaluation of perineal sensation and rectal sphincter tone, examination of the penis, size and location of the urethral meatus, urethral discharge, or evidence of stricture. The average volume for an adult testis is 25 mL or approximately 5 × 3 cm (testicular volume can be measured with an orchidometer or calipers). Very small or soft testes are usually associated with a decrease in germinal tissue mass due to either testicular failure or some abnormality in the hypothalamic–pituitary axis leading to hypogonadotropic hypogonadism. The epididymis is palpated to evaluate for swelling or tenderness due to epididymitis. The vas deferens should be evaluated by palpation and the spermatic cords palpated for the presence of a varicocele. Valsalva's maneuver can be used to accentuate a varicocele. A transrectal examination of the prostate is done for detecting prostatitis and cystic dilatation of the seminal vesicles. Normally, the seminal vesicles are not palpable and the prostate is firm.

Following the history and physical examination of both partners, an initial diagnosis should be made and initial laboratory and diagnostic tests are ordered. The history and examination may clearly point to one or more etiologies.

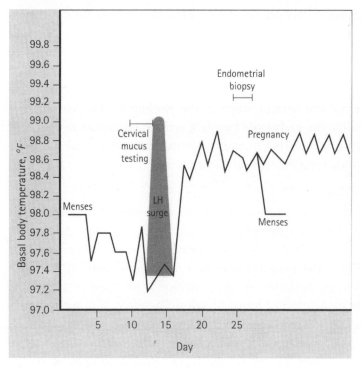

Figure 38-1 Basal body temperature (BBT) chart demonstrating a biphasic ovulatory pattern. BBT charts are an inexpensive, retrospective means of ovulation detection. Many clinicians believe that appropriate use of the BBT chart, which costs almost nothing, can yield useful results. For some couples, the BBT has teaching value. LH, luteinizing hormone. (Reproduced with permission from Buster JE. Diagnostic Evaluation of the Infertile Couple. Philadelphia: Current Medicine; 1999. Stenchever MA, Mishell DR Jr, eds. Atlas of Clinical Gynecology; vol 3.).

World Health Organization. *WHO Laboratory Manual for the Examination of Human Semen and Sperm–Cervical Mucus Interaction. Cambridge: Cambridge University Press; 1999*

Initial Laboratory and Diagnostic Tests

Although routine preobstetrical screening of infertile women is not mandatory, it is extremely helpful to screen for anemia and blood type, including Rh and antibody status. A RhoGAM may be needed following early spontaneous abortions or ectopic pregnancies. Women with a negative titer for rubella will require immunization and must wait 1 month prior to initiating therapy for infertility. Human immunodeficiency virus (HIV), hepatitis, and syphilis screening are essential in high-risk populations, those undergoing assisted reproductive techniques (ART), and those receiving cryopreserved gametes.

Evaluation and Documentation of Ovulation

Ovulatory factors of female infertility may be due to multiple causes (Speroff et al, 1999). These include polycystic ovary syndrome, oligomenorrhea, or amenorrhea associated with excessive weight loss or gain, eating disorders, thyroid abnormalities, and galactorrhea. If the menses are regular, spontaneous, and cyclic, adequate ovulation and follicle development should be assessed through multiple cycles. Basal body temperature charting, sonographic follicle monitoring, urinary LH detection, midluteal progesterone levels, and endometrial biopsy are used to evaluate ovulation and subsequent corpus luteum function.

BASAL BODY TEMPERATURE

Although much maligned, the basal body temperature chart is a useful and cost-effective index for evaluating ovulation. The temperature is taken upon awakening and before any activity. A biphasic chart characterized by a sustained increase of at least 0.4°F (0.22°C) for 12 to 15 days is consistent with ovulation and an adequate luteal phase length (**Fig. 38-1**). The day of ovulation is usually suggested by the day of the lowest temperature (nadir) and is followed by a sustained 0.4°F rise in temperature. However, significant variation in temperature may occur and it may be difficult to predict the time or presence of ovulation in some cycles. A luteal phase length of less than 11 days, as measured by basal body temperature recording, correlates with luteal phase defects diagnosed by endometrial biopsy. The temperature chart also serves as a visual reminder for the couple and physician as to the frequency and timing of intercourse and the timing of medications and studies in the infertility evaluation. It is our practice to write the various steps of the workup in the margins of a temperature chart and on the first consultation, giving the couple a written outline as to the steps that will be involved in their infertility workup. This reassures the couple that a plan has been established and will be carried out within a reasonable time frame.

SERUM PROGESTERONE (P4)

Serum progesterone levels obtained at midluteal phase evaluate the occurrence and adequacy of ovulation and corpus luteum function. Although the exact normal values for progesterone are disputed, most clinicians agree that a level of $\geq$10 ng/mL is indicative of adequate ovulation or luteinization (Hensleigh and Fainstat, 1979). Others suggest that three samples obtained in the luteal phase totaling 15 ng/mL constitute a normal ovulation. As progesterone is secreted in a pulsatile manner, a single low level may not indicate a defect of luteal function. Therefore, if progesterone is to be used as an index of ovulation, it should be used in multiple cycles or multiple samples obtained every other day during the luteal phase and averaged to yield a single result. Historically, a luteal phase defect is defined as a lag of more than 2 days in the histological development of the endometrium compared with the day of the cycle (presumably due to inadequate progesterone secretion or action) and can be found in up to 30% of isolated cycles of normal women. Only if found repeatedly is the defect thought to be a possible factor in infertility. Approximately 3 to 4% of infertile women will be diagnosed as having luteal phase defect and the incidence is approximately 5% in women with a history of recurrent abortions (Peters et al, 1992).

ENDOMETRIAL BIOPSY

Endometrial biopsy may also be used to confirm ovulation and diagnose a luteal phase defect. It is usually performed late in the cycle, 1 to 2 days before expected menstruation. It is recommended that the couple refrain from intercourse or use barrier contraception during the cycle that the endometrial biopsy is obtained. The sample of endometrium is obtained with a curette from the anterior or lateral wall of the uterine fundus. Dating of endometrium is best correlated with the timing of the ovulation as detected by sonography or LH timing rather than backdating from the onset of the subsequent menstrual cycle. It should also be noted that a delay in maturation of a single endometrial biopsy is a common finding, and therefore, must be repeated in another cycle before it may be interpreted as indicative of the presence of a luteal phase defect. The use of sonography or urinary LH monitoring may enhance the predictive value of both midluteal progesterone measurement and endometrial biopsy.

OTHER OVULATION DOCUMENTATION TESTING

Preovulatory transvaginal sonography is a highly useful tool for evaluating adequacy of folliculogenesis (**Fig. 38-2**), endometrial development and oocyte release. A triple-line endometrial pattern seen on sonography before ovulation is predictive of subsequent pregnancy (Serafini et al, 1994). It has been proposed that a considerable number of previously unexplained infertility may be due to dysfolliculogenesis (i.e., development of multiple small follicles that bring about premature or inadequate luteinization).

Regardless of the method chosen to assess adequate ovulation, we suggest that luteal abnormalities be detected by various methods in multiple cycles before instituting therapy. We determine serum TSH and prolactin in most women with infertility but in all women with oligomenorrhea,

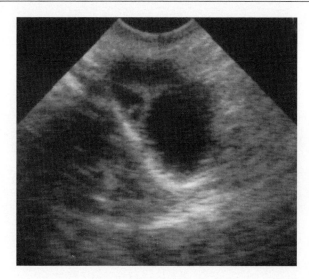

Figure 38-2 Transvaginal ultrasound shows a mature ovarian follicle.

amenorrhea, or galactorrhea. Serum androgens and androgen precursors (i.e., total testosterone and dehydroepiandrosterone sulfate [DHEAS]) are obtained only in hirsute women and gonadotropins (FSH and possibly LH) are obtained in women with amenorrhea. Furthermore, we suggest that day 3 FSH, estradiol, and inhibin B levels be obtained in women over the age of 35 to detect rises in FSH or estradiol or decline in inhibin B consistent with diminished ovarian reserve.

Treatment of Ovulatory Disorders

In women with ovulatory dysfunction with normal TSH, prolactin, and FSH (if indicated), ovulation induction can be initiated with clomiphene citrate (CC) in appropriate doses. Contraindications to CC include ovarian cysts >20 mm, organic intracranial lesions, pituitary macroadenomas, liver disease, uncontrolled thyroid or adrenal dysfunction, visual disturbances, and undiagnosed abnormal uterine bleeding. A standard approach to ovulation induction with CC is as follows: if necessary, induce menses with 10 mg medroxyprogesterone acetate for 5 days, after a negative pregnancy test result; initiate 50 mg of CC on days 3 to 7; commence urine LH testing on cycle day 10 to time intercourse or inseminations; measure serum progesterone level 7 days after LH spike to document ovulatory dose; in the absence of ovulation, increase daily dose of CC by 50 mg to a maximum daily dose of 150 mg; in the presence of ovulation, continue the ovulatory dose for 3 to 6 cycles with addition of sonogram monitoring, an ovulatory dose of human chorionic gonadotropin (hCG) when the follicle is mature, and intrauterine insemination (IUI) (Dodson and Haney, 1991).

If infertility is the result of anovulation caused by polycystic ovary syndrome (PCOS), ovulation can be induced, most commonly by administration of CC. If ovulation is not induced with CC alone, combined treatment with CC and metformin (if insulin resistant) (Arici et al, 1994), CC and gluco-corticoids (if serum androgen levels are elevated) (Nestler et al, 2002), or CC and bromocriptine (if prolactin levels are slightly elevated) (Lobo et al, 1982) may be successful. **Fig. 38-3** outlines a treatment algorithm for infertile couples with oligo-anovulation. In women who have not conceived after six ovulatory cycles, a diagnostic laparoscopy may be considered to evaluate for the presence of asymptomatic endometriosis or pelvic adhesions (Polson et al, 1987). Three cycles of gonadotropin therapy should then be initiated with estradiol and sonographic monitoring followed by hCG and IUI with washed husband's sperm. In addition, laparoscopic ovarian resection or ovarian drilling may result in ovulation and pregnancy in CC-resistant women with polycystic ovary syndrome (Marcoux et al, 1997; Campo, 1998; Kriplani et al, 2001). If pregnancy has still not been achieved, up to three

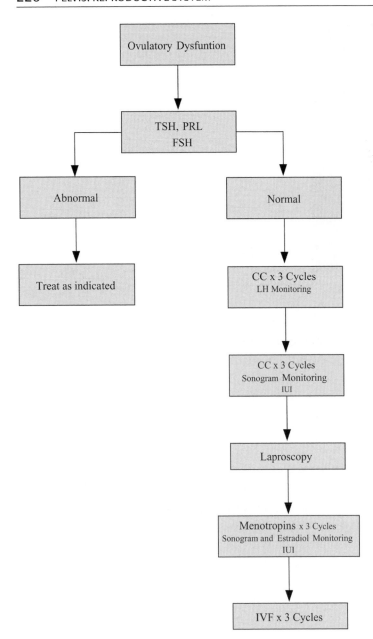

Figure 38-3 Treatment algorithm for infertile couple with oligo-anovulation. CC, clomiphene citrate; FSH, follicle-stimulating hormone; IUI, intrauterine insemination; IVF, in vitro fertilization; LH, luteinizing hormone; PRL, prolactin; TSH, thyroid stimulating hormone.

cycles of in vitro fertilization (IVF) should be offered to the infertile couple. Patients with a day 3 FSH >10 mIU/mL should have a repeat FSH and estradiol (familiarity with one's own laboratory threshold is important). With persistent elevation of these values, oocyte donation may be considered (**Fig. 38-4**).

Semen Analysis

A semen analysis should be obtained in all couples presenting with infertility. The specimen is obtained by masturbation into a sterile collection cup. Forty-eight to 72 hours of abstinence is recommended prior to analysis. The sample should be delivered to the laboratory within 1 hour of collection at body temperature. The test is essential despite a history of past paternity because

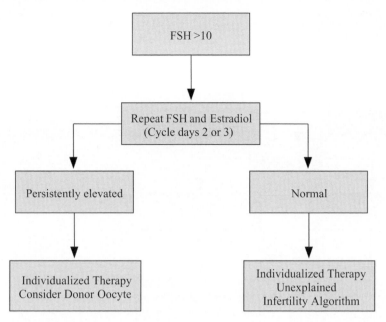

Figure 38-4 Treatment algorithm for infertile couple with elevated cycle day 3 follicle-stimulating hormone (FSH).

paternity may be in doubt in a troubled relationship. Frequently, one encounters the infertile couple who have had a normal postcoital test in the past and this has been interpreted as adequate evaluation of the male. However, the postcoital test does not substitute for a formal semen analysis. Reluctance to provide a sample may be due to hesitation or embarrassment about masturbation and can be overcome by the use of silicon condoms, which allow the man to produce a semen sample by intercourse. However, it should be noted that most condoms are made with latex and should not be used for collection purposes because latex may be toxic and most are also coated with nonoxynol-9, a detergent that disrupts cell membranes and is therefore a potent spermicide.

The semen analysis should have a volume of 2 to 5 mL, a concentration of 20 to 200 million sperm/mL with 50% directional motility, liquefaction at room temperature in 1 to 20 min, pH of 7.5 (range 7.0–8.031), and >14% normal by strict criteria (World Health Organization, 1999; Gunlap et al, 2001). There is a great variation from sample to sample in terms of volume, number, motility, and morphology and, in addition, there may be seasonal variation in these values. Approximately 90 days are required to produce spermatozoa. Therefore, it is recommended that if an abnormality is found, a repeat analysis be performed 2 to 3 months later to determine the presence of male factor. It is inappropriate to designate a male as infertile based upon a single semen analysis.

The use of IUI for the primary treatment of male factor infertility associated with severe oligospermia (<10 million/mL) or oligoasthenoteratospermia (decreased sperm density, decreased motility, and increased abnormal sperm forms) remains controversial because of extremely low pregnancy rates (Dodson and Haney, 1991; Arici et al, 1994). For couples with severe oligospermia or those with sperm-directed antibodies, IVF or IVF/intracytoplasmic sperm injection (ICSI; the direct injection of a single spermatozoon into the cytoplasm of an oocyte) may be a better choice. Endocrine evaluation, karyotyping, and screening for CF and Y chromosome microdeletions may be indicated (Najmabadi et al, 1996; Krausz et al, 1999, 2001). Couples with mild to moderate oligospermia, on the other hand, may be treated with IUI in conjunction with menotropins for controlled ovarian

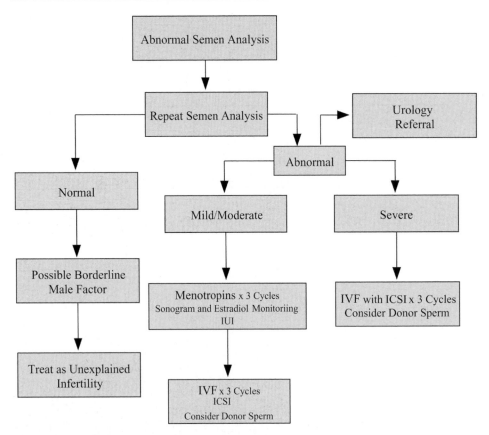

Figure 38-5 Treatment algorithm for infertile couple with male factor infertility. ICSI, intracytoplasmic sperm injection; IUI, intrauterine insemination; IVF, in vitro fertilization.

hyperstimulation prior to IVF. A treatment algorithm for male factor infertility is outlined in **Fig. 38-5.** In men with repeat abnormal semen analysis, an enhanced sperm penetration assay (SPA) as well as referral to a urologist specializing in male infertility may be considered. Persistent infertility can be treated with IVF with consideration of ICSI or the use of donor sperm.

Tubal-Uterine Evaluation

HYSTEROSALPINGOGRAPHY

HSG is an important tool in infertility evaluation. A history of PID, septic abortion, ruptured appendix, tubal surgery, or ectopic pregnancy alerts the physician to the possibility of tubal damage. The HSG provides information regarding the shape of the uterine cavity and patency of the fallopian tubes. It should be performed in the early follicular phase of the cycle, as soon as menstrual bleeding has ceased. This eliminates the risk of reflux of blood or performance of the procedure during early conception. The small chance of infection (1%) can be reduced by the following: (1) avoid performing the procedure in the presence of significant pelvic tenderness or adnexal mass suspected to be a tubo-ovarian complex; (2) preprocedure chlamydia and/or gonococcal screening; (3) prophylactic antibiotics (usually doxycycline 100 mg bid beginning the day before the procedure and continuing until the day after; and (4) Betadine application to the cervix before this procedure.

There is some evidence that an HSG itself is therapeutic and pregnancies have been reported following the procedure (Alper et al, 1986). In rare instances, HSG can result in an allergic reaction or infection. Women who are allergic to iodinated contrast or are suspected of having occult infections should not undergo this procedure; instead, the pelvis is evaluated by laparoscopy and chromotubation.

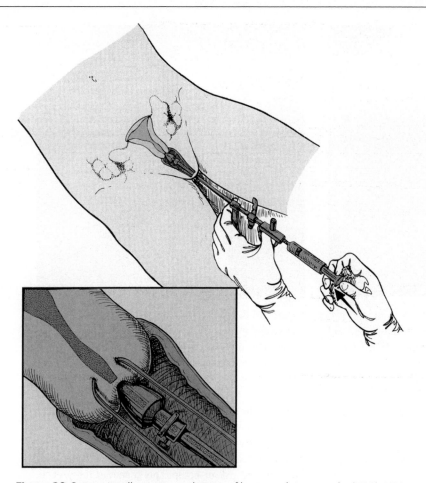

Figure 38-6 Drawing illustrating technique of hysterosalpingography (HSG). HSG provides information about the uterine cavity and fallopian tube patency. It is usually performed on cycle days 6 through 10. For most women, this is the time between the cessation of menstrual bleeding and ovulation. The cervix is cleansed with disinfectant. After stabilization with a tenaculum, and placement of the cannula, approximately 3 to 5 mL of radiopaque contrast is injected. This allows visualization of the endocervical canal, uterine cavity, and both tubes. (Reproduced with permission from Buster JE. Diagnostic Evaluation of the Infertile Couple. Philadelphia: Current Medicine; 1999: Fig. 9–17A, p 9.8. Stenchever MA, Mishell DR Jr, eds. Atlas of Clinical Gynecology; vol 3.)

HSG is performed under fluoroscopy and a minimal number of films are taken. Following an initial film, 3 to 5 mL contrast is slowly injected to visualize the uterine cavity. This is of special importance in DES-exposed women, many of whom have abnormalities of uterine contour. Cervical traction is often necessary to completely evaluate the uterine cavity. A small acorn tip is preferred over balloon-type catheters because the latter obstructs visualization of the cavity (**Fig. 38-6**). Another 5 mL contrast is injected to assess tubal patency. A follow-up film is obtained to evaluate peritubal adhesions (after 10 min when using water-soluble contrast or after 24 hours when using oil-based contrast). Use of a prostaglandin synthesis inhibitor 30 minutes prior to the procedure can decrease the pain associated with HSG (Owens et al, 1985).

In a retrospective review of 130 women reporting at least 1 year of unprotected intercourse without conception with a normal HSG, pelvic examination, historical screening for pelvic inflammatory disease, prolactin and thyroxine assays, postcoital test, confirmation of ovulation, and normal partner semen analysis, laparoscopy showed normal pelvic anatomy in only 42.3% (El-Yahia, 1994). Pelvic

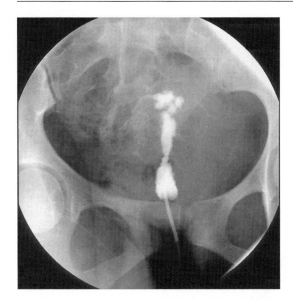

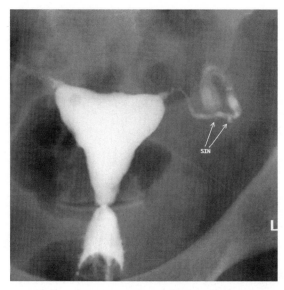

Figure 38-7 Chronic granulomatous endometritis. Twenty-nine-year-old woman with a positive PPD and 10-year history of primary infertility. Patient denied history of prior uterine instrumentation. The chest radiograph showed evidence of prior granulomatous disease with a Ranke complex. Hysterosalpingogram shows a markedly abnormal uterus with small capacity and multiple irregular filling defects most compatible with synechiae. Dilation and curettage were performed and revealed chronic granulomatous endometritis, and acid fast bacilli were identified by Fite's stain.

Figure 38-8 Salpingitis isthmica nodosa (SIN). Thirty-two-year-old woman with history of right salpingectomy for ectopic pregnancy. Hysterosalpingogram shows a normal uterine cavity and endocervical canal. The right fallopian tube is not opacified. The left fallopian tube has several diverticula along the isthmus (arrows) and is markedly dilated in the ampullary segment, consistent with hydrosalpinx. No free spillage of contrast into the peritoneal cavity is seen. SIN is an inflammatory condition of the fallopian tubes associated with infertility and an increased risk of ectopic pregnancy (Creasy et al, 1985). The diagnosis is best made radiographically at HSG, where the characteristic finding consists of multiple nodular diverticular spaces in close approximation to the true tubal lumen (By permission from Jenkins et al, 1993).

adhesions were found in 20.8%. Other abnormalities included pelvic endometriosis, PID, and uterine leiomyoma. Thus, in the presence of a normal HSG, the following is recommended: (1) laparoscopy not be performed until 3 months after a normal HSG because of the potential therapeutic effect of HSG; (2) laparoscopy be performed after a normal HSG if pregnancy has not occurred by 6 months to 1 year because of the high incidence of pelvic pathology; and (3) HSG using water-soluble contrast media has a therapeutic effect comparable to that described for oil-soluble contrast media (Cundiff et al, 1995). **Figs. 38-7** through **38-10** show examples of abnormalities seen on HSG.

SONOHYSTEROGRAPHY

Sonohysterography is ultrasonography of the uterus following injection of saline into the uterine cavity through a no. 8 pediatric Foley catheter with the balloon inflated in the cervix (**Figs. 38-11** and **38-12**). Sonohysterography is more sensitive than HSG in the identification of uterine polyps or myomata and causes less patient discomfort (Session et al, 1997; Soares et al, 2000).

Mild distal tubal disease may be amenable to laparoscopic tuboplasty, whereas moderate to severe tubal occlusion is most effectively managed with IVF (**Fig. 38-13**) (Schlaff et al, 1990). When a proximal tubal occlusion is evident on HSG, laparoscopy and hysteroscopy with tubal cannulation may be performed (**Fig. 38-14**). Uterine filling defects are evaluated with hysteroscopy and treated appropriately. Patients with a normal HSG and laparoscopy are treated according to the unexplained infertility algorithm (**Fig. 38-15**).

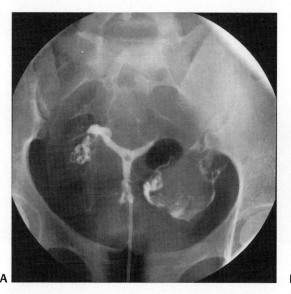
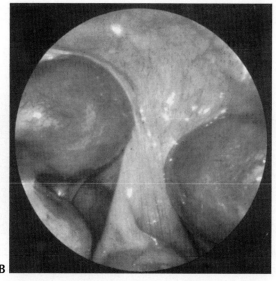

Figure 38-9 (A) Bicornuate uterus. Hysterosalpingogram (HSG) shows a deep fundal impression in the uterine cavity. The fallopian tubes are normal. There is free spillage of contrast material into the peritoneal cavity bilaterally. A bicornuate uterus cannot be distinguished from a septate uterus on the basis of the HSG alone. As the latter may be associated with a relatively high incidence of spontaneous abortion that may be overcome by surgical correction, certainty with regard to diagnosis is mandatory (Lavergne et al, 1996; Heinonen, 1997). Laparoscopy allows distinguishing these two entities. If the uterus is septated, during direct visualization the fundal surface is suggestive of a single myometrial mass, whereas the fundus is bilobular in the presence of uterine duplication. **(B)** Bicornuate uterus. Laparoscopyshows a band of fibrous tissue separating the cornua of the bilobar uterine fundus. A bicornuate uterus has a single cervix, a heart-shaped fundus, and two uterine cavities separated by myometrium. Conversely, a septate uterus has a single cervix, a flat fundus, and two uterine cavities separated by relatively avascular scar tissue. (See Color Plate 38–9B.)

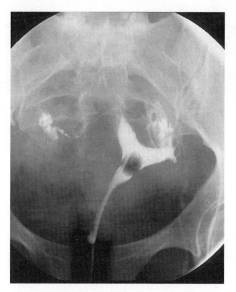

Figure 38-10 Arcuate uterus. Hysterosalpingogram shows prompt filling of both fallopian tubes with free spill into the peritoneum bilaterally. The intercornuate distance measures 33 mm. The distance from the inter-cornuate line to the contrast filling the uterine cavity at the fundus measures 7.8 mm. The arcuate uterus had no impact on reproduction (Raga et al, 1997).

TIMING OF TESTING

In the first month of evaluation, the use of condoms or barrier contraceptives is recommended. On day 1, the woman begins the basal body temperature recording. An HSG is scheduled for days 6 to 10 of the cycle to avoid menstruation and the possibility of radiation exposure to a potential embryo. Home urine LH testing is begun on days 10 through 18. A serum progesterone level is obtained 7 days after the LH surge. An endometrial biopsy is obtained on days 25 to 28, most accurately dated to LH surge. During this time, a semen analysis is also obtained.

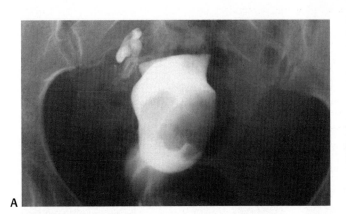
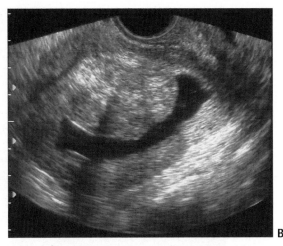

Figure 38-11 Leiomyomata. (**A**) Hysterosalpingogram: shows multiple filling defects in the uterine cavity consistent with the presence of leiomyomata. (**B**) Sonohysterography: Longitudinal view after saline infusion shows a large anterior wall leiomyoma.

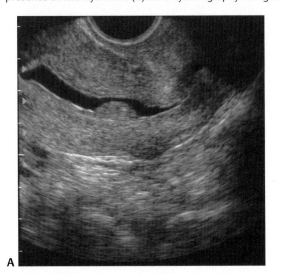
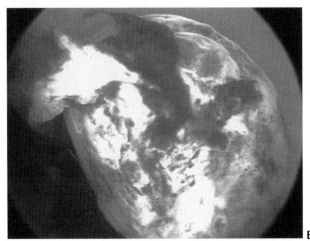

Figure 38-12 Polyps. (**A**) Sonohysterography: Longitudinal view after saline infusion sonography shows a smoothly marginated structure projecting from the posterior endometrial surface of the lower uterine body. This appears to extend from the basal layer of the endometrium and is consistent with a polyp. (**B**) Hysteroscopic polypectomy specimen. The histological diagnosis was benign endometrial polyp. (See Color Plate 38–12B.)

In the second month, a follow-up visit is scheduled between days 12 to 14 or following the LH surge, at which time a postcoital test is performed (if indicated). At this time, test results, HSG films, and other data are reviewed with the couple. Further evaluation may be indicated if all tests are normal, or laparoscopy is indicated if the HSG suggests tubal pathology. Hysteroscopy is optional unless uterine pathology is suggested on HSG.

Further Diagnostic Testing

LAPAROSCOPY

The next frequently done tests in infertility evaluation are laparoscopy and/or hysteroscopy. Laparoscopy is performed when all other tests have been normal or when there is reason to suspect intra-abdominal pathology (such as endometriosis or pelvic adhesions). Laparoscopy is scheduled in the early to midfollicular phase of the cycle to avoid disrupting a pregnancy or a well-vascularized corpus luteum. At this stage of the cycle, the thickness of the endometrium is low, allowing for accurate evaluation of the uterine cavity. If hysteroscopic surgery is planned because of abnormality seen on HSG (leiomyomata,

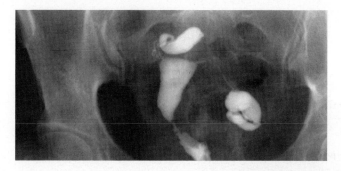

Figure 38-13 Bilateral large hydrosalpinges. Hysterosalpingogram shows anormal endocervical canal and a normal uterine cavity. Large bilateral hydrosalpinges are present.

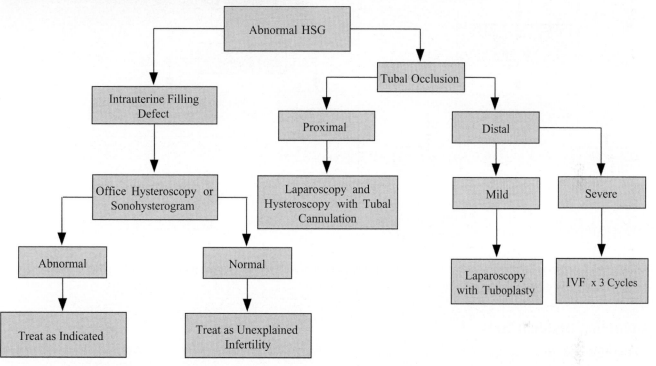

Figure 38-14 Treatment algorithm for infertile couple with uterotubal infertility diagnosed by an abnormal hysterosalpingogram. HSG, hysterosalpingography; IVF, in vitro fertilization.

adhesions, or septums), it may be useful to pretreat the patient with gonadotropin-releasing hormone (GnRH) analogs or oral contraceptive pills to reduce the height of the endometrium, thereby increasing visualization.

Most infertility procedures (lysis of adhesions, removal or ablation of endometriosis lesions, or tubal surgery) can be performed via the laparoscope by a reproductive endocrinologist or reproductive surgeon. Hysteroscopy usually requires dilation of the cervix and use of a distending medium such as Hyscon, sorbitol, glycine, or saline. Following this procedure, a cannula or catheter should be inserted into the cervix so that methylene blue or indigo carmine dye can be injected to evaluate tubal patency during laparoscopy.

Laparoscopy is performed under general anesthesia in a steep Trendelenburg position. A systematic and thorough evaluation is required in a planned and organized manner to rule out pelvic pathology, including evaluation of the undersurface of the ovaries. Photograph or video recording is helpful for documenting disease. In women who have a normal laparoscopy or who have undergone surgical correction of either endometriosis or adhesions, expectant management, or a more aggressive treatment for "unexplained infertility," may be pursued. Utilizing this algorithm, patients undergo three cycles of CC stimulation with sonographic monitoring, hCG, and IUI. If no pregnancy results, three cycles of gonadotropin therapy and IUI should be offered prior to proceeding to IVF.

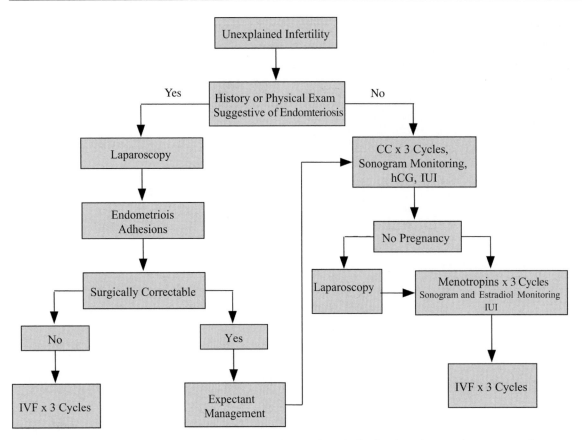

Figure 38-15 Treatment algorithm for infertile couple with unexplained infertility. hCG, human chorionic gonadotropin; IUI, intrauterine insemination; IVF, in vitro fertilization.

Additional Optional Tests

POSTCOITAL TESTING

A postcoital test has been advocated to evaluate the presence of cervical factors. Unfortunately, most poor postcoital tests are the result of improper timing. Most often, the test is performed on day 12 of the cycle, but if ovulation occurs earlier or later, the test often results in immobile sperm. It has been our observation that many so-called cervical factors have as their origin poor timing or inadequate follicle development with poor estrogen production. There is considerable lack of standardization in postcoital testing. We advocate that the test be done 24 to 36 hours prior to ovulation determined by urinary LH testing and that 0 to 4 hours elapse between intercourse and the examination. At that time, one should find an open cervix and clear cervical mucus with spinnbarkeit of 8 to 10 cm (length of stretch of the cervical mucus), five to 15 directionally motile sperm per high-power field, and the presence of ferning of the cervical mucus. Despite the manner in which the postcoital test is carried out, some investigators have suggested that it provides little information regarding potential fertility (Griffith and Grimes, 1990). Support for this contention comes from the finding of sperm in the peritoneal fluid at laparoscopy in patients having poor postcoital tests and the finding that 27% of fertile couples show either no sperm or less than one sperm per high-power field in their postcoital test (Asch, 1978). Nevertheless, at a minimum, a normal postcoital test provides information about the adequacy of coital technique. Our approach to cervical factor infertility is identical to our empirical approach to unexplained infertility, largely because of our abandonment of the postcoital test.

SPERM ANTIBODIES

Antisperm antibodies are found in <2% of fertile men and women in serum, sperm, and cervical mucus, and in 5 to 25% of infertile couples (Kutteh et al, 1992; Marshburn and Kutteh, 1994). Individuals selected for testing include those with conditions in which the blood–testis or excurrent ductal system is breached, such as testicular biopsy, vasectomy reversal, or obstructive lesions of the male ductal system. Sperm agglutination is frequently a result of genital tract infection due to prostatitis, urethritis, or epididymitis. These disorders should be treated with antibiotics before testing for sperm antibodies. The absence of motile sperm in midcycle cervical mucus after intercourse has been correlated with sperm-associated antisperm antibodies in approximately 50% of men (Mathur et al, 1984). As many as 17% of women in couples with unexplained infertility are found to have serum antisperm antibodies. Women with a history of frequent receptive anal or oral intercourse should be considered for antisperm antibody testing (Marshburn and Kutteh, 1994).

Clumping found on the standard semen analysis may also be consistent with antibodies. Specific tests for antisperm antibodies in cervical mucus, serum, and seminal plasma are available, and at present the Immunobead Assay is recommended. A direct assay is preferred in the male, whereas an indirect one is performed in the female. The significance of these tests in regard to infertility workup is not always clear because some couples have been known to conceive in the presence of high levels of antisperm antibodies. However, it is believed that decreased or impaired movement of sperm through genital tract secretions and failure of fertilization may be due to sperm antibodies. Patients with high levels of antibodies and prolonged infertility should be offered IVF with possible ICSI (Bates, 1997; Mardesic et al, 2000).

Summary

- Infertility affects about 10 to 15% of couples in the reproductive age group.
- The major causes of infertility are a male factor (30–40%), ovulatory dysfunction (15–20%), or tuboperitoneal disease (30–40%). No cause can be found in about 10%, whereas 20 to 40% may have multiple factors.
- Peak rate of conception in both men and women occurs at age 24 and begins to decline significantly after age 35 so that for every 5 years, the length of time for conception doubles.
- The incidence of impaired fertility also increases with advanced maternal age: 11.7% in women <25 years and 42.1% for women 35 years and older.

Further Reading

Abma JC, Chandra A, Mosher WD, et al. Fertility, family planning, and women's health: new data from the 1995 National Survey of Family Growth. Vital Health Stat 23 1997;19:1–114

Alper MM, Garner PR, Spence JEH, et al. Pregnancy rates after hysterosalpingography with oil- and water-soluble contrast media. Obstet Gynecol 1986;68:6–9

Arici A, Byrd W, Bradshaw K, et al. Evaluation of clomiphene citrate and human chorionic gonadotropin treatment: a prospective, randomized, crossover study during intrauterine insemination cycles. Fertil Steril 1994;61:314–318

Asch RH. Sperm recovery in peritoneal aspirate after negative Sims-Huhner test. Int J Fertil 1978; 23:57–60

Baird DD, Wilcox AJ. Cigarette smoking associated with delayed conception. JAMA 1985;253:2979–2983

Bates CA. Antisperm antibodies and male subfertility. Br J Urol 1997;80:691–697

Bolumar F, Olsen J, Boldsen J. Smoking reduces fecundity: a European multicenter study on infertility and subfecundity. The European Study Group on Infertility and Subfecundity. Am J Epidemiol 1996;143:578–587

Bolumar F, Olsen J, Rebagliato M, et al. Caffeine intake and delayed conception: a European multi-center study on infertility and subfecundity. European Study Group on Infertility Subfecundity. Am J Epidemiol 1997;145:324–334

Campo S. Ovulatory cycles, pregnancy outcome and complications after surgical treatment of polycystic ovary syndrome. Obstet Gynecol Surv 1998;53:297–308

Collins JA, Wrixon W, Janes LB, et al. Treatment-independent pregnancy among infertile couples. N Engl J Med 1983;309:1201–1206

Conway GS, Jacobs HS. *Acanthosis nigricans* in obese women with the polycystic ovary syndrome: disease spectrum not distinct entity. Postgrad Med J 1990;66:536–538

Creasy JL, Clark RL, Cuttino JT, et al. Salpingitis isthmica nodosa: radiologic and clinical correlates. Radiology 1985;154:597–600

Cundiff G, Carr BR, Marshbum PB. Infertile couples with a normal hysterosalpingogram: reproductive outcome and its relationship to clinical and laparoscopic findings. J Reprod Med 1995;40:19–24

Dodson WC, Haney AF. Controlled ovarian hyperstimulation and intrauterine insemination for treatment of infertility. Fertil Steril 1991;55:457–467

El-Yahia AW. Laparoscopic evaluation of apparently normal infertile women. Aust N Z J Obstet Gynaecol 1994;34:440–442

Fundamental considerations. In: Keller DW, Strickler RC, Warren JC, eds. Clinical Infertility. Norwalk, CT: Appleton-Century-Crofts; 1984:1–9

Gindoff PR, Jewelewicz R. Reproductive potential in the older woman. Fertil Steril 1986;46:989–1001

Gray RH. Epidemiology of infertility. Curr Opin Obstet Gynecol 1990;2:154–158

Griffith CS, Grimes DA. The validity of the post-coital test. Am J Obstet Gynecol 1990;162:615–620

Gunalp S, Onculoglu C, Gurgan T, et al. A study of semen parameters with emphasis on sperm morphology in a fertile population: an attempt to develop clinical thresholds. Hum Reprod 2001;16:110–114

Guzick D, Bradshaw KD, Grun B, et al. Factors affecting the probability of pregnancy in a cycle of donor insemination [abstract]. Proc Am Fert Soc 1986;35:170

Hammond EC. Smoking in relation to physical complaints. Arch Environ Health 1961;3:146–164

Heinonen PK. Reproductive performance of women with uterine anomalies after abdominal or hysteroscopic metroplasty or no surgical treatment. J Am Assoc Gynecol Laparosc 1997;4:311–317

Hembree WC, Zeidenberg P, Nahas GG. Marijuana's effect on human gonadal function. In: Nahas GG, ed. Marijuana, Chemistry, Biochemistry and Cellular Effects. New York; Springer-Verlag; 1976:521–532

Hendershot GE, Mosher WD, Pratt WF. Infertility and age: an unresolved issue. Fam Plann Perspect 1982;14:287–289

Hensleigh PA, Fainstat T. Corpus luteum dysfunction: serum progesterone levels in diagnosis and assessment of therapy for recurrent and threatened abortion. Fertil Steril 1979;32:396–400

James W. The causes of the decline in fecundability with age. Soc Biol 1979;26:330–334

Jenkins CS, Williams SR, Schmidt GE. Salpingitis isthmica nodosa: a review of the literature, discussion of clinical significance, and consideration of patient management. Fertil Steril 1993;60:599–607

Krausz C, Quintana-Murci L, Barbaux S, et al. A high frequency of Y chromosome deletions in males with nonidiopathic infertility. J Clin Endocrinol Metab 1999;84:3606–3612

Krausz C, Rajpert-De Meyts E, Frydelund-Larsen L, et al. Double-blind Y chromosome microdeletion analysis in men with known sperm parameters and reproductive hormone profiles: microdeletions are specific for spermatogenic failure. J Clin Endocrinol Metab 2001;86:2638–2642

Kriplani A, Manchanda R, Agarwal N, et al. Laparoscopic ovarian drilling in clomiphene citrate-resistant women with polycystic ovary syndrome. J Am Assn of Gynecol Laparoscopists 2001;8:511–518

Kutteh WH, McAllister D, Byrd W, et al. Anti-sperm antibodies: current knowledge and new horizons. Mol Androl 1992;4:183–193

Lavergne N, Aristizabal J, Zarka V, et al. Uterine anomalies and in vitro fertilization: what are the results? Eur J Obstet Gynecol Reprod Biol 1996;68:29–34

Lobo RA, Paul W, March CM, et al. Clomiphene and dexamethasone in women unresponsive to clomiphene alone. Obstet Gynecol 1982;60:497–501

Marcoux S, Maheux R, Berube S. Laparoscopic surgery in infertile women with minimal or mild endometriosis. Canadian Collaborative Group on Endometriosis. N Engl J Med 1997;337:217–222

Mardesic T, Ulcova-Gallova Z, Huttelova R, et al. The influence of different types of antibodies on in vitro fertilization results. Am J Reprod Immunol 2000;43:1–5

Marshburn PB, Kutteh WH. The role of antisperm antibodies in infertility. Fertil Steril 1994;61:799–811

Mathur S, Williamson HO, Baker ME, et al. Sperm motility on postcoital testing correlates with male autoimmunity to sperm. Fertil Steril 1984;41:81–87

Mosher WD, Pratt WF. Fecundity and infertility in the United States: incidence and trends. Fertil Steril 1991;56:192–193

Najmabadi H, Huang V, Yen P, et al. Substantial prevalence of microdeletions of the Y-chromosome in infertile men with idiopathic azoospermia and oligozoospermia detected using a sequence-tagged site-based mapping strategy. J Clin Endocrinol Metab 1996;81:1347–1352

Nestler JE, Stovall D, Akhter N, et al. Strategies for the use of insulin-sensitizing drugs to treat infertility in women with polycystic ovary syndrome. Fertil Steril 2002;77:209–215

Owens OM, Schiff I, Kaul AF, et al. Reduction of pain following hysterosalpingogram by prior analgesic administration. Fertil Steril 1985;43:146–148

Peters AJ, Lloyd RP, Coulam CB. Prevalence of out-of-phase endometrial biopsy specimens. Am J Obstet Gynecol 1992;166:1738–1745

Polson DW, Mason HD, Franks S. Bromocriptine treatment of women with clomiphene-resistant polycystic ovary syndrome. Clin Endocrinol (Oxf) 1987;26:197–203

Raga F, Bauset C, Remohi J, et al. Reproductive impact of congenital Mullerian anomalies. Hum Reprod 1997;12:2277–2281

Schlaff WD, Hassiakos DK, Damewood MD, et al. Neosalpingostomy for distal tubal obstruction: prognostic factors and impact of surgical technique. Fertil Steril 1990;54:984–990

Schwartz D, Mayaux MJ. Female fecundity as a function of age: results of artificial insemination in 2193 nulliparous women with azoospermic husbands. Federation CECOS. N Engl J Med 1982;306:404–406

Scott RT Jr, Hofmann GE. Prognostic assessment of ovarian reserve. Fertil Steril 1995;63:1–11

Serafini P, Batzofin J, Nelson J, et al. Sonographic uterine predictors of pregnancy in women undergoing ovulation induction for assisted reproductive treatments. Fertil Steril 1994;62:815–822

Session DR, Lee GS, Kelly AC. A comparison of pain tolerance during x-ray hysterosalpingography and sonohysterosalpingography. Albunex Study Group. Gynecol Obstet Invest 1997;43:116–119

Soares SR, Barbosa dos Reis MM, Camargos AF. Diagnostic accuracy of sonohysterography, transvaginal sonography, and hysterosalpingography in patients with uterine cavity diseases. Fertil Steril 2000;73:406–411

Speroff L, Glass RH, Kase NG. Clinical Gynecologic Endocrinology and Infertility. 6th ed. Baltimore: Lippincott Williams & Wilkins; 1999

Tietze C, Guttmacher AF, Rusin S. Time required for conception in 1727 planned pregnancies. Fertil Steril 1950;1:338–346

CHAPTER 39 Fallopian Tube Recanalization

Amanjit Gill and Lindsay Machan

Clinical Presentation

A 31-year-old Caucasian woman was evaluated for primary infertility. She had been unable to conceive despite 2 years of appropriately timed unprotected intercourse. She had regular menstrual cycles and denied any history of pelvic inflammatory, sexually transmitted, or systemic disease. Her husband's semen analysis was normal. Physical examination was normal and basal body temperature chart and luteal phase serum progesterone both confirmed ovulation.

Radiological Studies

A hysterosalpingogram (HSG) demonstrated a normal uterine cavity. There was no contrast opacification of either fallopian tube (**Fig. 39-1A**).

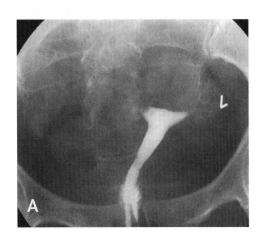

Figure 39-1 Therapeutic fallopian tube recanalization. (**A**) The initial hysterosalpingogram (HSG) demonstrates no opacification of either fallopian tube.

Diagnosis

Infertility due to bilateral proximal fallopian tube occlusion

Treatment Options and Treatment

Infertility due to proximal tubal occlusion can be treated by restoration of tubal patency or assisted reproductive technologies such as in vitro fertilization (IVF) or intracytoplasmic sperm injection (ICSI), bypassing the issue of tubal egg transport. Tubal occlusions can be repaired surgically or by transcervical fallopian tube recanalization (FTR). FTR is the only means of restoring tubal patency without laparotomy. Although FTR can be performed under fluoroscopic, sonographic, or endoscopic guidance, the highest technical success rate is achieved with fluoroscopic guidance. Assisted reproductive techniques are expensive, complex, and potentially stressful. They

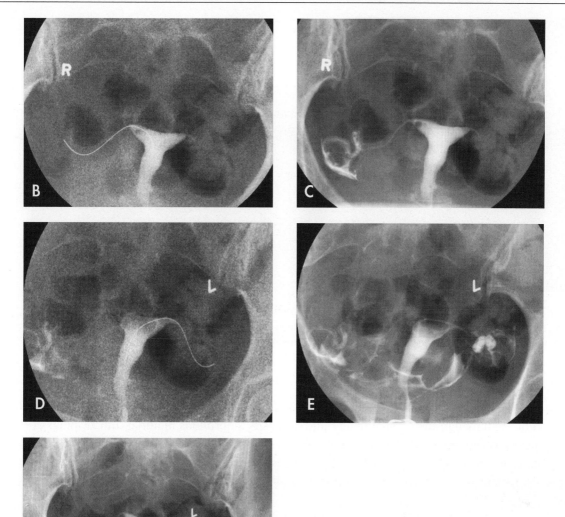

Figure 39-1 *(Continued)* (**B**) Recanalization of the right fallopian tube by passage of a 3F straight catheter and guide wire coaxially through a 5.5F catheter positioned at the cornu. (**C**) Salpingogram after recanalization shows a normal-appearing right fallopian tube. (**D**) Recanalization of the left fallopian tube with a 3F catheter and guide wire. (**E**) Salpingogram after recanalization shows a patent left fallopian tube. (**F**) The completion HSG shows bilateral fallopian tube opacification and peritoneal spill.

are indicated in patients with proximal fallopian tubal occlusion when the cause of infertility is multifactorial (e.g., advanced age of the woman, endometriosis, hormonal or ovarian abnormalities, and/or male factor infertility) or when procedures to restore tubal patency have failed. The American Society of Reproductive Technology recommends that in patients with cornual tube obstruction, fallopian tube cannulation be performed prior to institution of assisted reproductive techniques. However, in practice, often turf and economic considerations may determine which therapy the patient receives.

The patient described here underwent outpatient fluoroscopically guided FTR (see **Fig. 39-1**).

Discussion

Fallopian tube disease is the most common cause of female infertility. The most common test to evaluate the fallopian tubes is the HSG. In 10 to 25% of HSGs performed for infertility, contrast fails

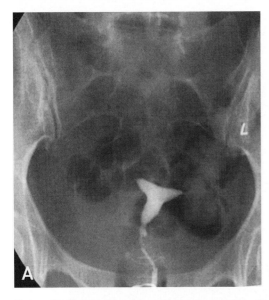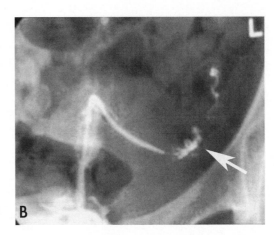

Figure 39-2 Fallopian tube occlusion due to salpingitis isthmica nodosa. (**A**) On the initial hysterosalpingogram, there is no contrast opacification of either fallopian tube. (**B**) The tube was patent at the cornu. The selective left salpingogram shows multiple diverticula in the isthmic region (arrow). These are typical for salpingitis isthmica nodosa.

to extend into the fallopian tubes. This may be due to inadequate injection pressure (technical factor); obstruction of the lumen in the cornual region due to spasm, amorphous material (mucus plugs), or tubal polyps; or cornual obstruction due to mural disease such as chronic salpingitis or previous surgery. The tubes may appear to be occluded proximally but the occlusion is due to lesions of the more distal segment by salpingitis isthmica nodosa, endometriosis, chronic salpingitis, or peritubal adhesions (**Fig. 39-2**).

In cases where a proximal tubal obstruction was diagnosed by HSG or laparoscopy, histology of the resected tubal specimens revealed no abnormality in 20% (obstruction presumably due to spasm), amorphous debris or minimal adhesions in 40%, and extensive fibrosis or salpingitis isthmica nodosa in 40%.

Selective salpingography performed after recanalization shows normal-appearing tubes in approximately one third of the patients. Approximately one third have patent tubes but the tubal anatomy and appearance of the peritoneal spill suggest peritubal adhesions. In the remainder, most demonstrate patent tubes with a focal dilation at the site of obstruction, tubal patency with salpingitis isthmica nodosa, or proximal patency and a distal hydrosalpinx.

Benefits and Potential Risks of FTR

Although FTR has been used for midtubal stenoses from salpingitis isthmica nodosa or occlusions occurring after tubal ligation reanastomosis, the principal indication is occlusion in the cornual region (the segment of the fallopian tube passing through the uterine wall).

Selective salpingography is valuable for differentiating spasm or transient obstruction from true tubal obstruction, identifying the etiology of an occlusion, and, frequently, demonstrating findings not evident at laparoscopy. In contrast to operative treatment of tubal occlusions, FTR is an outpatient procedure with virtually no recovery time or morbidity and has a high technical success rate. This is particularly important in this group of patients because infertility is not an illness.

Technique

Pretreatment assessment by an infertility specialist or gynecologist includes verification of appropriately timed unprotected intercourse for at least 1 year, confirmation of ovulation, physical examination, and assessment of male partner fertility. If the physical examination reveals an abnormality, the patient undergoes a pelvic ultrasound and laparoscopy with assessment of tubal patency by methylene blue injection. If the physical examination is normal, an HSG is obtained. If a tubal abnormality is demonstrated, some specialists proceed with selective salpingography at the same sitting. (For a detailed discussion of infertility evaluation, refer to Chapter 38.)

The fallopian tube recanalization procedure is performed on an outpatient basis during the first 5 days after the menstrual bleeding has stopped. Antibiotic prophylaxis (doxycycline 100 mg PO twice a day) is started on the evening prior to or on the morning of the procedure and continued for 3 to 5 days post-procedure. Informed consent should include the discussion of the possibility of ectopic pregnancy, tubal perforation, vasovagal reaction, idiosyncratic reaction to the contrast agent, and adnexal infection. The patient should arrange for someone to drive her home after the procedure because she will have received sedation and analgesia.

Premedication consists of intravenous midazolam (Versed) 2 mg and fentanyl 100 μg. As distention of the uterus can be very uncomfortable, additional amounts of analgesia may be required.

For the procedure, the patient is placed in a lithotomy position and foam padding is used to elevate the buttocks. Foam pads placed beneath the knees are also preferable to stirrups. The perineum is prepped with Betadine (povidone iodine) and sterile draped. A warmed vaginal speculum is inserted and the uterine cervix is also prepped with Betadine. The cervix is then sprayed with topical Xylocaine and the cervical os is cannulated. HSG is performed to reconfirm proximal tubal occlusion. Cannulation of the cervical os can be done with a tenaculum forceps and Tenacath (Cook Gynecology, Spencer, IN), a Sovak Hysterograph vacuum cup (Cook Incorp., Bloomington, IN), or an endocervical balloon catheter (Cook Incorp., Bloomington, IN).

A multipurpose-shaped catheter is coaxially inserted through the cervical cannula (e.g., a Thurmond–Rosch Fallopian Recanalization Kit, Cook Incorp., Bloomington, IN) and the ostium of the occluded tube is catheterized. Difficulty in advancing an angled catheter into a cornu because of uterine flexion or angulation can usually be overcome by applying traction on the cervix with a tenaculum placed at the 12 o'clock position. This will straighten the uterine cavity.

A selective salpingogram is obtained by injecting contrast into the tubal ostium. If the selective salpingogram confirms proximal tubal occlusion, a 3F straight catheter is inserted coaxially through the multipurpose catheter and the obstruction is probed with a 0.014 in. guide wire. Once the guide wire crosses the obstruction, it is followed with the 3F catheter. The guide wire is removed and contrast is injected through the 3F catheter to check patency of the distal tube.

Alternatively, the obstruction can be crossed with a 0.035 in. hydrophilic angled Glide wire (Terumo Medical Corporation, Tokyo, Japan). After crossing the obstruction, the guide wire is removed and contrast is injected through the catheter to confirm distal tubal patency.

After recanalizing one side, the same sequence of steps is repeated for the contralateral occlusion. A completion HSG may then be obtained through the cervical cannula to document tubal patency. The tube that was recanalized first may not opacify on the completion HSG. This is due to spasm and does not warrant repeated catheterization.

POST-PROCEDURE CARE

The patient is observed for 60 minutes after the procedure. The intraprocedure findings and results are reviewed with the patient and her husband. The patient is also appraised of the possibility of vaginal spotting or pelvic cramping over the subsequent 1 to 2 days. The pain responds well to medication used for menstrual cramps. The patient is asked not to use tampons for any vaginal bleeding till her next cycle and to avoid intercourse for 24 hours.

Outcome

Technical success is achieved in 71 to 100% of patients with proximal tubal occlusion, 44 to 77% with occlusion after surgical reversal of tubal ligation, and 77 to 82% with occlusion due to salpingitis isthmica nodosa. Failure to engage the tubal ostium is most often due to severe flexion or angulation of the uterine cavity but may also be due to a congenital abnormality, uterine leiomyomata, or polyps. Inability to advance a catheter through an obstruction may be due to tubal scarring from salpingitis, endometriosis, or surgery.

Reported pregnancy rates vary, with an average of ~30%. The highest pregnancy rate of 58% was reported after an average follow-up of 1 year. This was observed in women who had been recommended tubal microsurgery or in vitro fertilization for documented, isolated proximal tubal obstruction. All pregnancies were intrauterine. A randomized prospective study comparing FTR to other therapies has not been done and is not likely to be possible. Allowing for this limitation, published pregnancy rates in comparable patient cohorts are very similar to those for tubal micro-surgery and assisted fertility techniques. Approximately 25% of tubes opened by FTR will reocclude by 6 months. If the patient is not pregnant by that time, the tubes should be reevaluated and reopened if necessary.

Complications

- *Tubal perforation:* The fallopian tube is a thick, muscular structure and does not perforate easily. The incidence of perforation is 2% and no adverse sequelae have been reported. No additional monitoring or treatment is required. Perforation is visualized as free contrast into the peritoneal cavity. A submucosal perforation is more common and appears as an extraluminal pooling of contrast or venous intravasation.
- *Ectopic pregnancy:* Tubal pregnancies occur in 3% of patients after FTR. The risk of tubal pregnancy is increased in the presence of tubal mucosal abnormalities or peritubal adhesions.
- *Pelvic infection:* Pelvic infection following fallopian tube recanalization has not been reported.
- *Radiation exposure:* The absorbed radiation dose to the ovaries from this procedure is 0.85 cGy, a dose that is acceptable for women of reproductive age. In contrast to the fertilized gamete, the ovum (before fertilization) is relatively radioresistant. In addition, the procedure is performed during the follicular phase of the menstrual cycle to ensure that the patient is not pregnant. The radiation dose also depends upon the equipment used and the number of radiographs obtained. At our institution, pulsed fluoroscopy is used and the fluoroscopic images are stored to document different steps of the procedure. Radiographs are obtained only when diagnostic information from an HSG or selective salpingogram is required.

PEARLS AND PITFALLS_____

- Fallopian tube disease is the most common cause of female infertility.
- The fallopian tubes fail to opacify in 10 to 25% of HSGs performed for infertility. The etiology includes technical factors, cornual spasm, mucus plugs or polyps, mural tubal disease, and after surgery.
- Technical success of transcervical fallopian tube recanalization is between 71 and 100% for proximal tubal occlusion, 44 and 77% for occlusion post–tubal ligation reversal surgery, and 77 and 82% for salpingitis isthmica nodosa.

- Published pregnancy rates are comparable to those after tubal microsurgery and assisted fertility techniques.

Further Reading

Houston JG, Machan LS. Salpingitis isthmica nodosa: technical success and outcome of fluoroscopic transcervical fallopian tube recanalization. Cardiovasc Intervent Radiol 1998;21:31–35

Maubon AJ, De Graef M, Boncoeur-Martel MP, et al. Interventional radiology in female infertility: technique and role. Eur Radiol 2001;11:771–778

Papaioannou S, Afnan M, Coormarasamay A, et al. Long-term safety of fluoroscopically guided selective salphingography and tubal catheterization. Hum Reprod 2002;17:370–372

Papaioannou S, Afnan M, Girling AJ, et al. Diagnostic and therapeutic value of selective salphingography and tubal catheterization in an unselected infertile population. Fertil Steril 2003;79:613–617

Pinto AB, Hovsepian DM, Wattanakumtomkul S, et al. Pregnancy outcomes after fallopian tube recanalization: oil-based versus water-soluble contrast agents. J Vasc Interv Radiol 2003;14:69–74

Thurmond AS. Imaging of female infertility. Radiol Clin North Am 2003;41:757–767

Thurmond AS. Pregnancies after selective salphingography and tubal recanalization. Radiology 1994;190:11–13

Thurmond AS, Brandt KR, Gorrill MJ. Tubal obstruction after ligation reversal surgery: results of catheter recanalization. Radiology 1999;210:747–750

Thurmond AS, Machan LS, Maubon AJ, et al. A review of selective salphingography and fallopian tube recanalization. Radiographics 2000;20:1759–1768

Thurmond A, Maubon A, Rouanet JP. Tubal diseases: from diagnosis to intervention. J Radiol 2001;82: 1857–1863

Zagoria RJ. Transcervical fallopian tube recanalization. Appl Radiol 1995;24:34–39

CHAPTER 40 Transcervical Lysis of Intrauterine Adhesions

Vishvanath C. Karande

Clinical Presentation

A 32-year-old woman was evaluated for secondary infertility of 2 years' duration. Her menstrual cycles were regular, but she noticed that lately they had become scant and lasted for only 2 days. Her past history was significant for two elective terminations of pregnancy, each in the first trimester. On both occasions, dilatation and curettage were reported as having been uncomplicated. Her past medical history was otherwise unremarkable. Physical examination was normal. The infertility workup of the couple was otherwise negative.

Radiological Studies

A hysterosalpingogram (HSG) was obtained and demonstrated obliteration of two thirds of the uterine cavity (**Fig. 40-1A**). Some contrast was seen in the lower uterine segment and in the right cornu. The right fallopian tube was demonstrated to be patent. The left fallopian tube was not visualized.

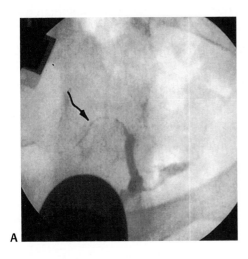

A

Figure 40-1 Intrauterine adhesions (Asherman's syndrome). (**A**) Hysterosalpingogram shows obliteration of two third's of the uterine cavity by adhesions. There is faint opacification of the right fallopian tube (arrow). The left tube is not visualized.

Diagnosis

Intrauterine adhesions (Asherman's syndrome)

Treatment

The intrauterine adhesions (IUAs) were mechanically lysed with 2 mm microlaparoscopy scissors (US Surgical Corporation, Norwalk, CT). These stainless steel scissors are a part of the Auto Suture Minisite laparoscopic reusable instrument set and are designed for use as an accessory during laparoscopy. They have a flush-port, which is used for irrigation purposes during laparoscopy (**Fig. 40-2**). They are stronger than the scissors used during hysteroscopy and therefore easily cut through adhesions. The scissors are inserted into the uterine cavity through the central channel of a routinely used cervical cannula (Conceptus, San Carlos, CA). For the purpose of delineating

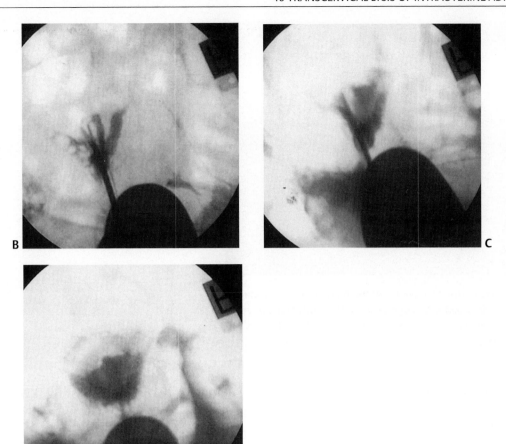

Figure 40–1 *(Continued)*. (**B,C**) Images showing progress of lysis of the intrauterine adhesions. (**D**) Uterine cavity configuration appears at the end of the procedure.

the adhesions during the procedure, radiographic contrast is injected through the flush-port by an assistant.

The procedure begins in the lower portion of the uterine cavity. The adhesions were then systematically lysed until the cavity had a relatively normal appearance (**Figs. 40-1B-D**). As the adhesions were lysed, contrast could be seen entering the left fallopian tube, which was subsequently demonstrated to be patent. The cervical cannula was then inserted into the uterine cavity and its balloon gently overinflated to further separate the adhesions. Flimsy adhesions can be lysed using the balloon alone, without resorting to use of the scissors. At the end of the procedure, a 14F pediatric Foley catheter was inserted into the uterine cavity and left in place for 3 days.

The patient was treated with doxycycline 100 mg twice daily for 3 days for infection prophylaxis. She was also given Premarin 1.25 mg (Wyeth-Ayerst, Philadelphia, PA) twice daily for 30 days to promote healing. Provera 10 mg (Pharmacia Upjohn, Kalamazoo, MI) once daily was added for the last 10 days of Premarin therapy. An HSG (not shown) obtained 1 month later showed a normal-appearing uterine cavity.

Discussion

The commonest factor antecedent to IUA is endometrial curettage during or shortly after an elective pregnancy termination. Other factors include evacuation of a hydatiform mole, cesarean section, myomectomy, diagnostic curettage, pelvic irradiation, and genital tuberculosis. IUA may be of three types: (1) multiple avascular strands of fibrous tissue between the anterior and posterior uterine walls, (2) vascularized and dense adhesions, which may contain inactive endometrium or

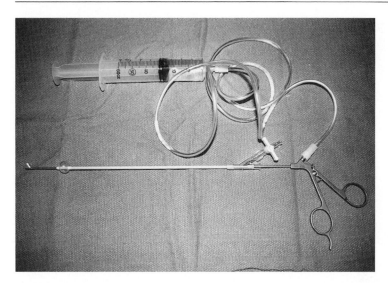

Figure 40-2 Instruments used for lysis of intrauterine adhesions. The micro-laparoscopy scissors are inserted through the central channel of a Conceptus Soft Seal Cervical Catheter. Contrast medium is injected through the flush-port of the hollow scissors.

myometrium, or (3) muscular adhesions where there is no endometrial basalis. The first two types are amenable to treatment, with a relatively good prognosis. Muscular adhesions carry an extremely poor prognosis because there is no viable endometrium. In such cases, no endometrial stripe is seen on ultrasound.

When the diagnosis of IUA is made with HSG, the patient is usually treated surgically via operative hysteroscopy under general anesthesia. The above-described technique makes it possible for the adhesions to be treated at the time of diagnosis, in one sitting. The cost savings are obvious because the expense of the operating room and general anesthesia are avoided. In addition, possible complications of hysteroscopy such as fluid overload and electrolyte imbalance are avoided. A major advantage of this technique is that it offers depth perception regarding completeness of the resection because the uterine cavity assumes a normal, triangular shape. In addition to lysis of uterine adhesions, this technique can be used for resection of a uterine septum.

Prior to the procedure, detailed informed consent must be obtained describing possible risks and complications, which include bleeding, infection, and uterine perforation with possible bowel injury. The amount of radiation exposure is well within safe limits and this should be explained to the patient as well. The procedure can generally be performed with a paracervical block alone. In apprehensive patients, it is prudent to utilize intravenous sedoanalgesia, a combination of fentanyl (Elkins-Sinn, Cherry Hill, NJ) and midazolam (Versed, Roche Laboratories, Nutley, NJ). In these cases, the patient's vital signs and oxygen saturation should be monitored continuously.

Precautions are necessary during this fluoroscopically guided procedure. The scissor handles should be carefully maintained in the plane of the uterine cavity. This ensures that the blades open and close in the plane of the cavity so that only the adhesions are lysed and the blades do not burrow into the myometrium. The procedure is quick and quite painless. However, if the myometrium is entered, there is some pain and an immediate extravasation of contrast into the myometrium. If this happens, one needs to wait for a few minutes for the extravasated contrast to clear into the circulation before proceeding with the rest of the lysis.

Unlike hysteroscopy, where large volumes of fluid are used to distend the uterine cavity, with fluoroscopic resection, low volumes of contrast medium are used and the cavity is therefore relatively flat (less distended). It is therefore easy to stay in the proper plane by maintaining the scissor handles (and therefore the blades) in the plane of the cavity. If the scissors need to be rotated during the procedure, the jaws must be closed prior to rotation. If the scissors are rotated with the jaws open, the patient will experience discomfort.

PEARLS AND PITFALLS_____

- Endometrial curettage is the commonest causative factor for intrauterine adhesions.
- With the technique described, intrauterine adhesionss can be treated at the time of diagnosis, avoiding a second, usually more expensive, surgical procedure.
- Microlaparoscopy scissors or the balloon from the cervical cannula can be used for the lysis.

Further Reading

Karande VC, Gleicher N. Resection of uterine septum using gynecoradiological techniques. Hum Reprod 1999;14:1226–1229

Karande V, Levrant S, Hoxsey R, et al. Lysis of intrauterine adhesions using gynecoradiologic techniques. Fertil Steril 1997;68:658–662

Karande VC, Pratt DE, Balin MS, et al. What is the radiation exposure to patients during a gynecoradiologic procedure? Fertil Steril 1997;67:401–403

Schenker JG. Etiology of and therapeutic approach to synechia uteri. Eur J Obstet Gynecol Reprod Biol 1996;65:109–113

CHAPTER 41 Uterine Cervix Dilation

Kevin W. Dickey

Clinical Presentation

A 32-year-old woman was evaluated for primary infertility. During the preceding workup, an attempt at endometrial biopsy was unsuccessful because of a suspected cervical stenosis. She was referred to interventional radiology for hysterosalpingography (HSG) and possible intervention.

Radiological Studies

HSG was performed with a balloon catheter and showed a retroflexed uterus with a narrowed cervical canal and two contrast-filled outpouchings (**Fig. 41-1**). The fallopian tubes were obstructed.

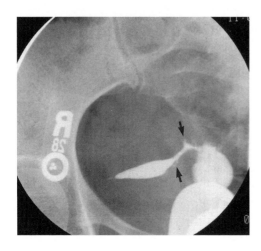

Figure 41-1 Hysterosalpingogram shows a narrowed, retroflexed endocervical canal with abnormal contrast filled outpouchings consistent with false passages (arrows). The fallopian tubes do not opacify.

Diagnosis

Uterine cervical stenosis; false passages created by previous instrumentation

Treatment Options

The use of rigid instruments to find the true lumen, especially within a uterus that is flexed, is prone to creation of false passages or repeated entry into those already created. Transabdominal ultrasound may be used to guide a rigid or semimalleable instrument through the cervical canal, although false passages can be difficult to identify. Visualization with hysteroscopy is limited in a severely narrowed cervical canal. With fluoroscopically assisted guide wire and catheter methods, the true cervical canal as well as any false passage or stenosis can be visualized. Once these abnormalities are demonstrated, they can be crossed and dilation can then be performed for treatment.

Treatment

Prior to the procedure, the patient was given an intravenous dose of doxycycline 100 mg. During the procedure, conscious sedation was administered using fentanyl (Elkins-Sinn, Cherry Hill, NJ) and

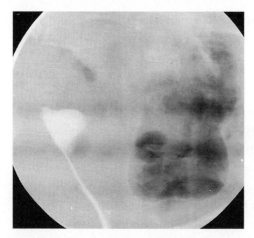

Figure 41-2 Under fluoroscopic guidance, a 5F Berenstein glide catheter has been advanced into the uterine cavity over a 0.035 in. J-tipped guide wire.

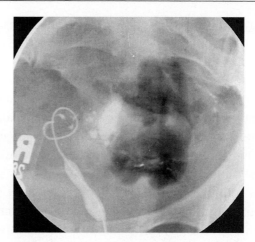

Figure 41-3 A 6 mm × 2 cm angioplasty balloon is used to dilate the narrowed and damaged cervical canal.

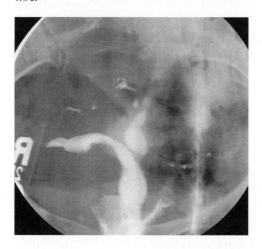

Figure 41-4 Postdilation hysterosalpingogram shows a wider cervical canal and less filling of false channels. This patient also underwent bilateral fallopian tube recanalization.

midazolam (Versed, Roche Laboratories, Nutley, NJ). With the patient on the fluoroscopic table in the lithotomy position, a speculum was inserted into the vagina. Under direct visualization, a 6F 23 cm long sheath was inserted into the cervix and water-soluble contrast material injected. The endocervical canal was opacified and the lesions identified (**Fig. 41-1**). Under fluoroscopic guidance, a 65 cm 5F Berenstein glide catheter (Boston Scientific, Inc., Natick, MA) and 0.035 in. 3 mm J-wire (Cook Incorp., Bloomington IN), were manipulated across the abnormally narrowed segment and past the false passages, into the uterine cavity (**Fig. 41-2**). The glide catheter was then exchanged for a 6 mm × 2 cm angioplasty balloon and the stenotic endocervical canal was dilated (**Fig. 41-3**). Upon completion of the dilation, an HSG was performed (**Fig. 41-4**). This patient subsequently underwent bilateral fallopian tube recanalization. She was discharged after a 1-hour recovery period. Two months after the dilation and fallopian tube recanalization, she underwent successful intrauterine insemination and gave birth to a healthy, full-term infant.

Discussion

Abnormalities of the exocervical os and endocervical canal are uncommon. When present, these can impede the diagnostic workup and treatment of infertility. The most common abnormalities are stenosis and false passage. A stenosis can be caused by previous cone biopsy, infection, and subsequent scarring, or may be congenital as in women who had in utero diethylstilbestrol (DES) exposure. False passage is the result of previous instrumentation of the endocervical canal, especially in the presence of a uterus that is ante- or retroflexed.

The normal diameter of the nulliparous cervical canal is 5 to 6 mm. Cervical stenosis that is not severe enough to cause hematometra has been associated with infertility. These endocervical lesions make it difficult to obtain an endometrial biopsy or provide a safe conduit for intrauterine insemination or embryo transfer. Under imaging guidance, traversing a tortuous and damaged endocervical canal is less traumatic and, in selected cases, more successful than the use of traditional methods of cannulating the cervix.

In a small study involving 15 women, Dickey et al (1996) performed cervical dilation in an outpatient setting. In two of the patients, an external drain (6 French All-Purpose Drainage catheter, Boston Scientific, Natick, MA) was placed to stent the cervical canal for a period of 4 weeks. In two patients, a sheath or catheter was left in place for immediate endometrial biopsy (as part of the workup for infertility). Of the 15 women treated, four conceived and three of the four carried pregnancies to term. The fourth woman had a spontaneous abortion at 8-week gestation. Abusheikha et al (1999) have subsequently published data in support of cervical dilation for cervical stenosis in preparation for in vitro fertilization–embryo transfer (IVF-ET). Although no large study has been performed, it appears that in selected patients, the effect of dilation can last for at least 6 months.

An additional study by Dickey and colleagues (2002) demonstrated the utility of cervical dilation techniques in the evaluation and treatment of women with postmenopausal bleeding. In this setting, endometrial biopsy is essential to the workup. Cervical stenosis may occur in these women due to atrophy or scarring. As is seen in the premenopausal population, instrumentation without imaging guidance can lead to failure of cannulation of the uterine cavity and the creation of false passages. Fluoroscopically guided crossing of the endocervical canal and balloon dilation can provide the necessary conduit for the gynecologist to perform an endometrial biopsy or hysteroscopy. This dilation procedure is usually performed in the operating room immediately prior to the gynecological procedure. In this small series, 13 of 14 postmenopausal women underwent successful transvaginal cervical dilation and all of them subsequently had a successful endometrial biopsy and/or hysteroscopy.

Abnormalities of the endocervical canal can be treated with dilation using fluoroscopy and a few standard tools of interventional practice. The true cervical lumen must be identified by contrast opacification of the uterine canal before dilation can be performed. The dilation may aid in the workup of infertility by providing a conduit for biopsy, may aid in infertility treatment by augmenting successful insemination or embryo transfer (techniques of assisted fertilization), or may provide safe passage for sperm transfer in unassisted fertilization. Moreover, this technique can be utilized in postmenopausal women to facilitate endometrial biopsy in the presence of a stenotic cervix. The amount of discomfort experienced during the procedure is easily controlled with conscious sedation, and the infection risk is minimal.

PEARLS AND PITFALLS

- Marked ante- or retroflexion of the uterus can make non-image-guided cervical canal instrumentation difficult and can lead to false passages and the development of stenoses.
- Using fluoroscopy and standard angiographic tools, the damaged cervical canal can be traversed and dilated.
- The true cervical lumen must be identified by contrast opacification of the uterine canal before dilation is performed.

Further Reading

Abusheikha N, Lass A, Akagbosu F, et al. How useful is cervical dilatation in patients with cervical stenosis who are participating in an in vitro fertilization-embryo transfer program? The Bourn Hall experience. Fertil Steril 1999;72:610–612

Dickey KW, Rao ST, Asis MC, et al. Transvaginal balloon dilation of the stenotic cervix in post-menopausal women: an aid to biopsy and curettage. J Vasc Interv Radiol 2002;13(Ann Meeting Suppl):S25

Dickey KW, Zreik T, Hsia H, et al. Transvaginal uterine cervical dilation with fluoroscopic guidance: preliminary results in patients with infertility. Radiology 1996;200:497–503

Luesley DM, Redman CWE, Buxton EJ, et al. Prevention of post–cone biopsy cervical stenosis using a temporary cervical stent. Br J Obstet Gynaecol 1990;97:334–337

Schmidt G, Fowler W. Cervical stenosis following minor gynecologic procedures on DES-exposed women. Obstet Gynecol 1980;56:333–335

Zreik TG, Dickey KW, Keefe DL, et al. Fluoroscopically guided cervical dilatation in patients with infertility. J Am Assoc Gynecol Laparosc 1996;3(Suppl 4):S56

SECTION IV
Retroperitoneum

CHAPTER 42 Nephrostomy and Ureteral Stenting
Carl F. Beckmann

Clinical Presentation

A 71-year-old man was seen at another hospital because of urinary retention. Transurethral resection of the prostate and bone scan established the diagnosis of a differentiated prostatic adenocarcinoma metastatic to the sacrum. Diethylstilbestrol, 1 mg/day was prescribed.

When first seen at our hospital, he had a 2-week history of decreased force and caliber of the urinary stream, occasional right flank pain, frequency, and dysuria. Blood urea nitrogen was 61 mg/dL and creatinine was 3.5 mg/dL. Cystoscopy revealed a small, contracted urinary bladder and a trigone full of tumor. The ureteral orifices could not be identified. He experienced an episode of septicemia, which responded to antibiotic therapy.

Radiological Studies

An excretory urogram was obtained and revealed bilateral distal ureteral obstruction (**Fig. 42-1**).

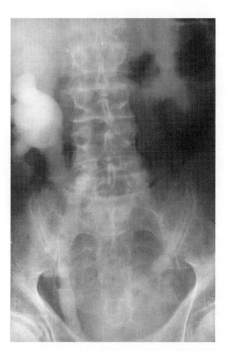

Figure 42-1 A 60-minute film from an intravenous pyelogram shows distal ureteral obstruction with bilateral hydronephrosis and hydroureter.

Diagnosis

Stage D carcinoma of the prostate and bilateral ureteral obstruction

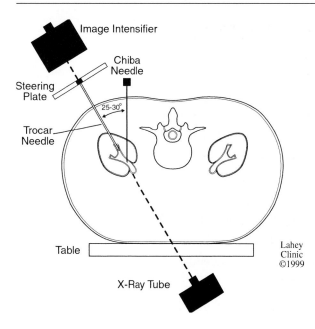

Figure 42-2 Schematic drawing showing access to the renal collecting system for nephrostomy catheter placement. A 22 gauge Chiba needle has been inserted into the renal pelvis using ultrasonography or fluoroscopy. The trocar needle is placed into a posterior calyx under fluoroscopic guidance. (Reprinted with permission of Lahey Clinic, Burlington, MA.)

Treatment

The patient was referred for bilateral nephrostomy catheter placement. With the patient in the prone position, the dilated right renal pelvis was easily localized using ultrasonography, and a 22 gauge Chiba needle (DCHN-22–20.0, Cook Incorp., Bloomington, IN) was advanced into the renal pelvis in perpendicular fashion. The initial aspirate of urine was sent for culture, and the renal collecting system was opacified with contrast. The second, posterolateral puncture site was selected in the posterior axillary line below the twelfth rib. After administration of local anesthesia, a small skin incision was made and an 18 gauge trocar needle (DTN-18–15.0, Cook Incorp.) was inserted into a middle minor infundibulum using a steerable plate (ANH-300, Cook Incorp.) under fluoroscopic guidance (**Fig. 42-2**). After passage of a Benson wire (TSFB-35–145-BH, Cook Incorp.), a 5F fascial dilator was advanced into the renal pelvis. At this point, the soft Benson wire was exchanged for a stiff Amplatz wire (46–523, Boston Scientific, Watertown, MA) and after further dilation of the tract to 10F, an 8.5F nephrostomy catheter (ULT 8.5-38–25-P-4S-NCL, Cook Incorp.) was inserted into the renal pelvis. Because of the history of septicemia, a nephrostomy catheter was also inserted on the left side, in the same manner (**Fig. 42-3**). The urine cultures were sterile. Renal function improved and the blood urea nitrogen dropped to 35 mg/dL and creatinine to 1.4 mg/dL.

Three days later, he underwent bilateral ureteral stent placement. The nephrostomy catheter was removed over an LLT guide wire (TSFNB-35–145, Cook Incorp.). Using a J-shaped 5F catheter (P5.0-35–65-M-NS-0, Cook Incorp.), the ureter was entered and the distal ureteral obstruction was crossed. After exchange of the LLT wire for a 0.035 in. Amplatz wire (46–523; Boston Scientific), an 8.5F ureteral stent (UTSSW-8.5-26-AMP-RH, Cook Incorp.) was placed and subsequently a nephrostomy catheter was reinserted. The procedure was then repeated for the opposite side. One day later, the urine was clear and bilateral nephrostograms confirmed patency of the stents. The nephrostomy catheters were removed.

The patient tolerated this procedure well and remained afebrile but continued to have leakage of urine from both nephrostomy sites. He also experienced right flank pain. Sonography showed a severe right hydronephrosis and a moderate left hydronephrosis. The hydronephrosis was believed to result from back pressure from the contracted bladder, with the stents transmitting the elevated bladder pressure into the kidneys. After insertion of a Foley balloon catheter into the bladder, the stents functioned well (**Fig. 42-4**) and the back pain resolved.

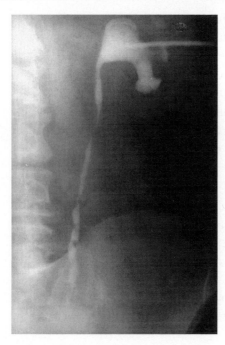

Figure 42-3 Left nephrostogram: the nephrostomy has been inserted through a midcalyx to facilitate subsequent placement of a ureteral stent.

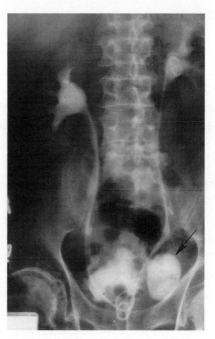

Figure 42-4 Intravenous pyelogram obtained after placement of a Foley catheter into the bladder. Both ureteral stents are patent. The bladder is contracted and a large left-sided diverticulum is present (arrow).

The patient underwent radiotherapy to the prostate followed by bilateral orchiectomy with an excellent result. The bladder Foley was removed. He was managed with bilateral double-J stents, which were exchanged cystoscopically every 3 to 6 months. Intravenous pyelography 8 years after the first ureteral stent placement continued to show decompressed upper tracts and no appreciable bladder outflow obstruction.

Discussion

The usual indication for nephrostomy placement is to provide drainage for a distal obstruction. In patients with malignancy and unilateral distal ureteral obstruction, we place a nephrostomy only if signs of renal failure or infection are present. Most of these patients undergo ureteral stent placement at a later time. However, if the latter treatment fails, the patient will have to be managed with percutaneous nephrostomy tubes for life, with all of the problems associated with external tubes and drainage bags. In obstructed kidneys, the success of nephrostomy catheter placement approaches 100% (Farrell and Hicks, 1997). However, it can be difficult in patients with a decompressed collecting system and in those who have distal leaks.

Clotting parameters (platelets, prothrombin, partial thromboplastin time) should be checked and, if necessary, corrected before nephrostomy placement. Pretreatment with antibiotics is important. For patients in whom there is a low index of suspicion for urinary tract infection, our practice is to give 1 g cefazolin intravenously after the patient arrives in the radiology department. In patients with a high index of suspicion for urinary tract infection (i.e., those with fever, urinary diversion conduit, or infectious renal calculi), a combination of broad-spectrum antibiotics is given, such as ampicillin and gentamycin or ampicillin and levaquin. If the urine culture is positive, the choice of antibiotics is based upon those results.

It is useful to use a fluoroscopic C-arm for placement of a nephrostomy catheter (see **Fig. 42-2**). With the patient in the prone position, the renal pelvis can be localized using ultrasonography or by fluoroscopy after intravenous contrast injection. The ideal course of the nephrostomy catheter is from the posterior axillary line below the twelfth rib into a posterior calyx or minor infundibulum, usually in the lower pole of the kidney. Because the long axis of the posterior calyx and minor infundibulum correspond to the avascular plane, a nephrostomy catheter threaded along this course should avoid the major vessels (Zagoria and Dyer, 1999). In addition, this course avoids the pleural space and prevents kinking of the catheter when the patient is lying on the back.

In our experience, nephrostomy catheter placement can be best achieved utilizing the "double-needle" technique (see **Fig. 42-2**). The initial access with a 22 gauge needle inserted into the renal pelvis in perpendicular fashion permits excellent opacification of the collecting system and facilitates accurate puncture of the desired calyx and/or infundibulum under fluoroscopy (with an 18 gauge trocar needle) in a manner not possible with ultrasonography. An alternative method for the posterolateral puncture that is preferred by some is a 22 gauge needle of a Neff percutaneous access set (NPAS-100, Cook Incorp.).

For drainage, we use self-retaining Cope-loop-nephrostomy catheters, which are less prone to dislodgment. The newer nephrostomy catheters have a larger inner to outer diameter ratio and they are less likely to kink.

Subsequent conversion of a nephrostomy catheter to an internal stent is frequently requested in patients with distal obstruction. The stent may be used to open a ureter obstructed by a benign stricture or by cancer or to protect the ureter while it heals after surgery or percutaneous dilation. Thus the use of a stent may be short term, as in patients with benign diseases, or long term, as in patients with cancer. For antegrade ureteral stent placement, ideally, the nephrostomy access should be via a middle or upper pole calyx (see **Fig. 42-3**). During passage of the guide wire and insertion of the stent, this approach permits the pushing forces to be directed toward the ureter and bladder. On the other hand, if the nephrostomy is through a lower pole calyx or infundibulum, the pushing forces will be directed cephalad. This problem can sometimes be overcome by advancing the stent through a transrenal peel-away introducer sheath (PLVTW-10-38-30, Cook Incorp.) that extends into the ureter.

To pass a stent through an obstructed ureter, careful fluoroscopic guidance is necessary. We use a combination of a slightly curved 5F polyethylene catheter and a soft, straight guide wire or glide wire to cross the obstruction. Once the guide wire and catheter are in the bladder, the guide wire is exchanged for a heavy-duty Amplatz wire, which is used for ureteral stent placement. Dilation of the narrowed segment with an angioplasty balloon will facilitate insertion of the stent. The new percutaneously introduced stents have significant improvements, including a higher internal to external diameter ratio and numerous large side holes along the length of the stent. They are made of a low-friction material, permitting easy passage of a guide wire. The first such stent was the Amplatz stent, which is made of soft C-flex material and is introduced over an inner stiffening catheter that is removed after repositioning the stent. Further improvement is the addition of a hydrophilic coating. Percuflex is a material with similar characteristics.

Antegrade placement of a stent is frequently possible even after the retrograde approach fails. Placement of a ureteral stent transmits the intravesical pressure to the ureter and renal pelvis (Watson, 1997). Therefore, bladder outflow obstruction will interfere with proper functioning of the stent and will need to be treated (Hubner et al, 1992).

Plentiful intake of fluids should be encouraged in these patients to ensure adequate urine output and thus decrease the chance of stent obstruction. Patients should be made aware that pain or decreased urine output or both may indicate stent obstruction. The greatest risk associated with an indwelling stent is infection, and urine cultures should be obtained frequently. Indwelling stents

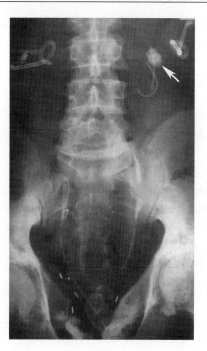

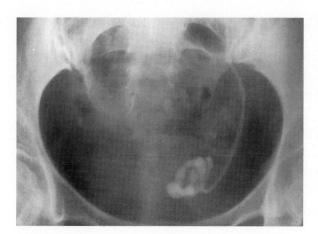

Figure 42-5 Marked incrustation of the distal ureteral stent 4 months after extracorporal shock wave lithotripsy. This 45-year-old woman had the ureteral stent placed prior to undergoing extracorporal shock wave lithotripsy for a 1.5 cm left renal calculus.

Figure 42-6 Fragmentation of the "forgotten stents" and stone formation around an intrapelvic stent fragment (arrow). This 75-year-old man with carcinoma of the prostate had bilateral polyurethane ureteral stents placed 18 months earlier but was lost to follow-up. He presented with fragmentation of the forgotten stents. Bilateral nephrostomy catheters are in place.

should be changed every 3 months to prevent occlusion caused by buildup of incrustation (**Figs. 42-5** and **42-6**) (Somers, 1996). This complication is more common in patients with a propensity to form stones. Some of these stents will degrade and fragment if left in place for a long time (see **Fig. 42-6**) (Somers, 1996).

Complications

Complications are relatively uncommon. In a series of 454 nephrostomies, massive hematuria or pararenal hematoma or both requiring blood transfusions occurred in 2.8% of patients (Farrell and Hicks, 1997). Septicemia occurred in 0.9% and pneumothorax in 0.2%. Complications requiring catheter exchange within 30 days occurred in 2.6% of patients: The nephrostomy catheters were either dislodged or blocked and kinked or there was leakage of urine along the nephrostomy catheter requiring placement of a larger catheter.

PEARLS AND PITFALLS_____

- The fluoroscopically guided double-needle technique permits excellent collecting system opacification and facilitates accurate puncture of the desired calyx/infundibulum with an 18 gauge trocar needle for nephrostomy catheter placement.

- The two main complications of percutaneous nephrostomy placement are bleeding and septicemia. These can be avoided if the procedure is performed when clotting parameters are normal and with adequate antibiotic coverage.
- Antegrade ureteral stent placement is facilitated by a renal entry site in a middle or upper pole calyx.
- Bladder outflow obstruction interferes with proper ureteral stent function and should be treated before placement of the stent.
- Ureteral stents should be exchanged every 3 months to prevent occlusion and encrustation.

Further Reading

Farrell TA, Hicks ME. A review of radiologically guided percutaneous nephrostomies in 303 patients. J Vasc Interv Radiol 1997;8:769–774

Hubner WA, Plas EG, Stoller ML. The double-J ureteral stent: in vivo and in vitro flow studies. J Urol 1992;148(2 Pt 1):278–280

Somers WJ. Management of forgotten or retained indwelling ureteral stents. Urology 1996; 47:431–435

Stables DP, Ginsberg NJ, Johnson ML. Percutaneous nephrostomy: a series and review of the literature. AJR Am J Roentgenol 1978;130:75–82

Watson G. Problems with double-J stents and nephrostomy tubes. J Endourol 1997;11:413–417

Wickbom I. Pyelography after direct puncture of the renal pelvis. Acta Radiol 1954;41:505–512

Zagoria RJ, Dyer RB. Do's and don't's of percutaneous nephrostomy. Acad Radiol 1999;6:370–377

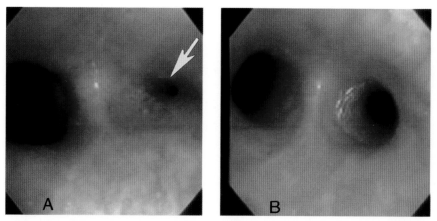

Figure 8-3 (**A**) Bronchoscopic view before and (**B**) after stent placement. Prior to stenting, there is near-total collapse of the right main stem bronchus (arrow). Following stent placement, it is wide open. A stent was previously placed in the left main stem bronchus. (See Figures 8–3A and 8–3B, page 35.)

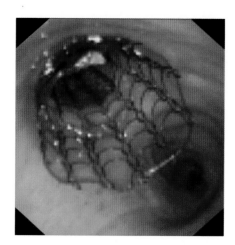

Figure 8-7(B) Covered Ultraflex stent used to seal a bronchoesophageal fistula after stent deployment. (See Figure 8–7B, page 40.)

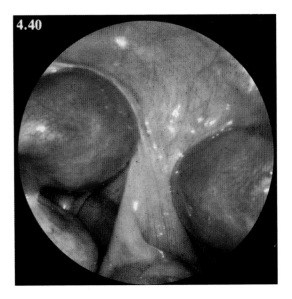

Figure 38-9 (**B**) Bicornuate uterus. Laparoscopyshows a band of fibrous tissue separating the cornua of the bilobar uterine fundus. A bicornuate uterus has a single cervix, a heart-shaped fundus, and two uterine cavities separated by myometrium. Conversely, a septate uterus has a single cervix, a flat fundus, and two uterine cavities separated by relatively avascular scar tissue. (See Figure 38–9B, page 231.)

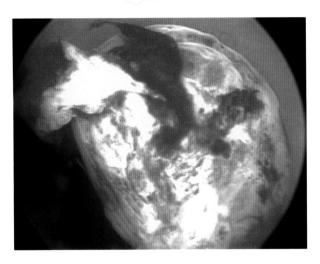

Figure 38-12 Polyps. (**B**) Hysteroscopic polypectomy specimen. The histological diagnosis was benign endometrial polyp. (See Figure 38–12B, page 232.)

CHAPTER 43 Ureteral Occlusion for Urinary Leaks

Christopher P. Molgaard

Clinical Presentation

A 75-year-old woman with a history of endometrial carcinoma presented with the complaint of urine leakage from the vagina. The endometrial carcinoma had been treated with total abdominal hysterectomy and pelvic radiation therapy 23 years earlier. Five years prior to her current problem, she had tumor recurrence at the vaginal apex that was treated with intracavitary radiation to the upper vaginal vault. Physical examination revealed a 7 cm mass at the apex of the vagina and urine leaking from the vagina.

Radiological Studies

Computed tomography of the pelvis (not shown) demonstrated a soft tissue mass at the vaginal apex. On cystography (**Fig. 43-1**) there was leakage of contrast from the bladder into the vagina.

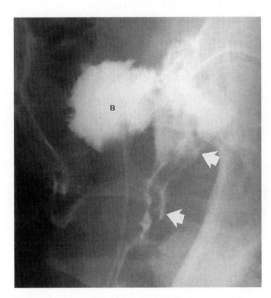

Figure 43-1 Cystogram shows the vesicovaginal fistula. Contrast is seen leaking from the bladder (b) into the vagina (arrows).

Diagnosis

Vesicovaginal fistula

Treatment Options

Surgical urinary diversion to a stoma for eliminating urinary flow through the fistula was not possible because of the recurrent pelvic neoplasm and history of radiation therapy involving bowel loops in the pelvis. Therefore, permanent urinary diversion via bilateral nephrostomy catheters was performed together with occlusion of the ureters.

261

Methods for percutaneous occlusion of the ureters include the translumbar clip and transrenal embolization. Percutaneous translumbar occlusion is performed by placement of a metallic clip directly on the ureter via a large caliber translumbar sheath. Placement of embolic material in the ureter is a more widely used and technically simpler approach. All such patients have a nephrostomy in place, which allows transrenal access to the ureter. Materials that have been used for this purpose include stainless steel coils and gelatin sponge pledgets (Gelfoam, Upjohn, Kalamazoo, MI) detachable balloons, ureteral plugs, tissue adhesives, and electrocautery with a radio frequency catheter. Transrenal occlusion with Gianturco coils (Cook Incorp., Bloomington, IN) and Gelfoam, was chosen because of the high technical success rate, relative ease of placement, and low complication rate.

Treatment

Bilateral percutaneous nephrostomy catheters were placed using a standard technique (see Chapter 42). The catheters were left to external drainage for 3 days. Because this did not completely "dry up" the fistulous drainage, we elected to proceed with ureteral embolization. The nephrostomy catheter was removed over a guide wire, and a 9F sheath was placed in the renal pelvis. A 5F angiographic catheter and a soft-tipped guide wire were manipulated from the renal pelvis into the distal ureter. The guide wire was removed and a nest of 6 mm Gianturco coils was placed in the distal ureter. Multiple Gelfoam pledgets were then placed within the nest of coils. At the superior end of the nest, two 12 mm coils were placed; these were purposely oversized relative to the ureteral diameter to prevent proximal migration of the coils. The coil placement was continued until there was no antegrade flow of contrast into the bladder through the embolized segment of ureter. Eight coils were used in each ureter. At the conclusion of the ureteral occlusion a nephrostomy catheter was inserted and left to gravity drainage. There was marked decrease in the urine leakage with near complete perineal dryness for approximately 2 months. The patient then noted an increase in urine leakage from the vagina and decreased output from her right nephrostomy. The nephrostogram showed a kink in the catheter and some contrast passage into the bladder through the coiled segment of the distal ureter (**Fig. 43-2**). Additional coils were placed in both ureters until there was no further flow into the bladder (**Fig. 43-3**).

Following the repeat embolization, there was no further urine leakage and complete perineal dryness. The nephrostomy catheters were exchanged every 8 weeks. The patient remained asymptomatic from her vesicovaginal fistula until her death, 16 months after her initial ureteral embolization.

Discussion

Urinary fistulas due to trauma or other benign etiology are often cured by temporary urinary diversion with nephrostomy catheters, ureteral stents, bladder catheters, and local surgical repair. Vesicovaginal or ureterovaginal fistulas associated with pelvic malignancy and radiation therapy are usually not adequately treated by catheter diversion and local surgery. Surgical diversion with ileal loop formation can be attempted in the appropriate patient. However, because of advanced and often recurrent malignancy, sequelae of radiation therapy, overall poor health, and advanced age, many patients are not suited for surgical management. In these patients, percutaneous ureteral occlusion with urinary diversion via nephrostomy catheters can be of great benefit in ameliorating the psychological and physical discomfort of continuous urinary incontinence.

There are several methods for percutaneous ureteral occlusion. Percutaneous ureteral clipping involves the placement of a large-caliber sheath into the retroperitoneum via a flank approach. The ureter is grasped and a metallic clip is placed on it to obstruct the flow of urine, which is diverted via nephrostomy catheters. The procedure is effective but requires a custom-made metallic clip and large-caliber translumbar tract directly to the ureter for placement of the clip.

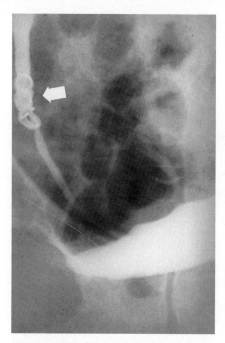

Figure 43-2 A right nephrostogram shows contrast flowing through the nest of coils (arrow) into the distal ureter and bladder.

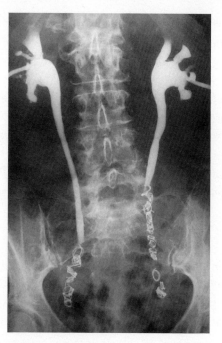

Figure 43-3 Bilateral nephrostograms obtained following placement of additional coils demonstrate complete occlusion of the ureters with no further contrast flow into the bladder.

The transrenal approach to the ureter via a standard nephrostomy tract obviates the need for a second percutaneous puncture. From this approach, detachable balloons, tissue adhesive, Gianturco coils with Gelfoam pledgets, and other occluding devices may be placed in the ureter. Although detachable balloons and tissue adhesives can effectively occlude the ureter, they have a tendency to migrate with the ureteral peristalsis and in 30 to 45% of cases reintervention in needed to maintain ureteral occlusion.

Ureteral occlusion with Gianturco coils and Gelfoam pledgets has multiple advantages over the other methods. These materials are readily available and most vascular/interventional radiologists have experience in using them. The procedure is effective and the reintervention rate to maintain ureteral occlusion is low. Coils should be oversized relative to the diameter of the ureter to prevent coil migration if the proximal ureter dilates due to nephrostomy tube dysfunction.

The mechanism of ureteral occlusion by coils and gelatin sponge pledgets is different from that of the vascular system (where thrombosis is induced). Laboratory studies of ureteral embolization have shown that in the acute phase, the occlusion is caused by physical obstruction of the ureteral lumen by the coil and Gelfoam nest together with some kinking of the ureter as the oversized coils attempt to assume their helical shape. Subsequently, a stricture develops at the site of coil deposition, leading to long-term occlusion.

Complications

Complications associated with ureteral embolization are rare. Asymptomatic coil migration into the renal pelvis and passage of coils into the bladder or through the fistula have been reported. Complications related to the nephrostomy are also uncommon. These include bleeding associated with nephrostomy placement, catheter kinking or leakage, and urinary tract infection. Catheter-related complications can be minimized by exchanging the catheter at a minimum of every 3 months.

PEARLS AND PITFALLS

- Transrenal ureteral occlusion with diverting nephrostomy should be considered in patients with vesico- or ureterovaginal fistulas associated with advanced or recurrent pelvic malignancy and history of radiation therapy.
- Ureteral occlusion with coils and Gelfoam pledgets is safe and effective and is easily performed via a standard nephrostomy access.
- Coils should be oversized relative to the diameter of the ureter to prevent migration into the renal pelvis or the bladder.
- Nephrostomy catheters should be changed at least every 3 months because catheter occlusion may be associated with recurrent urinary leakage as a result of increased ureteral pressure.

Further Reading

Bing KT, Hicks ME, Figenshau RS, et al. Percutaneous ureteral occlusion with use of Gianturco coils and gelatin sponge, I: swine model. J Vasc Interv Radiol 1992;3:313–317

Farrell TA, Wallace M, Hicks ME. Long-term results of transrenal ureteral occlusion with use of Gianturco coils and gelatin sponge pledgets. J Vasc Interv Radiol 1997;8:449–452

Farrell T, Yamaguchi T, Barnhardt W, et al. Percutaneous ureteral clipping: long-term results and complications. J Vasc Interv Radiol 1997;8:453–456

Schild HH, Gunther R, Thelen M. Transrenal ureteral occlusion: results and problems. J Vasc Interv Radiol 1994;5:321–325

CHAPTER 44 Symptomatic Renal Cyst

Fah Sean Leong and Carl F. Beckmann

Clinical Presentation

A 62-year-old woman with a left renal cyst was evaluated for intermittent left flank pain that had been present for 4 years. Two years earlier, her urologist had placed a left ureteral stent. However, the left flank pain persisted. She denied urinary tract infections, gross hematuria, or difficulty with voiding. Multiple ultrasound scans performed during the previous 4 years documented a stable-appearing left parapelvic renal cyst.

Radiological Studies

Computed tomography (CT) of the abdomen (not shown) 4 months prior to referral showed a 4 cm left renal parapelvic cyst that appeared to be partially obstructing the lower pole collecting system. On renal ultrasonography, the parapelvic cyst measured 3 × 4 cm and there was some caliceal dilation (**Fig. 44-1**).

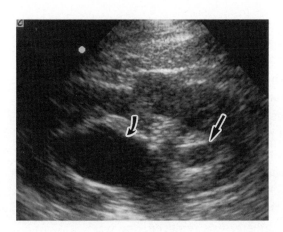

Figure 44-1 A 62-year-old patient with intermittent left flank pain. Ultra-sonography shows a 3 × 4 cm parapelvic cyst (curved arrow) with some caliceal dilation (straight arrow).

Diagnosis

Partially obstructing left parapelvic renal cyst

Treatment

The cyst appeared to be partially obstructing the lower pole collecting system and was considered to be the cause of her symptoms. Therefore, cyst aspiration and sclerotherapy were undertaken. The patient was placed in the prone position on the angiography table and 100 mL Omnipaque 300 was injected intravenously to opacify the collecting system. Under ultrasound guidance, a ring needle (DLPN-40–25-Ring, Cook Incorp., Bloomington, IN) was advanced into the cyst in perpendicular fashion. A 5F pigtail catheter was then inserted into the cyst over a guide wire. Approximately 100 mL of straw-colored fluid was drained and a sample sent for cytological examination. Diluted contrast (100 mL) was instilled into the cavity. Images were obtained for evaluation of the cyst wall in the

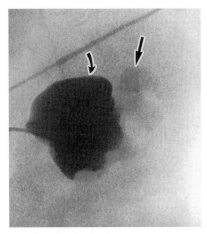

Figure 44-2 After intravenous injection of contrast material and needle opacification of the cyst with 100 mL of dilute contrast material, a sharply defined, smoothly outlined, lobulated cyst is demonstrated (curved arrow). There is dilation of the intrarenal collecting system (straight arrow).

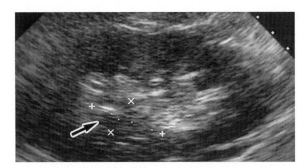

Figure 44-3 Ultrasonography 7 months after aspiration and sclerosant therapy shows no residual cyst. An area of heterogeneous echo texture (straight arrow) in the renal sinus was noted to correspond to the region of the obliterated cyst.

anteroposterior, posteroanterior, right and left decubitus, and cross-table lateral projections. These demonstrated a sharply defined, smoothly outlined, lobulated cyst (**Fig. 44-2**) and dilation of the intrarenal collecting system. The dilute contrast was aspirated through the catheter and 5 mg bupivacaine hydrochloride, 0.5%, was instilled for anesthetic purposes and was subsequently aspirated. Doxycycline (250 mg) was instilled into the cyst cavity for sclerotherapy. No immediate complications were noted. Cytological examination of the cyst fluid revealed no tumor cells.

One month later, she was reevaluated for persistent left flank pain. Ultrasonography revealed reaccumulation of some fluid in the left parapelvic cyst. A second aspiration and sclerotherapy were performed. After placement of a 5F pigtail catheter, only 35 mL of clear yellow fluid was aspirated. The cyst cavity was filled with 15 mL of absolute alcohol, and the patient was slowly rotated 360 degrees. After 20 minutes, the alcohol was aspirated, and the catheter was removed. She was symptom free at 7 months follow-up. Renal ultrasonography showed complete decompression of the cyst (**Fig. 44-3**). An area of heterogeneous echo texture was present in the renal sinus corresponding to the obliterated cyst.

Discussion

Only a few benign renal cysts are thought to cause symptoms such as flank discomfort, possibly because of partial obstruction of the collecting system. Rarely, there may be severe pain due to torsion of a pedunculated cyst, hypertension caused by renovascular ischemia, proteinuria secondary to renal vein compression, or polycythemia and jaundice (Hartman, 1989). It is for these rare causes that treatment of benign cysts is indicated.

Puncture of a renal cyst is performed under ultrasound guidance with the patient in the prone position and using a posterior or posterolateral access below the twelfth rib. During cyst puncture, the renal hilum and larger hilar vessels should be avoided. For the initial puncture, we use a 22 gauge Chiba needle (DCHN-22–20, Cook, Incorp.) or a ring needle (DLPN-40–25-Ring, Cook, Incorp.). Over a guide wire, this is exchanged for a 5F pigtail catheter. The cyst is then aspirated, and the aspirate is sent for cytological evaluation (Amis et al, 1987). Cystography is performed by injecting diluted contrast material (50% dilution of Omnipaque 300) at a volume not to exceed the volume of the aspirated cyst fluid, and images of the cyst wall are obtained in several projections. If the criteria of a benign renal cyst are met (e.g., smooth cyst walls, clear cyst aspirate), we proceed with sclerotherapy.

The indwelling pigtail catheter should be checked for free in- and outflow before the sclerosant is injected. This ensures that the sclerosant can be removed after coating and inactivating the secreting cells inside the cyst cavity. Pain can be severe after sclerotherapy and should be anticipated and treated appropriately. Injection of a small amount of 0.5% bupivacaine hydrochloride into the cyst cavity, which is then aspirated before injecting the sclerosant, may help to alleviate the pain. Most patients manage well at home, but some require mild analgesics.

The renal cysts usually reaccumulate after aspiration alone. Only one of 20 cysts treated by aspiration showed a 50% or greater reduction in size by ultrasonography after 3 months (Ohkawa et al, 1993). If a recurrence is to be prevented, sclerosis of the cyst wall is necessary. The risk of reaccumulation after sclerotherapy depends upon the size of the cyst and the amount of sclerosant injected. To maximize the effect of the sclerosing agent, prior aspiration of the cyst is necessary.

Various sclerosing agents have been used to obliterate cysts. These include absolute alcohol, povidone iodine, doxycycline, and minocycline. Presently, the most commonly used sclerosing agent is absolute alcohol. Ideally, to prevent a recurrence, the volume of absolute alcohol instilled should be equal to 12 to 25% of the cyst volume. In one series of 34 renal cysts treated with absolute alcohol, there was only one recurrence where a small cyst volume replacement was used (3.7% of cyst volume) (Bean, 1981). All others were treated with 95% alcohol in a volume equal to 12% or more of the cyst volume. Another study using 95% alcohol showed that those with a diameter >10 cm (5/23 patients) recurred after an average of 3 months (Hobarth and Kratzik, 1991). Bean found that after 1 to 3 minutes of contact with absolute alcohol, the epithelial cell lining of the cyst became fixed and nonviable (Bean, 1981). The cyst capsule is penetrated only after a prolonged contact (4–12 hours). To prevent complications, the absolute alcohol should be aspirated after 20 minutes (Ozgur et al, 1988).

Doxycycline is an alternative to tetracycline as a medicinal sclerosant, with a similar mechanism of action. It has been used for pleurodesis in the treatment of patients with malignant pleural effusions and for sclerosis of lymphoepithelial cysts (Robinson et al, 1993; Lustig et al, 1998).

Ohkawa et al used minocycline, a long-acting tetracycline, as a sclerosing agent in doses of 100 to 200 mg to treat 154 renal cysts, with good results (Ohkawa et al, 1993). After 3 months, 69 cysts were no longer demonstrable, 49 showed a 50% or greater reduction in size, and only eight were unchanged or had slightly increased in size. No severe adverse effects were reported. Fever and pain developed in 12.8% of patients.

Povidone iodine sclerotherapy of symptomatic renal cysts in five patients was reported by Phelan et al (1999). An 8F Cope-loop-nephrostomy tube was placed percutaneously into the renal cyst and left in place for 3 to 5 days, during which the patient self-administered 5 mL of a 50:50 solution of povidone iodine, which remained in the cyst cavity for 5 minutes. This procedure was performed twice a day. The cyst was aspirated dry before and after instillation of the sclerosant. The tube was removed when the measured cyst fluid volume was <10 mL in a 24-hour period. Four of the five patients had complete resolution of the cyst. One patient had considerable reduction in the diameter of the cyst (from 15 to 5 cm). All patients had resolution of symptoms. Two patients had documented resolution of a segmental hydronephrosis that was secondary to obstruction by parapelvic cysts.

Complications

Complications of cyst puncture occur in 2 to 4% of patients. These include hemorrhage, pneumothorax, infection, and sterile flank abscess. Renal cysts in the upper pole are associated with a higher

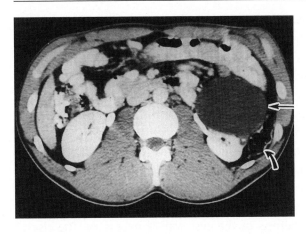

Figure 44-4 Computed tomographic (CT scan of a patient with a large left renal cyst (straight arrow) and posterolateral location of the descending colon (curved arrow). Percutaneous lateral access to the left renal cyst requires either CT guidance or a combination of fluoroscopic and ultrasound guidance to avoid puncturing the colon.

incidence of complications; they may require a puncture above the twelfth and sometimes above the eleventh rib for access. Such a high puncture is associated with complications in up to 12% of patients. These include: pneumothorax, hydrothorax, or even laceration of the lung. Such punctures should be performed in expiration and under fluoroscopic guidance. Whenever possible, the access site should remain below the twelfth rib.

A previous CT will help to define the spatial relationship between the kidney and adjacent colon, which lie in the retroperitoneal space. This is particularly important in patients who have had surgery in the abdominal cavity or the retroperitoneal space (especially surgery involving the colon, adrenal glands, kidneys, spleen, and pancreas) because the relationship between large and/or small bowel and the targeted kidney may be altered. Therefore, in such patients the renal cysts should be targeted by either CT guidance or a combination of ultrasonography and fluoroscopic guidance to prevent inadvertent perforation of a hollow viscus (**Fig. 44-4**).

Complications associated with the use of alcohol as a sclerosant include leakage outside the cyst, particularly into the renal collecting system, which can result in extensive tissue sloughing.

PEARLS AND PITFALLS_____

- Renal cysts are very common but rarely cause symptoms.
- Symptomatic renal cysts may manifest with pain, hypertension, proteinuria, and polycythemia.
- Cysts treated by simple aspiration usually recur. Cyst aspiration followed by sclerotherapy provides durable results.
- The most commonly used sclerosing agent is absolute alcohol. The injection volume of alcohol used for sclerotherapy should equal 12 to 25% of the cyst volume.
- In large cysts, multiple sclerotherapy treatments are often necessary.

Further Reading

Amis ES Jr, Cronan JJ, Pfister RC. Needle puncture of cystic renal masses: a survey of the Society of Uroradiology. AJR Am J Roentgenol 1987;148:297–299

Bean WJ. Renal cysts: treatment with alcohol. Radiology 1981;138:329–331

Hartman DS. Renal cystic disease. Armed Forces Institute of Pathology. Atlas of Radiologic–Pathologic Correlations, fascicle 1. Philadelphia: WB Saunders; 1989

Hobarth K, Kratzik C. Percutaneous sclerosing of kidney cysts with alcohol [in German]. Urologe A 1991;30:189–190

Lustig LR, Lee KC, Murr A, et al. Doxycycline sclerosis of benign lymphoepithelial cysts in patients infected with HIV. Laryngoscope 1998;108:1199–1205

Ohkawa M, Tokunaga S, Orito M, et al. Percutaneous injection sclerotherapy with minocycline hydrochloride for simple renal cysts. Int Urol Nephrol 1993;25:37–43

Ozgur S, Cetin S, Ilker Y. Percutaneous renal cyst aspiration and treatment with alcohol. Int Urol Nephrol 1988;20:481–484

Phelan M, Zajko A, Hrebinko RL. Preliminary results of percutaneous treatment of renal cysts with providone-iodine sclerosis. Urology 1999;53:816–817

Robinson LA, Fleming WH, Galbraith TA. Intrapleural doxycycline control of malignant pleural effusions. Ann Thorac Surg 1993;55:1115–1121

CHAPTER 45 Staghorn Calculus

Christoph Wald and Carl F. Beckmann

Clinical Presentation

A 43-year-old woman was seen in the walk-in clinic with complaints of chronic back and left flank pain. Urine analysis revealed hematuria and the hematocrit was 33%. Other laboratory values including serum creatinine were normal.

Radiological Studies

An abdominal radiograph demonstrated a large staghorn calculus in the left kidney (**Fig. 45-1**). The left renal collecting system was partially obstructed on intravenous pyelography.

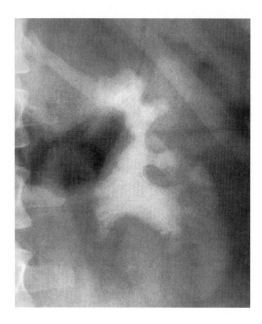

Figure 45-1 Radiograph of the left kidney shows a large staghorn calculus. The upper pole projects above the twelfth rib.

Diagnosis

Large staghorn calculus

Treatment

The large calculus was considered suitable for percutaneous nephrolithotomy followed by extracorporal shock wave lithotripsy (ESWL).

After induction of general anesthesia, cystoscopy was performed with the patient in the supine position. This showed a normal bladder and normal ureteral orifices. A 7F balloon occlusion catheter (OB/11.5/7/65, Boston Scientific, Watertown, MA) was advanced into the left renal pelvis through the ureter. A Foley catheter was placed in the bladder for drainage after removal of the cystoscope. The patient was then placed in prone position and the collecting system around the staghorn calculus was opacified via the balloon occlusion catheter. The occlusion balloon is very cautiously inflated

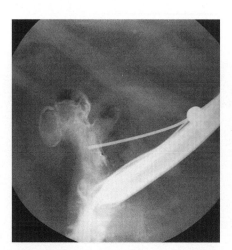

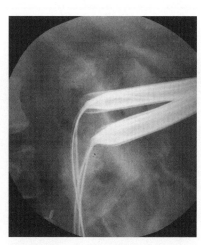

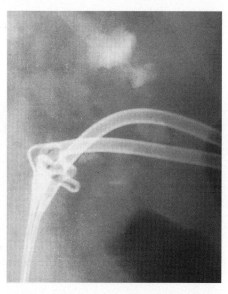

Figure 45-2 Using the lower pole sheath and dilator, the kidney has been levered inferiorly, permitting puncture of the upper pole infundibulum from below the twelfth rib.

Figure 45-3 A second 30F sheath has been placed in the upper pole. Dilators and "working" and "safety" wires are in place.

Figure 45-4 Upon completion of the percutaneous nephrolithotomy procedure, two 18F Malecot nephrostomy/stent catheters have been placed in the renal pelvis. Residual calculus fragments are present.

under fluoroscopic visualization only if retrograde opacification is inadequate. Under fluoroscopy the lower pole infundibulum close to the posterior calyx was punctured from the left posterior axillary line using an 18 gauge trocar needle (DTN-18–15, Cook Incorp., Bloomington, IN) and Amplatz needle holder with silicone inserts (# 90000, Cook Urological Co., Spencer, IN). A Benson guide wire (Cook Incorp.) was inserted followed by placement of a 5F Kumpe catheter (HNBR5.0-38-40-P-NS-KMP, Cook Incorp.) in the renal pelvis for directional control.

The Benson guide wire and catheter were advanced into the distal ureter. The Benson wire was then exchanged for a stiff Amplatz "working" wire (Cook Incorp.), which was advanced into the distal ureter. Fascial dilators (up to 12F) were used to enlarge the tract. Through a 10F sheath, a second, soft-tipped guide wire ("safety" wire) was placed in the distal ureter. Over the stiff working wire, the tract was dilated from the skin to the renal pelvis using an Amplatz renal dilator set (Cook Incorp.), and subsequently, a 30F sheath was advanced into the lower pole collecting system. The sheath was stiffened by inserting the 30F Amplatz dilator and then carefully pushed cranially under fluoroscopy, thus levering the entire kidney caudally so that the upper pole infundibulum projected below the twelfth rib. An 18 gauge trocar needle was then placed in the upper pole infundibulum without violation of the pleural space (**Fig. 45-2**). After dilation of the second tract, another 30F Amplatz sheath and safety wire were inserted through the upper pole (**Fig. 45-3**).

Through the accesses provided, the urologist was able to remove 90% of the staghorn calculus using ultrasonic fragmentation. Several caliceal fragments could not be removed (**Fig. 45-4**). An 18F Malecot nephrostomy catheter/stent (08278, Cook Urological) was placed through each access. The patient subsequently underwent ESWL for the remaining fragments.

Discussion

Percutaneous nephrolithotomy alone or in combination with ESWL has obviated the need for surgery in the vast majority of patients with renal stone disease. First described in 1976 by Fernström and Johansson, this technique has become widely accepted and is a safe procedure. The indications and contraindications for percutaneous nephrolithotomy are listed in **Table 45-1**.

Table 45-1   Indications and Contraindications for Percutaneous Nephrolithotomy

Indications

Large-volume calculi (>2.5 cm), e.g., staghorn calculi

Calculi proximal to an infundibular stenosis or in a caliceal diverticulum

Calculi impacted in the proximal ureter

Calculi in dilated lower pole calyces (because fragments cannot be cleared after ESWL)

Cystine and calcium oxalate monohydrate calculi that are refractory to ESWL

Unusual anatomy, such as a horseshoe kidney in which the calculus cannot be targeted by ESWL

Nonradiopaque uric acid calculi

Stone disease in the presence of high-grade ureteral stricture or obstruction

Contraindications

Uncorrected coagulopathy

Active urinary tract infection

Obesity (specifications for the fluoroscopic table are the limiting factor)

Unusual body habitus in which the distance from the skin to the collecting system exceeds the length
   of instruments/sheaths used

ESWL, extracorporal shock wave lithotripsy.

In patients with large-volume calculi (e.g., staghorn calculus), ESWL is likely to yield an excessive amount of fragments/debris that cannot be excreted spontaneously through the ureter. Therefore, in such patients, the main objective is the percutaneous removal of as much calculus volume as possible. Often, access to a lower pole calyx (below the twelfth rib) combined with a flexible nephroscope permits sufficient debulking of the calculus. However, in some patients, two or even three percutaneous nephrostomies are necessary to provide satisfactory access to the lower, middle, and upper pole calices.

An intercostal approach, usually to the middle and upper pole, is associated with complications from violation of the pleural space (in ~12% of the patients). We prefer the technique first described by Karlin and Smith (1989), in which the kidney is displaced inferiorly (below the twelfth rib) when multiple punctures are required for patients with large staghorn calculi. However, this technique is often not possible in patients who have scarring from prior renal surgery. Fortunately, in most of the latter patients, the posterior costophrenic sulcus is also scarred permitting a safe intercostal approach. Thus, in such patients, we prefer to puncture above the twelfth rib for percutaneous nephrolithotomy or nephrostomy placement, to avoid traversing the dense scar tissue usually associated with prior renal surgery.

Outcome

Smith et al (1990) from our institution reviewed the success rates of various therapeutic algorithms for 376 patients treated for complex renal calculi. ESWL monotherapy was associated with a success rate of only 36%, whereas primary percutaneous nephrolithotomy was successful in 83% of patients. The combination of these two modalities yielded a 93% therapeutic success. Hence, percutaneous nephrolithotomy is our choice for primary therapy in patients with complex calculi, followed by ESWL, if necessary.

Complications

The most commonly encountered complications include renal hemorrhage, renal pelvic and ureteral tears, injury to adjacent organs, including colonic perforation, and transgression of the pleural space with resulting pneumo- or hydrothorax, fever, and sepsis.

PEARLS AND PITFALLS_____

- Because of the large calculus burden, staghorn calculi should be treated first by percutaneous nephrolithotomy, followed by ESWL.
- A higher success rate is achieved if percutaneous nephrolithotomy is followed by ESWL for treatment of staghorn calculi.
- Pneumothorax occurs in ~12% of patients after puncture above the twelfth rib. However, puncture above the twelfth rib is usually safe in patients that have previously undergone ipsilateral renal surgery.
- The risk of pneumothorax can be avoided by displacing the kidney downward and performing a second puncture at the upper pole calyx from below the twelfth rib.

Further Reading

Eisenberger F, Fuchs G, Miller K, et al. Extracorporal shockwave lithotripsy (ESWL) and endourology: an ideal combination for the treatment of kidney stones. World J Urol 1985;3:41

Fernström I, Johansson B. Percutaneous pyelolithotomy: a new extraction technique. Scand J Urol Nephrol 1976;10:257–259

Karlin GS, Smith AD. Approaches to the superior calix: renal displacement technique and review of options. J Urol 1989;142:774–777

Moskowitz GW, Lee WJ, Pochaczevsky R. Diagnosis and management of complications of percutaneous nephrolithotomy. Crit Rev Diagn Imaging 1989;29:1–12

Nieh PT, Roth RA, Beckmann CF. Percutaneous removal of renal calculi. In: Libertino JA, ed. Reconstructive Urologic Surgery. St. Louis: Mosby-Year Book; 1998:73–81

Picus D, Weyman PJ, Clayman RV, et al. Intercostal-space nephrostomy for percutaneous stone removal. AJR Am J Roentgenol 1986;147:393–397

Roth RA, Beckmann CF. Complications of extracorporal shock-wave lithotripsy and percutaneous nephrolithotomy. Urol Clin North Am 1988;15:155–166

Segura JW. Role of percutaneous procedures in the management of renal calculi. Urol Clin North Am 1990;17:207–216

Segura JW. The role of percutaneous surgery in renal and ureteral stone removal. J Urol 1989;141:780–781

Segura JW, Patterson DE, LeRoy AJ, et al. Percutaneous removal of kidney stones: review of 1,000 cases. J Urol 1985;134:1077–1081

Smith JJ III, Hollowell JG, Roth RA. Multimodality treatment of complex renal calculi. J Urol 1990;143:891–894

Young AT, Hunter DW, Castaneda-Zuniga WR, et al. Percutaneous extraction of urinary calculi: use of the intercostal approach. Radiology 1985;154:633–638

CHAPTER 46 Accidentally Ligated Ureter

Christoph Wald and Carl F. Beckmann

Clinical Presentation

A 36-year-old woman underwent abdominal hysterectomy for benign disease at another institution. The operation was complicated by laceration of the urinary bladder, which was surgically repaired. During the postoperative period, she continued to have left flank pain. Intravenous pyelography (IVP) 5 weeks after surgery revealed obstruction of the left collecting system. She was referred for further management.

Radiological Studies

Percutaneous nephrostomy was performed in the routine fashion to decompress the left renal collecting system (see Chapter 42). The nephrostogram showed a dilated left pelvocaliceal system and tortuosity of the ureter (**Fig. 46-1**). There was an abrupt blockage of contrast flow in the distal ureter, close to the bladder (**Fig. 46-2**).

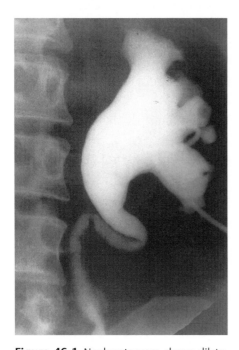

Figure 46-1 Nephrostogram shows dilatation of the left renal pelvis and calyces.

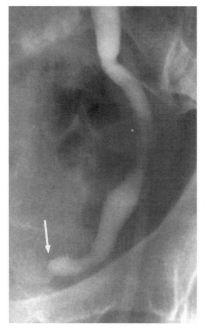

Figure 46-2 The distal left ureter is abruptly occluded near the ureteropelvic junction (arrow).

Diagnosis

Accidentally ligated ureter

Treatment

The abrupt termination of the contrast column in the distal ureter was presumed to be from accidental ligation of the ureter at the time of hysterectomy. Urine cultures were sterile. Two days after placement of the percutaneous nephrostomy, the distal ureter was balloon dilated.

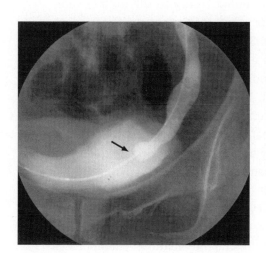

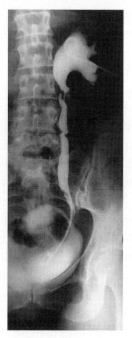

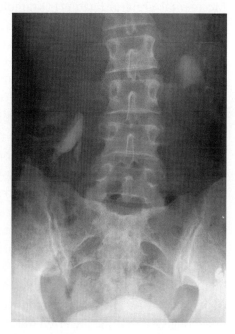

Figure 46-3 A guide wire is across the stricture (arrow).

Figure 46-4 Nephrostogram obtained after balloon dilatation of the stricture and insertion of a ureteral stent. A nephrostomy catheter is in the left renal pelvis.

Figure 46-5 A 10-minute film from an intravenous urogram obtained 3 months after ureteral dilatation and stenting shows no obstruction. The ureter is of a normal size and the calices are well-defined.

With the patient in the prone position on the angiographic table, the nephrostomy catheter was removed over a Benson wire (TSFB-35–145 BH, Cook Incorp., Bloomington, IN). A 5F soft-tipped catheter with a J-shaped hook was inserted into the renal pelvis and advanced into the proximal ureter. Using a combination of the catheter and a J-shaped Lunderquist wire for torque control (HSF-38–125-THG, Cook Incorp.), the tortuous proximal ureter was negotiated to the level of obstruction. The Lunderquist wire was then exchanged for a Terumo glide wire (46–165, Boston Scientific, Watertown, MA), which was used to cross the distal ureteral obstruction. Once the obstruction was crossed, the Lunderquist wire was reinserted and the stricture was dilated with a 5 mm high-pressure angioplasty balloon (Blue Max, Boston Scientific, Watertown, MA) (**Fig. 46-3**). (Although a Lunderquist wire was used in this case, we usually prefer a stiff Amplatz wire [THSB-38–145-AES-BH, Cook Incorp.].)

Subsequently, an 8.5F ureteral stent (UTSSW-8.5–26-AMP-RH, Cook Incorp.) was inserted in an antegrade fashion followed by placement of an 8.5F nephrostomy catheter (**Fig. 46-4**). The nephrostomy drainage was clear the next day and the catheter was clamped (i.e., placed to internal drainage). This was well tolerated overnight, without pain. The nephrostomy was removed the following day, and the patient was discharged. Six weeks later, the ureteral stent was removed cystoscopically. The patient remained asymptomatic. Excretory urography obtained 3 months later showed continued patency of the distal ureter (**Fig. 46-5**).

Discussion

Benign ureteral strictures can be congenital or acquired. Acquired, iatrogenic strictures are relatively uncommon but can occur following ureteroscopy (accidental ureteral perforation) or pelvic surgery (accidental ureteral ligation) (Kramolowsky, 1987; Polat et al, 1997). Postoperative anastomotic strictures may occur after dismembered pyeloplasty, ureteroenterostomy, and ureteroneocystostomy. A stricture can also occur after percutaneous removal of impacted ureteral calculi and after ureterolithotomy (Beckmann et al, 1989). Additional risk factors for the development of ureteral strictures are retroperitoneal surgery (secondary to ischemic injury to the ureter), radiation therapy, thermal damage from electrohydraulic lithotripsy, and inflammatory disease such as tuberculosis (Ford et al, 1984; Miller, 1986; Lytton et al, 1987; Weinberg et al, 1987).

Accidental ligation of the ureter during pelvic surgery is a relatively rare occurrence and is usually treated surgically. Percutaneous treatment with balloon dilation has been successful in several reported cases (Reimer and Oswalt, 1981; Kaplan et al, 1982; Neumeyer, 1990). Successful retrograde recanalization of the ureter by placement of ureteral stents has also been described (Witherington and Shelor, 1980). Typically, absorbable suture material is used during pelvic surgery; therefore, it is advisable to wait at least 20 days after the surgery before attempting to dilate a ligated ureter (Kaplan et al, 1982). By this time, the suture will have been absorbed and balloon dilation can be easily performed.

Ureteral strictures can be treated in a retrograde fashion via cystoscopic placement of the dilation balloon or in an antegrade fashion through a nephrostomy tract. The middle or upper pole renal collecting system is the preferred route of access in percutaneous ureteral interventions. This approach permits the catheter and guide wire to be directed down toward the bladder and will greatly facilitate crossing a narrowed segment. Balloon size is selected according to the measured or estimated size of the normal ureter above or below the stricture. In the distal ureter, typically we dilate with a 4 to 6 mm diameter balloon (12–18F). In the proximal ureter, an 8 to 10 mm diameter balloon (24–30F) is more commonly used (i.e., for the treatment of ureteropelvic junction strictures).

Outcome

During the past 20 years, we have seen four patients with an accidentally ligated ureter. We were able to successfully dilate the ureter in all patients. In simple ureteral ligation with absorbable suture material, the success rate of percutaneous treatment is high. However, if damage to the ureter is extensive (i.e., transection, laceration, or vascular damage), percutaneous treatment is less likely to be successful and surgical repair is frequently indicated (Polat et al, 1997).

In a series of 72 patients treated for acquired benign ureteral strictures, the cause, length, and duration of the stricture were important determinants of the primary success of percutaneous treatment (Beckmann and Roth, 1995). Treatment was successful in eight of 10 patients with strictures or occlusions following minimal ureteral trauma during ureteroscopy. The success rate for dilatation of chronic strictures is lower. Chronic anastomotic strictures after ureteroenterostomy, ureteroneocystostomy, or secondary ureteropelvic junction strictures after dismembered pyeloplasty were successfully dilated in only 60% of patients. Strictures of less than 3 months' duration could be treated successfully in 86% of patients, whereas the success rate was only 59% for strictures that had been present for longer than 12 months. Strictures less than 2 cm in length were successfully treated in 72% of patients compared with 42% if longer than 2 cm. The latency period for strictures to recur after treatment appears to correlate with the duration of the stricture before treatment. Thus patients initially treated for chronic ureteral strictures should be observed for a longer period of time.

Percutaneous dilation should be considered the initial treatment modality for acquired benign ureteral strictures and obstructions, such as those occurring after accidental ligation. This procedure is considerably less traumatic and reduces morbidity and length of hospitalization when compared with open surgical reconstruction. Percutaneous treatment of strictures, even when unsuccessful, does not preclude a subsequent successful surgical repair.

PEARLS AND PITFALLS_____

- An accidentally ligated ureter can be treated percutaneously with a high success rate.
- Dilatation should be delayed for a minimum of 20 days from the time of injury to permit absorption of suture material.
- Percutaneous dilation should be the treatment of first choice for benign ureteral strictures. Even if unsuccessful, it does not preclude later surgical repair.
- Etiology, length, and chronicity are important determinants of the success of dilatation in acquired ureteral strictures.
- Patients treated for chronic strictures (>12 months' duration) need to be observed for an extended period to permit timely recognition of late recurrence.

Further Reading

Beckmann CF, Roth RA. Dilatation of benign ureteric strictures [abstract]. Cardiovasc Intervent Radiol 1995;18(Suppl 1):S92

Beckmann CF, Roth RA, Bihrle W III. Dilation of benign ureteral strictures. Radiology 1989;172:437–441

Ford TF, Parkinson MC, Wickham JE. Clinical and experimental evaluation of ureteric dilatation. Br J Urol 1984;56:460–463

Kaplan JO, Winslow OP Jr, Sneider SE, et al. Dilation of a surgically ligated ureter through a percutaneous nephrostomy. AJR Am J Roentgenol 1982;139:188–189

Kramolowsky EV. Ureteral perforation during ureterorenoscopy: treatment and management. J Urol 1987;138:36–38

Lytton B, Weiss RM, Green DF. Complications of ureteral endoscopy. J Urol 1987;137:649–653

Miller RA. Endoscopic surgery of the upper urinary tract. Br Med Bull 1986;42:274–279

Neumeyer K. Percutaneous treatment of benign ureteric stenosis and fistulae. Fortschr Roentgenstr 1990;152:708–712

Polat O, Gul O, Aksoy Y, et al. Iatrogenic injuries to ureter, bladder and urethra during abdominal and pelvic operations. Int Urol Nephrol 1997;29:13–18

Reimer DE, Oswalt GC Jr. Iatrogenic ureteral obstruction treated with balloon dilation. J Urol 1981;126:689–690

Weinberg JJ, Ansong K, Smith AD. Complications of ureteroscopy in relation to experience: report of survey and author experience. J Urol 1987;137:384–385

Witherington R, Shelor WC. Treatment of postoperative ureteral stricture by catheter dilation: a forgotten procedure. Urology 1980;16:592–595

CHAPTER 47 Caliceal Diverticulum Calculi

Carl F. Beckmann

Clinical Presentation

A 31-year-old woman with a history of urinary tract infections was seen at another hospital for intermittent left flank pain. The workup demonstrated a calculus in a caliceal diverticulum. She underwent extracorporal shock wave lithotripsy twice, but not all fragments were passed. One year later, she continued to experience left flank pain and was referred for percutaneous removal of the retained fragments.

Radiological Studies

An abdominal radiograph showed multiple stone fragments over the lower pole of the left kidney (**Fig. 47-1A**). On excretory urography, these fragments were localized to a caliceal diverticulum. On computed tomography (CT), the caliceal diverticulum appeared to be posterolateral to a posterior calyx in the mid to lower portion of the left kidney (**Fig. 47-1B**). The retained fragments appeared to layer.

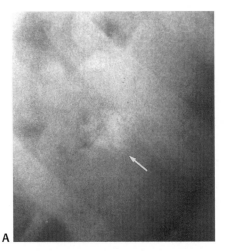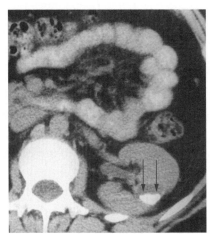

A   B

Figure 47-1 Thirty-one-year-old woman with persistent left flank pain 1 year after extracorporal shock wave lithotripsy for calculi in a caliceal diverticulum. (**A**) Closeup section from an abdominal radiograph shows calculi in the inferolateral aspect of the left kidney (arrow). (**B**) Image from an abdominal computed tomographic scan shows layering of the fragments in a posterolateral caliceal diverticulum (arrows).

Treatment

Under general anesthesia, with the patient in the lithotomy position, a 7F occlusion balloon catheter was placed in the left ureter via the cystoscope. The catheter tip was advanced above the ureteropelvic junction. The patient was then placed in the prone position. The occlusion balloon was inflated and the renal collecting system opacified with contrast. The inflated occlusion balloon was gently withdrawn until it occluded the ureteropelvic junction. The collecting system was then carefully distended. Using C-arm fluoroscopy, the caliceal diverticulum was punctured with a biliary ring needle (DPLN-40–25-ring, Cook Incorp., Bloomington, IN) from a skin access site in the left posterior axillary line. The caliceal diverticulum was opacified with contrast (**Fig. 47-1C**). The needle puncture

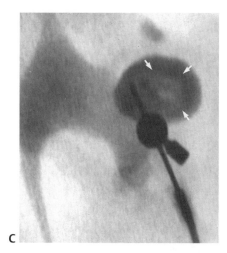
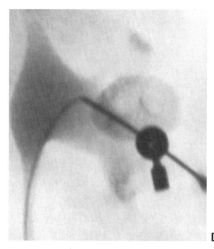

C

D

Figure 47-1 (*Continued*) (**C**) With the patient prone (image reversed for comparison), the posterolateral calyx has been punctured and opacified with contrast. The central filling defect represents the calculi within the caliceal diverticulum (arrows). (**D**) The puncture needle has been advanced into the corresponding infundibulum and a guide wire passed into the ureter (image reversed for comparison).

was then extended into the adjacent infundibulum (**Figs. 47-1D** and **Fig. 47-2A**). A soft-tipped guide wire (Benson wire, TSFB-35–145 BH, Cook Incorp.) was advanced through the renal pelvis into the distal ureter and subsequently exchanged for a stiff "working" wire (Amplatz wire, THSF-38–145-AES-BH, Cook Incorp.). The tract was then dilated to 10F, and a second guide wire (Benson wire) was inserted through a 10F sheath to serve as a "safety" wire.

A balloon dilatation catheter (Amplatz Tractmaster, TMS/10–12/7/40, Boston Scientific, Watertown, MA) was inserted over the working wire to create a 30F tract into the renal pelvis through the caliceal diverticulum. A 30F sheath was inserted over the inflated balloon catheter and the tip positioned in the renal pelvis (**Fig. 47-2B**). Under direct nephroscopic visualization, the 30F sheath was withdrawn until its tip was in the caliceal diverticulum, and the calculi were then removed (**Fig. 47-2C**). The lining of the caliceal diverticulum and of the connecting isthmus was fulgurated. At the termination of the procedure, a 22F Foley catheter was inserted into the renal pelvis through the caliceal diverticulum to serve as a nephrostomy (**Fig. 47-2D**). It was left in place for 6 weeks. On follow-up evaluation, the patient was asymptomatic and free of calculi. A small, residual caliceal diverticulum remained.

Discussion

Caliceal diverticula are urothelium-lined cavities situated peripherally at the corticomedullary junction. They are connected to the renal collecting system by a narrow isthmus. Caliceal diverticula are found in 0.4% of individuals (Middleton and Pfister, 1974; Timmons et al, 1975). Although the majority of caliceal diverticula do not cause symptoms, they can be a nidus for calculus formation and infection in 9.5 to 35% of such individuals. The latter can result in the occlusion of the narrow isthmus. Chronic or recurrent pain, pyonephrosis, and progressive renal damage can develop in these patients, necessitating intervention.

For caliceal diverticula containing calculi, percutaneous treatment is superior to extracorporal shock wave lithotripsy as poor drainage from the diverticulum prevents spontaneous passage of the calculus fragments. Percutaneous treatment is less invasive and spares more tissue than the conventional surgical approaches.

Most caliceal diverticula are related to the upper or lower pole calices (Wulfsohn, 1980) and are amenable to percutaneous treatment. If the caliceal diverticulum is related to the middle calices,

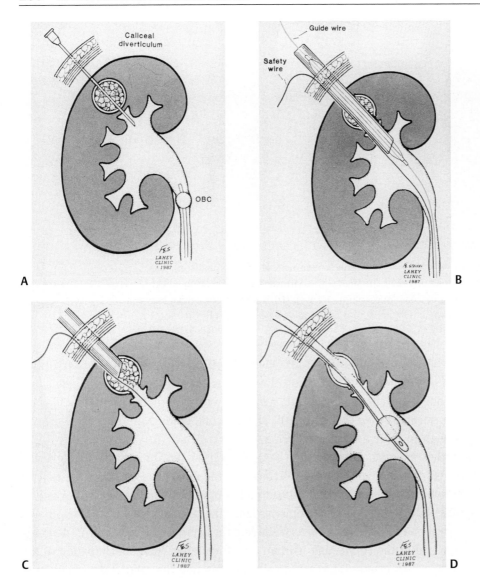

Figure 47-2 Schematic drawings illustrating the technique for percutaneous removal of calculi from an upper pole caliceal diverticulum. (**A**) After inflation of the occlusion balloon catheter (OBC) and retrograde opacification of the collecting system, percutaneous puncture is performed through the caliceal diverticulum into the associated infundibulum. Two guide wires are passed through the renal pelvis into the ureter and the tract is balloon dilated, creating a 30F tract through the caliceal diverticulum into the renal pelvis. (**B**) A 30F working sheath is then inserted over the inflated balloon. (**C**) The tip of the working sheath is withdrawn into the caliceal diverticulum for the removal of the calculi. (**D**) After the calculi have been removed, a 22F Foley catheter is inserted through the caliceal diverticulum into the renal pelvis to serve as a nephrostomy. (Reprinted with permission of the Lahey Clinic, Burlington, MA.)

percutaneous treatment should be reserved for those located posteriorly (Ruckle and Segura, 1994). When the diverticulum is located ventrally, direct puncture and subsequent tract dilatation can cause vascular injury because of the intervening renal parenchyma. CT helps to define the spatial relationship between the caliceal diverticulum and corresponding infundibulum.

Hulbert et al (1986) described a percutaneous technique in which the caliceal diverticulum is punctured directly, and a large nephrostomy tract is created into the caliceal diverticulum for the removal of calculi followed by the placement of a large nephrostomy tube, which leads to obliteration of the diverticulum. This technique is difficult and often unsuccessful. Difficulties arise when the diverticular neck is occluded or narrowed to such a degree that the guide wire cannot be advanced into the renal pelvis or ureter.

Often not enough length of guide wire can be anchored in the caliceal diverticulum to afford sufficient traction for dilatation of the tract. The guide wire can dislodge, making dilatation of the tract impossible. To overcome this problem, we advance the puncture needle from the caliceal diverticulum into the adjacent infundibulum thereby creating an infundibulostomy (Roth and Beckmann, 1998). In this way, the guide wire can be advanced into the ureter thereby facilitating subsequent tract dilatation.

An upper pole caliceal diverticulum usually requires a puncture above the twelfth rib and sometimes even above the eleventh rib. Such a high puncture can result in a pneumo- or hydrothorax or lung laceration in up to 12% of patients. These punctures should be performed in expiration and under careful fluoroscopic guidance. If at all possible, the access should be below the twelfth rib.

Outcome

Percutaneous treatment renders 80 to 95% of patients free of calculi and nearly 100% of patients free of symptoms and infections (Shalhav et al, 1998; Donnellan et al, 1999). The creation of a large tract (30F) through a small caliceal diverticulum leads to erosion of the uroepithelial lining. This process can be enhanced by additional fulguration. Subsequent stenting with a large caliber nephrostomy tube results in formation of granulation tissue resulting in obliteration of small caliceal diverticula. We have treated 10 stone-filled caliceal diverticula utilizing this technique. Six have remained obliterated on follow-up pyelography. Larger caliceal diverticula usually remain open. In two large series, after percutaneous treatment, the caliceal diverticula were obliterated in 76% of patients (Shalhav et al, 1998).

PEARLS AND PITFALLS_____

- Caliceal diverticula occur in up to 0.4% of individuals and are a nidus for stone formation and infection in 9.5 to 35% of such individuals.
- Calculi in caliceal diverticula can be difficult to manage by extracorporal shock wave lithotripsy because the fragments created cannot pass through the narrow isthmus.
- Percutaneous treatment is feasible for the calculi-filled caliceal diverticulum associated with the upper or lower pole calices. If associated with middle calices, the diverticulum should be posterior or posterolateral to the collecting system.
- A CT scan should be used to define the spatial relationship between the caliceal diverticulum and adjacent infundibulum.

Further Reading

Donnellan SM, Harewood LM, Webb DR. Percutaneous management of caliceal diverticular calculi: technique and outcome. J Endourol 1999;13:83–88

Hulbert JC, Reddy PK, Hunter DW, et al. Percutaneous technique for the management of caliceal diveticula containing calculi. J Urol 1986;135:225–227

Middleton AW Jr, Pfister RC. Stone-containing pyelocaliceal diverticulum: embryonic, anatomic, radiologic and clinical characteristics. J Urol 1974;111:2–6

Roth RA, Beckmann CF. Renal caliceal diverticula. In: Libertino JA, ed. Reconstructive Urologic Surgery. 3rd ed. St. Louis: CV Mosby; 1998:137–140

Ruckle HC, Segura JW. Laparoscopic treatment of a stone-filled, caliceal diverticulum: a definitive, minimally invasive therapeutic option. J Urol 1994;151:122–124

Shalhav AL, Soble JJ, Nakada SY, et al. Long-term outcome of caliceal diverticula following percutaneous endosurgical management. J Urol 1998;160:1635–1639

Timmons JW, Malek RS, Hattery RR, et al. Caliceal diverticulum. J Urol 1975;114:6–9

Wulfsohn MA. Pyelocaliceal diverticula. J Urol 1980;123:1–8

CHAPTER 48 Retrorenal Colon

Saadoon Kadir

Clinical Presentation

A 42-year-old woman was referred for nephrostomy placement. She had undergone reimplantation of the left ureter and insertion of a stent. The stent had dislodged, resulting in obstruction of the renal collecting system.

Radiological Studies

Radiographs of the abdomen demonstrated the dislodged ureteral stent with the distal end lying above the ureterovesicular anastomosis (**Fig. 48-1**). In preparation for nephrostomy insertion, the patient was placed in the prone position and a 22 gauge Chiba needle was used to opacify the obstructed collecting system via a direct puncture of the renal pelvis. The stent that was coiled in the renal pelvis was used as target. A lower pole calyx was then selected for the placement of a nephrostomy through the left posterior axillary line. Lidocaine was injected and the 22 gauge injection needle was left in place for identification of the access route. During the attempt to fluoroscopically align the lower pole calyx and the 22 gauge needle in the posterior axillary line, a section of the air-filled colon was seen posterior to the mid and lower portions of the kidney, which precluded a safe access (**Fig. 48-2**). To further delineate the anatomy, the patient was taken for computed tomography (CT). Images obtained in the prone position confirmed the presence of colon behind the mid and lower portions of the left kidney (**Fig. 48-3**). She subsequently underwent cystoscopic retrieval of the migrated stent.

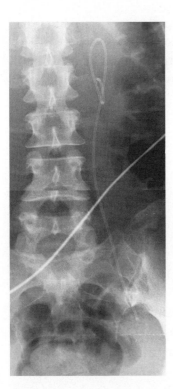

Figure 48-1 Abdominal radiograph shows a left ureteral stent that has migrated proximally into the renal pelvis. Gas-filled colon is seen adjacent to the lower pole of the kidney.

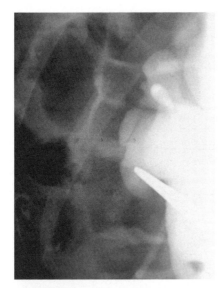
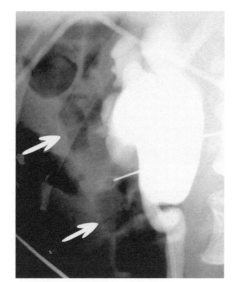
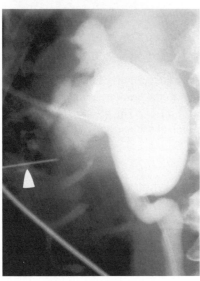

Figure 48-2 Images from the antegrade pyelogram in varying left posterior oblique projections with patient in the prone position show colonic gas (arrows) overlying the lower pole. Arrowhead points to the 22 gauge needle used for lidocaine injection along the typical nephrostomy tract.

Diagnosis

Retrorenal colon precluding nephrostomy placement

Discussion

Depending upon the age and body habitus of an individual, variable segments of the ascending and descending colon may pass behind segments of the kidneys. The overall incidence of a retrorenal colon has been reported to be between 1.9% on supine abdominal CT examinations to 10% in the prone position (Hopper et al, 1987). In most cases, the lateral one third of the renal circumference is affected but the colon was behind the posteromedial surface of the kidney in 4.7% of patients studied (Hopper et al, 1987). Prone CT examinations in patients undergoing percutaneous diskectomy showed a 0.29% incidence at the L4–L5 disk level and below (Helms et al, 1989). This is usually below the lower poles of the kidneys. In another study, colon was found to be present behind the lower renal poles in 1.7% on the right side and 0.7% on the left side (Prassopoulos et al, 1994). This overall incidence appears to be more in keeping with the nephrostomy practice experience.

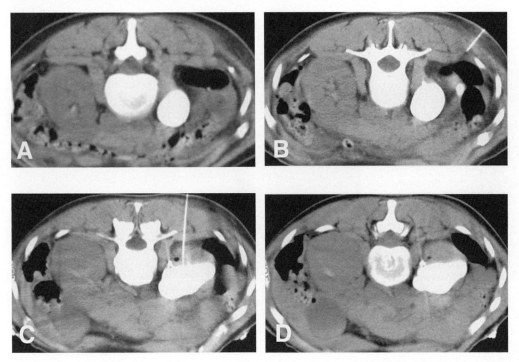

Figure 48-3 Contiguous computed tomographic images through the lower and midportions of the kidneys with the patient in the prone position show the gas-filled colon posterior to the lower pole of the left kidney. (**B**) Image shows the 22 gauge needle used for lidocaine injection (same as in **Fig. 48–2**). (**C** and **D**) show the 15 cm length, 22 gauge needle used for contrast opacification of the renal pelvis (**C**) and location of colon posterolateral to the kidney.

The risk of an inadvertent puncture of the colon may be higher when fluoroscopic guidance is used for renal collecting system access. Ultrasound guidance may avoid this problem because the presence of air readily identifies the colon. However, in practice, attention to the essentials of the procedure can also avoid such a complication when using fluoroscopic guidance (see Chapter 42).

Colon injury has been reported to occur after percutaneous renal surgery and nephrostomy placement. Individuals at risk include younger, lean body habitus males or older persons and those with mobile kidneys (Vallancien et al, 1985; Gerspach et al, 1997). Segments most likely to be affected are the ascending and descending colon in proximity to the lower pole of the kidney, colon that is distended with gas, and an access that is excessively lateral (Vallancien et al, 1985; Hopper et al, 1987; Prassopoulos et al, 1994). There appears to be a slight predisposition for the left side. Colonic injury has also been observed after percutaneous access to the middle calices.

Recognition of Injury to the Retrorenal Colon

Colonic laceration can result in an abscess formation of a colonephric or colocutaneous fistula. Rarely, there is intraperitoneal spillage of colonic contents resulting in peritonitis. During the procedure, colonic injury may be recognized by contrast opacification of the colonic lumen. An unrecognized injury may manifest post-procedure with either mild, nonspecific signs and symptoms such as low grade fever, abdominal or flank pain, ileus, and leucocytosis or with severe symptoms such as severe abdominal pain, peritonitis, sepsis, abscess, fecaluria, pneumaturia, or colonic hemorrhage (Vallancien et al, 1985; Gerspach et al, 1997). Symptoms may manifest within hours of the procedure or several days later.

Management of Colonic Injury

Most injuries can be managed conservatively with drainage of the colon or pericolonic space and the kidney. However, intraperitoneal injuries in association with colon perforation necessitate surgical intervention, whereas hemorrhage may be managed by interventional radiological methods.

Transcolonic passage of the 22 gauge needle is unlikely to cause serious complications such as an abscess or fistula, provided there is satisfactory urinary decompression via a functioning nephrostomy, and antibiotic coverage is initiated promptly. Inadvertent transcolonic catheter placement is treated as follows:

1. Ensure adequate renal drainage/decompression of the collecting system. The presence of a urinary obstruction may contribute to the formation of or sustaining a colonephric fistula. Either a double-J ureteral stent is placed through the existing tract or a second nephrostomy catheter is inserted via a safe route. In addition, a bladder catheter is inserted.

2. Once urinary drainage is ensured, the transcolonic catheter is withdrawn into the colon and left in place for ~2 to 3 weeks. This allows the tract to mature before the catheter is removed. A mature tract prevents spillage of intraluminal colonic materials and consequent infection. An alternative surgical method is to remove the catheter and insert a drain into the pericolonic space (Gerspach et al, 1997).

3. Appropriate antibiotics for a broad coverage should be initiated and continued until the tract is mature or the catheter is removed.

PEARLS AND PITFALLS_____

*   A retrorenal colon occurs in a small number of individuals and may be inadvertently injured during a percutaneous renal procedure.
*   Gas distention of the colon increases the risk of inadvertent injury.
*   Careful fluoroscopic assessment of the colon-kidney relationship will avoid this complication.
*   Preprocedure assessment by CT with the patient in the prone position or ultrasound guidance for the procedure may prevent inadvertent colonic injury.

Further Reading

Gerspach JM, Bellman GC, Stoller ML, et al. Conservative management of colon injury following percutaneous renal surgery. Urology 1997;49:831–836

Helms CA, Munk PL, Witt WS, et al. Retrorenal colon: implications for percutaneous diskectomy. Radiology 1989;171:864–865

Hopper KD, Sherman JL, Luethke JM, et al. The retrorenal colon in the supine and prone patient. Radiology 1987;162:443–446

Prassopoulos P, Gourtsoyiannis N, Cavouras D, et al. Interposition of the colon between the kidney and the psoas muscle: a normal anatomic variation studied by CT. Abdom Imaging 1994;19:446–448

Vallancien G, Capdeville R, Veillon B, et al. Colonic perforation during percutaneous nephrolithotomy. J Urol 1985;134:1185–1187

CHAPTER 49 Percutaneous Biopsy

Kamran Ali and Khaled K. Toumeh

Clinical Presentation

An adrenal mass was detected on chest computed tomography (CT) in a 61-year-old man with squamous cell carcinoma of the lung. A magnetic resonance (MR) examination that was performed at another hospital showed no signal dropout on out-of-phase images, which would have been diagnostic for an adenoma. Because the nature of this lesion was indeterminate, an adrenal biopsy was performed for establishing the diagnosis and for staging.

Radiological Studies

An abdominal CT examination showed the large left adrenal mass (**Fig. 49-1**). On the noncontrast examination, the lesion measured >20 Hounsfield units (HU).

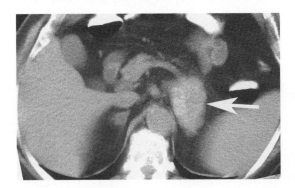

Figure 49-1 Computed tomographic scan of the abdomen shows a large left adrenal mass (arrow).

Diagnosis

Suspected adrenal metastasis from squamous cell carcinoma of the lung

Biopsy Procedure

Prebiopsy laboratory studies including coagulation parameters were within the normal range. The patient was kept NPO after midnight for the day of the procedure. Intravenous Versed and morphine were used for conscious sedation.

The biopsy was performed with the patient in the prone position. The skin entry site was localized with the aid of a biopsy grid, and the skin was then prepped and sterile draped. Local anesthetic was injected and a coaxial system consisting of a 19 gauge core biopsy needle introducer and 20 gauge Chiba needle was used to obtain tissue samples (**Fig. 49-2**). Three passes were made. In addition, a core biopsy was performed through the 20 gauge introducer needle. After the procedure, the patient was transferred to the short-term recovery unit for observation. There were no post-procedural complications and he was discharged home after 6 hours.

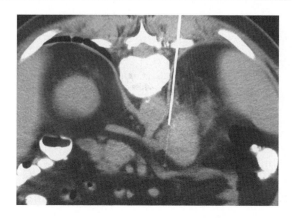

Figure 49-2 With the patient in the prone position, a 19 and 20 gauge coaxial needle biopsy system is directed into the adrenal tumor from a posterior approach.

Discussion

Several noninvasive methods have been developed to aid in differentiating between malignant and benign (i.e., adenomas) adrenal lesions. Nonenhanced CT has been used to characterize adrenal masses. A measurement of ≤10 HU has been the usual threshold for describing an adrenal lesion as an adenoma. On contrast-enhanced CT, a 50% contrast washout after 10 minutes has been used to differentiate between benign and malignant lesions. Because most adrenal masses are detected on contrast-enhanced CT and unenhanced images are not available, attenuation values in the mass are measured immediately postinjection (dynamic images obtained 60 to 80 seconds after intravenous contrast administration) and 10 minutes later. A contrast washout of ≥50% from the lesion correlates highly with benignity. Percent washout is calculated as follows:

$$1- (\text{HU on delayed images/HU on dynamic images}) \times 100.$$

On MR, the concept of chemical shift imaging has been used to differentiate adenoma from a metastatic focus. Utilizing T1-weighted images, in-phase and out-of-phase gradients are applied. Because of their intracellular lipid content, adrenal adenomas drop in signal on out-of-phase images **(Fig. 49-3)**. Positron emission tomography (PET) has also been used to differentiate benign and malignant adrenal lesions. After injection of fluorine-18 fluorodeoxyglucose (FDG), increased glucose utilization in malignant adrenal masses results in an increased uptake of FDG. Benign lesions do not demonstrate increased FDG uptake (Mayo-Smith et al, 2001). The negative predictive value of PET is around 90% for the detection of metastatic non-small cell lung cancer.

Despite these noninvasive imaging modalities, some lesions cannot be characterized accurately, making an adrenal biopsy necessary for establishing a diagnosis. Mayo-Smith et al (2001) have described an algorithm for the workup of adrenal masses in oncologic patients. Biopsy of an adrenal mass is recommended in one of two scenarios: (1) if a lesion measures >10 HU on noncontrast CT and does not demonstrate signal dropoff on T1-weighted chemical shift MR images, and (2) if the lesion demonstrates >30 HU with a washout of <50% after a 10-minute delay on contrast-enhanced CT.

CT is the modality of choice for adrenal biopsy. Silverman et al (1993) retrospectively analyzed 97 patients undergoing 101 biopsies. A diagnostic sample was obtained in ~86%. The accuracy of image-guided biopsy was 96%, the sensitivity was 93%, and the negative predictive value was 91%.

Technique

A coaxial technique using a core biopsy needle is most advantageous. The larger, outer needle is advanced into the lesion making a single skin puncture. Several passes can then be made with an inner needle in a coaxial fashion, and multiple biopsy specimens are obtained rapidly. Placement of

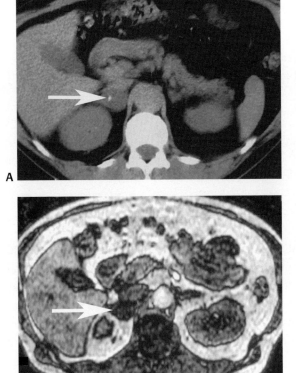

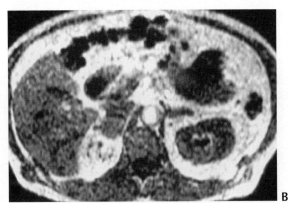

Figure 49-3 Computed tomographic (CT) and magnetic resonance (MR) images from another patient with no known malignancy show the characteristics of an adrenal adenoma. (**A**) CT shows a 3 cm, lower attenuation mass with a small parenchymal calcification (arrow). (**B,C**) MR images obtained in the in-phase (**B**) and out-of-phase (**C**) sequences. Benign adenomas are rich in intracellular fat and show a loss of signal in the out-of-phase sequences as the water and fat protons signals cancel each other. The appearance on the T1 out-of-phase image is typical for a benign adenoma (arrow).

the outer needle is less traumatic than having to perform multiple skin punctures. In addition, because of its larger diameter, such a needle can be torqued through a greater amount of lesion tissue (Hopper et al, 2000). The use of automated biopsy guns allows the acquisition of tissue cores with little shear or tissue fragmentation.

In our practice, we utilize a 19 and 20 gauge coaxial needle biopsy system (19 gauge × 10.2 cm coaxial introducer needle, MD Tech, Gainesville, FL; 20 gauge × 15 cm Super Core II Biopsy Instrument, MD Tech; 20 gauge × 15 cm Temno Chiba, Allegiance Healthcare Corp., McGaw Park, IL). Often, we use a 20 gauge core biopsy needle to obtain core specimens in addition to the fine needle aspirations.

Patient positioning is very important for the procedure. Placing the patient in the prone position may not always be feasible because in this position, ventilation of the lower lobes increases, causing inferior migration of the diaphragm. The position often preferred is the decubitus with the ipsilateral side down. This reduces ventilation in the dependent lung and causes upward migration of the diaphragm on that side, decreasing the risk of pneumothorax. If the patient can only be in the prone position, caudal angulation of the gantry can be used to avoid the posterior costophrenic sulcus (Arellano et al, 2000). An anterior approach has also been used for left adrenal lesions. This often traverses the stomach and tail of the pancreas and increases the risk of pancreatitis. The anterior approach should be employed only if another, safer approach fails or cannot be used. For right adrenal lesion, a transhepatic approach has also been used.

There are few contraindications for adrenal biopsy. These include coagulopathies, lesion inaccessibility, and an uncooperative patient. The procedure is usually performed on an outpatient basis. After the procedure, the patient is observed for ~6 hours and discharged home if there are no complications.

Complications

Complications occur in fewer than 5% of adrenal biopsies. Welch et al (1994) reported a 3% incidence of complications after percutaneous adrenal biopsy over a 10-year observation period. Potential complications include a pneumothorax if the pleural space is traversed during a posterior approach, bleeding extending to around the kidney, and hepatic bleeding if the transhepatic approach is used. Precipitation of an acute hypertensive crisis can occur during biopsy of an unsuspected pheochromocytoma.

PEARLS AND PITFALLS_____

- Adrenal biopsy is performed for diagnosis of indeterminate lesions and for treatment planning purposes.
- The procedure is most commonly performed under CT guidance.
- The use of a coaxial system permits multiple passes through a single skin puncture. Both fine needle aspiration for cytology and tissue core biopsies can be obtained.

Further Reading

Arellano RS, Boland GW, Mueller PR. Adrenal biopsy in a patient with lung cancer: imaging algorithm and biopsy indications, technique and complications. AJR Am J Roentgenol 2000;175:1613–1617

Hopper KD, Singapuri K, Finkel A. Body CT and oncologic imaging. Radiology 2000;215:27–40

Mayo-Smith WW, Boland GW, Noto RB, et al. State-of-the-art adrenal imaging. Radiographics 2001;21:995–1012

Price RB, Bernardino ME, Berkman WA, et al. Biopsy of the right adrenal gland by the transhepatic approach. Radiology 1983;148:566

Silverman SG, Mueller PR, Pinkney LP, et al. Predictive value of image-guided adrenal biopsy: analysis of results of 101 biopsies. Radiology 1993;187:715–718

Welch TJ, Sheedy PF, Stephens DH, et al. Percutaneous adrenal biopsy: review of a 10-year experience. Radiology 1994;193:341–344

CHAPTER 50 Adrenal Pseudotumor

Saadoon Kadir

Clinical Presentation

A 44-year-old woman was referred for biopsy of a left adrenal mass that was incidentally discovered at another institution during an evaluation for abdominal symptoms.

Radiological Studies

An image from the noncontrast abdominal computed tomography (CT) obtained at the referring institution is shown in **Fig. 50-1**. The adrenal area was reassessed by repeating the abdominal CT with the patient in the prone position (**Fig. 50-2**). In addition, supine images were obtained after oral contrast ingestion (**Fig. 50-3**).

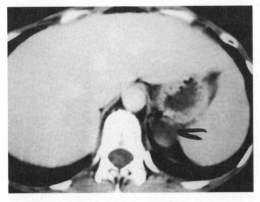

Figure 50-1 Noncontrast abdominal computed tomographic image from the referring institution shows an inhomogeneous mass in the region of the left adrenal gland.

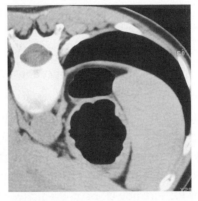

Figure 50-2 Repeat computed tomography with the patient in the prone position. Distension of this structure by air confirms it to be a pseudotumor caused by the stomach.

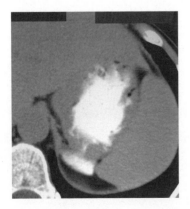

Figure 50-3 Supine image after oral contrast. Oral contrast is also present in the portion of the stomach that masqueraded as a mass.

Diagnosis

Left adrenal pseudotumor from nondistended stomach

Discussion

Pseudotumors in the region of the adrenal glands may be due to normal structures occurring in that region or from masses arising from extra-adrenal tissues. On the left side, normal structures that may simulate a mass include the stomach and blood vessels; in particular, dilated veins in patients with splenic vein occlusion and portal hypertension. Tumors or conditions that may simulate a left adrenal mass include a hematoma, rare bronchogenic cyst, neurogenic lesions, pancreatic tail, and other retroperitoneal lesions. On the right side, normal structures that may simulate a mass include the gallbladder and colon. Retroperitoneal hematoma or neoplasms may occasionally simulate a right adrenal lesion.

Although most adrenal masses have a CT attenuation similar to that of adjacent organs, some tumors may have a lower attenuation. This is most likely due to a higher fat content. Tumors with high fat content include myelolipoma, adrenal carcinoma, and occasional adenomas and pheochromocytomas.

Administration of oral contrast and imaging in the prone or decubitus position can usually differentiate a true left adrenal mass from a pseudotumor caused by the nondistended stomach. Such pseudotumors usually have the same density as other adjacent organs and in the prone position, air distends the stomach thereby readily identifying this to be a normal structure.

Percutaneous biopsy of the adrenal gland serves to provide a diagnosis in masses that cannot be characterized by noninvasive methods. Because biopsy of the left adrenal gland may be attempted from an anterior approach, a pseudotumor must be excluded before proceeding.

PEARLS AND PITFALLS

- Adrenal pseudotumors are uncommon and can occur on either side. These should be excluded prior to attempting a biopsy.
- On the left side, the nondistended gastric fundus may masquerade as an adrenal mass.
- Imaging in the decubitus or prone position can usually distinguish a left adrenal pseudotumor caused by the nondistended stomach from a true adrenal mass.

Further Reading

Brady TM, Gross BH, Glazer GM, et al. Adrenal pseudomasses due to varices: angiographic-CT-MRI-pathologic correlations. AJR Am J Roentgenol 1985;145:301–304

Hedayati N, Cai DX, McHenry CR. Subdiaphragmatic bronchogenic cyst masquerading as an adrenal incidentaloma. J Gastrointest Surg 2003;7:802–804

Karstaedt N, Sagel SS, Stanley RJ, et al. Computed tomography of the adrenal gland. Radiology 1978;129:723–730

Papanicolaou N, Pfister RC. Adrenal pseudotumor: gallbladder simulating a right adrenal mass. J Comput Tomogr 1985;9:171–172

Paul JG, Brosman S, Rhodes D. Pseudotumor of adrenal gland. Urology 1976;7:112–114

Schaner EG, Dunnick R, Doppmann JL, et al. Adrenal cortical tumors with low attenuation coefficients: a pitfall in computed tomography diagnosis. J Comput Assist Tomogr 1978;2:11–15

Schwartz JM, Bosniak MA, Megibow AJ, et al. Right adrenal pseudotumor caused by colon: CT demonstration. J Comput Assist Tomogr 1988;12:153–154

SECTION V
Miscellaneous

CHAPTER 51 Conscious Sedation for the Interventional Radiologist

Mohammad Maroof

Over the past decade, there has been rapid growth in the volume and variety of interventional radiology procedures. As these are performed more frequently and become more complex and time consuming, there has been a concurrent increase in the demand for sedoanalgesia (combined use of sedatives and analgesic drugs) to make these procedures more acceptable. The sedoanalgesia required for interventional radiology is of a level that keeps the patient calm, tranquil, and drowsy, perhaps even with closed eyes, but able to respond to verbal commands. This state of cortical depression is known as conscious sedation. The new Joint Commission on Accreditation of Healthcare Organizations (JCAHO) regulations contain recommendations made by the American Society of Anesthesiologists (ASA) (JCAHO Revision of anesthesia standards, 2001; Practice Guidelines, 2001). The revised standards include new language pertaining to the definition of sedation/ analgesia (**Table 51-1**).

Providing conscious sedation in the interventional radiology suite can be especially challenging because the patients requiring conscious sedation are frequently very ill. Other factors making conscious sedation difficult include: (1) access to the patient is limited because of the presence of x-ray equipment in the restricted space, (2) low-level lighting makes clinical observation of the patient difficult, and (3) the person(s) providing conscious sedation must often stand remote from the patient. Despite these limitations, the patients must be treated with the same level of vigilance and monitoring as those in the operating room setting.

Guidelines for the Conscious Sedation Provider

The American Nursing Association (ANA) and ASA provide conscious sedation practice standards and set certification criteria for both anesthesiologists and nonanesthesiologists (Practice Guidelines, 1996). The ANA guidelines state that a registered nurse (RN) may provide conscious sedation for patients during diagnostic, therapeutic, or surgical procedures provided it is permitted under state law and the following criteria are met (Holzman et al, 1994):

1. Conscious sedation by an RN is allowed as per institutional policy.
2. Medications are selected and ordered by a qualified anesthetist.
3. The RN would at no time leave the patient unattended or compromise monitoring while providing conscious sedation.
4. The RN should have sufficient training in conscious sedation.
5. Specific guidelines must be followed for monitoring drug administration.
6. There should be protocols in place for dealing with complications arising during the administration of conscious sedation.

Anesthesiologists are not responsible for the administration of conscious sedation in all cases. However, they should help in the formulation of conscious sedation policies and identification of at-risk patients in whom conscious sedation care may require the expertise of an anesthesiologist. This includes (Gilbertson, 1999):

1. Patients classified as ASA class 5 (see **Table 51-2**)
2. Patients that have required fiberoptic intubation in the past.
3. Patients with a history of difficult airway management or intubation.
4. Patients with a Mallampatti airway grade III or IV (see **Table 51-3**).

Table 51-1 Guidelines and Regulations: Key Components of JCAHO[a] Standards

ASA and JCAHO Continuum of Sedation			
Minimal	**Moderate**	**Deep**	**General**
Sedation	Sedation/analgesia	Sedation/analgesia	Anesthesia
Anxiolysis	Conscious sedation		
Responds normally to verbal commands	Responds purposefully to verbal commands/light touch	Responds purposefully to repeated or painful response/stimuli ? airway maintained	No reflex withdrawl

[a] JCAHO, Joint Commission on Accreditation of Healthcare Organizations

Table 51-2 American Society of Anesthesiologists Physical Status Classification

Class 1 Healthy patient, no medical problems
Class 2 Mild systemic disease
Class 3 Severe systemic disease, but not incapacitating
Class 4 Severe systemic disease that is a constant threat to life
Class 5 Moribund, not expected to live 24 hours, irrespective of operation

Table 51-3 The Four Classes of Oropharynx, Grouped According to Visualized Structures (Mallampatti, 1985)

Class I   Soft palate, fauces, uvula, anterior and posterior tonsillar pillars
Class II Soft palate, fauces, uvula
Class III Soft palate, base of uvula
Class IV Soft palate only

Preprocedure Assessment

Conscious sedation allows patients to undergo diagnostic and therapeutic procedures in a comfortable and safe manner. Safe conscious sedation requires a thorough preprocedure assessment, including the medical history and physical examination. Because of the nature of the drugs used for conscious sedation, the respiratory system is the one most likely to be influenced. This may require airway management. Therefore, head and neck mobility should be assessed and the airway classified based on the oropharyngeal structures (Mallampatti criteria, see **Table 51-3**), and the dentition status should be documented.

Laboratory workup is ordered as deemed necessary as well as judicious use of referrals to bring the patient into optimal condition. Anesthesia consultation is specifically needed for patients with limited head or neck movement, abnormal craniofacial anatomy, and morbid obesity (Gilbertson, 1999). Assessment of potential risk is necessary based on physical status. The most commonly used system for risk stratification is the ASA Physical Status Classification (**Table 51-2**). Finally, the conscious sedation plan must be tailored individually to suit the patient's needs and the procedures to be performed.

Clotting Parameters

Clotting parameters should be determined in patients with suspected abnormalities of clotting function, clinically apparent bleeding disorders, significant liver disease, 3 malabsorption, and those who are on anticoagulants. Risk versus benefit must be weighed realistically and close communication

with the referring physician must guide the decision to undertake an invasive procedure (and conscious sedation) in a coagulopathic patient.

Hypertension

The adequacy of blood pressure (BP) control is also of concern. Hypertension contributes to hematoma formation. Uncontrolled hypertension is defined as diastolic pressure greater than 100 mm Hg (Spies et al, 1991). The most important preventive measure for avoiding hypertension-related problems is to instruct patients to take their antihypertensive medications before the procedure, with the exception of diuretics. In cases with persistent BP elevation (>180/100 mm Hg), drugs for rapid control include:

Nifedipine (10 mg sublingually or chewed, may be repeated at 20-minute intervals for up to a total dose of 20–30 mg)
Labetalol (increments of 5–10 mg given by slow intravenous injection, up to an initial dose of 20 mg)
Esmolol (titrate dose upward by 50 μg/kg/min to a maximum of 300 μg/kg/min).

Adequate sedation may also lower the BP. Inadequate pain relief and bladder distension may contribute to hypertension and tachycardia. Use of opioids and urinary catheter placement before lengthy procedures can avoid such causes of hypertension and associated procedural interruptions.

Diabetes

Ideally, diabetics should be scheduled for morning procedures because this avoids prolonged fasting in patients who are at risk for symptomatic variations in blood glucose levels. Hirsch (1997) has described algorithms for the management of diabetics undergoing interventional radiology procedures. All diabetics should have their blood glucose levels checked as they arrive for the procedure. Type 1 (previously called insulin dependent) diabetics require insulin to avoid ketogenesis. Most such patients should not take their usual morning short-acting insulin before the procedure. Nonketotic hyperosmolar state may present a problem, especially in elderly, debilitated type 2 diabetics with poor intake. Fluid replacement with 0.9% saline is the most important treatment until urine output increases and hypotension is treated.

Nil Per Orally Guideline

Nil Per Orally (NPO) status should be carefully explained to the patient and documented. As suggested by the current ASA guidelines, patients should have had nothing to eat or drink for at least 6 hours before the procedure, with the exception of clear liquids, which are allowed up to 2 hours before the procedure. The only exception is for the administration of all oral cardiac, pulmonary, and antihypertensive medications. These should be taken at their regular scheduled times with sips of water. For emergency procedures, where the 6-hour wait cannot be implemented, the risk and benefits of a non-NPO status must be assessed on an individual basis.

Room Preparation

Ideally, the interventional radiology suite should be equipped for conscious sedation like a standard operating room with suction, oxygen, and nitrous oxide available. A dedicated phone line for the anesthesia team to be used for laboratory communication and management of emergencies is essential. Emergency equipment for cardiopulmonary resuscitation, including defibrillator and materials for surgical airway access, should be readily available. Because the room lights are often

dimmed during fluoroscopy, adequate spotlighting should be available for maintaining the anesthesia record and to observe monitors.

Conduct of Conscious Sedation

PATIENT POSITIONING

Because procedures can be lengthy, it is essential to make the patient comfortable before beginning the sedation. A comfortable air or foam mattress and a device for good head and neck positioning are needed. No amount of conscious sedation can substitute for careful patient positioning. Because the patient may return for multiple treatments, continued patient acceptance is important.

INTRAVENOUS ACCESS

For major cases, two intravenous lines should be available. In adult patients, one of these must be 18 gauge or larger. To maximize the distance between the fluoroscopy unit and conscious sedation provider, intravenous lines are prepared with two extension tubings. In one line, a stopcock or infusion port close to the patient can be used for continuous infusion. The second line can be used for bolus injections through a port furthest from the image intensifier to minimize radiation exposure to the conscious sedation provider. All lines should be labeled clearly.

MONITORING

As outlined by the ASA task force for nonanesthesiologists, this includes monitoring important physiological parameters such as ventilation, circulation, oxygenation, and level of consciousness. Clinical assessment through observation of chest excursion and auscultation is often successful in detecting early ventilatory depression. Because such close clinical observation or auscultation may not be possible during most interventional radiology procedures, capnography becomes very useful. Any alteration in the capnogram waveform or activation of the apnea alarms warrants immediate clinical assessment of the patient's ventilation.

Blood pressure assessment is essential either manually or through an automated device. Proper BP cuff positioning and device setting are important because improper cuff placement and prolonged or too frequent cycling by the automated device can lead to complications such as ulnar and radial nerve paresthesia, compartment syndrome, or superficial thrombophlebitis.

Heart rate and rhythm are monitored continuously using lead V5 for detecting ischemia in patients with known coronary artery disease, and lead II for detecting dysrythmias. Although there are no studies proving conclusively the utility of continuous electrocardiographic (EKG) monitoring and patient outcome, it is generally accepted that patients with ASA class 3 or higher or patients with a history of cardiovascular disease undergoing conscious sedation require EKG monitoring.

Clinical observation may not detect hypoxemia until the oxygen saturation has fallen below 85% and in some cases to 70%. Because conscious sedation requires the administration of drugs (benzodiazepines and narcotics) known to have the potential for respiratory depression, particularly when used in combination, pulse oximetry should be used routinely for the detection of hypoxemia. Besides continuous observation, oxygen saturation should be recorded every 10 minutes.

Vital signs (BP, respiratory rate, quality of respiration, heart rate, and level of responsiveness) should be recorded every 10 minutes and airway patency should be checked at frequent intervals. Although a 10-minute-interval recording may suffice for the majority of patients undergoing conscious sedation, more frequent monitoring is needed in patients classified as ASA 3 and higher and those undergoing intricate procedures of longer duration. Of note is that the clinical observation of the patient using the senses (eyes, ears, fingers, and even nose) gathers more information than the monitors of modern technology (Hirsch, 1997). Therefore, it is strongly emphasized that clinical

observation should always accompany monitoring with equipment during administration of conscious sedation. **Fig. 51-1** shows the anesthesia monitoring form that we use.

Drugs Used for Conscious Sedation

The importance of understanding the pharmacology of the drugs used during conscious sedation cannot be overemphasized. The main drugs used are benzodiazepines and opioids. Occasionally, barbiturates, propofol, and droperidol are also used. Regardless of the drugs, one must take into consideration factors such as advanced age, chronic obstructive pulmonary disease (COPD), liver and renal disease, altered protein binding, hypovolemia, and poor ventricular function, which markedly increase drug sensitivity. Brief pharmacology of some of the commonly used drugs is discussed in the following sections. For more detailed information, see Stoelting (1999).

CHLORAL HYDRATE

This is a commonly used sedative for infants and young children in a dose of 25 to 50 mg/kg administered orally or per rectum 30 to 60 minutes prior to a procedure. It may be repeated once for a total maximal dose of 120 mg/kg or 1 g. Important to remember is its long half-life (10 hours in toddlers) and the total dose should not exceed 2 g/24 hours. Although it has minimal respiratory effects, it should be used with caution in patients with sleep apnea because it may cause severe airway obstruction. As with all sedative drugs, close supervision is mandatory, especially during patient transportation.

PENTOBARBITAL

This has minimal respiratory depression if used alone and is long acting (4–6 hours). The usual dose is 1 to 3 mg/kg/IV or a single dose of 2 to 6 mg/kg administered orally, per rectum, or intramuscularly. The onset of action is 1 minute for intravenous administration and 10 to 15 minutes for intramuscular injection. The duration of action is 1 to 4 hours for intramuscular and 15 minutes for intravenous administration.

BENZODIAZEPINES

This group of drugs has been used most extensively for its anxiolytic, anterograde amnesic, and sedative effects. In addition, benzodiazepines offer cardiopulmonary stability in the commonly used dosage and have a reliable, specific antagonist—flumazenil. These drugs act through the inhibitory neurotransmitter in the central nervous system called gamma-aminobutyric acid (GABA). By attaching themselves to the GABA receptors, benzodiazepines enhance the affinity of the receptors to GABA resulting in central nervous system (CNS) depression. Both diazepam (Valium) and midazolam (Versed) have been used. However, midazolam has largely replaced diazepam because of its short half-life of ~3 hours as compared with the nearly 40-hour half-life of diazepam. Furthermore, midazolam injection is painless.

Midazolam, when used in the doses of 0.05 to 0.15 mg/kg (or 1 mg IV slowly q 2–3 minutes for a maximum dose of 5 mg), provides excellent anxiolysis and anterograde amnesia without causing hypotension or respiratory depression. This dose is sufficient for short procedures (elimination half-life is 2.5 hours). For longer procedures, it may be carefully repeated in doses of 0.5 to 1.0 mg to the desired effect. The usual total dose is between 2.5 and 5.0 mg. In elderly patients, lower doses should be used. The hypotension and respiratory depression seen with larger doses (>0.2 mg/kg) is greater than that with similar doses of diazepam. Although the CNS effects of midazolam are usually rapid, individual patient variability exists. It is therefore recommended that the calculated dose of midazolam be administered in small increments to avoid oversedation. If oversedation does occur, flumazenil may be administered in a titrated dose to achieve the desired effect. For complete reversal of the

UNIVERSITY OF NORTH CAROLINA HOSPITALS
Chapel Hill, North Carolina 27514
**SEDATION/ANALGESIA ASSESSMENT AND PROCEDURE
RECORD – MIM #21**
Date:_____

NPO since:_____ ID confirmed: _____

History and Physical Exam:
Allergies/Adverse Drug Reactions:_____

Comorbidities:
☐ Diabetes ☐ Anxious ☐ Respiratory Disease ☐ Renal Disease ☐ Special Precautions: _____
☐ Hypertension ☐ Substance Abuse ☐ Communicable Disease ☐ Sleep Apnea _____
☐ Seizure Disorder ☐ Cardiac Disease ☐ Bleeding Disorder ☐ Snoring ☐ Other: _____
☐ Pregnant ☐ Exposure to Communicable Disease

*Baseline Sedation Scale Score:_____ Mental Status: _____ Previous Sedation/Anesthesia Problems:_____

BP_____ P _____ R _____ T _____ Pain Score**_____ Baseline O_2 SAT:_____

Wt_____ Ht. _____ ☐ Actual ☐ Reported. Labs – Creat:_____ PT: _____ PTT: _____ Other: _____ ☐ NA

Routine/Current Medications:_____
_____
_____
_____

☐ Taken in last 8 hours:_____
Does patient/caregiver have any additional needs, problems, questions?_____

HPI/Indication _____
Airway Exam: ☐ normal ☐ abnormalities_____
Pulmonary Exam: ☐ normal ☐ abnormalities_____
Cardiac Exam: ☐ normal ☐ abnormalities_____
Other _____
_____

☐ Anesthesiology Consultation Indicated For: History of previous airway or sedation problem ☐ yes ☐ no Known airway abn or tumor ☐ yes ☐ no
Known medical or psychiatric instability ☐ yes ☐ no

Airway Class: Circle Appropriate Image

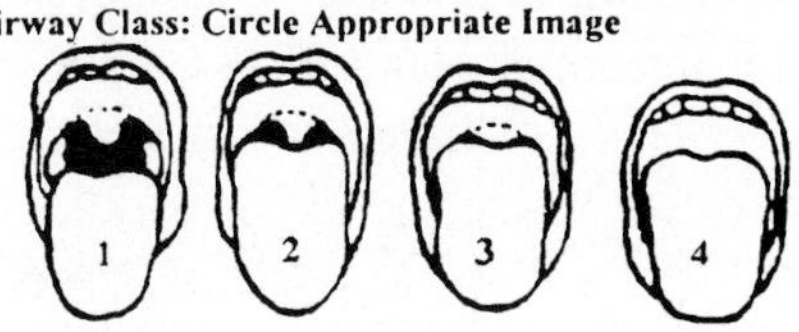

1 2 3 4

ASA Physical Status Class: I II III IV V
I A healthy patient
II A patient with mild systemic disease
III A patient with severe systemic disease
IV A patient with severe systemic disease that is a constant threat to life
V A moribund patient not expected to survive without the procedure

Sedation Plan:
☐ Sedation medication ordered
☐ Monitoring per policy/protocol
☐ Recovery per policy/protocol
☐ Options and risks of sedation discussed with patient/family
☐ Informed consent for procedure and sedation obtained

MD Signature_____**ID**_____

Quality – Safety checks:
Position: _____
Grounding Pad   ☐Yes ☐No ☐N/A, site_____
Safety strap on   ☐Yes ☐No ☐N/A
Oxygen   ☐Yes ☐No   Crash Cart/Ventilation kit   ☐Yes ☐No
Oxygen saturation monitor ☐Yes ☐No   Blood pressure monitoring capability ☐Yes ☐No
Bag Valve Mask   ☐Yes ☐No   Intravenous line (option of the operator) ☐Yes ☐No
Suction available   ☐Yes ☐No   EKG monitor/defibrillator available   ☐Yes ☐No
                                          (Required for patients with cardiac history)

Procedure Data:
Location: _____   Procedure: _____
Physician: _____   Procedure operator: _____
Procedure start time: _____   Procedure end time: _____
Monitoring start time: _____   Monitor end time: _____

Monitor signature/title:_____   ** Use Pain Scale (0-10), Face 0-5, or describe.

HD 5005 Rev 3/01, 6/01, 7/01, 1/02 Lawson 001211

Figure 51-1 Anesthesia monitoring form used at Memorial Hospital, Chapel Hill, NC.

benzodiazepine effect, a flumazenil dose of 0.5 mg may be necessary. An initial dose of 0.1 to 0.2 mg given intravenously, followed by 0.1 mg every 60 seconds up to 0.5 to 1.0 mg may be effectively used. Additional doses of flumazenil may have to be administered because the activity of flumazenil is short, lasting 30 to 60 minutes. Midazolam, being amnesic (anterograde), necessitates that any post-procedural instructions be discussed in the presence of an accompanying person. Also, the patient should be provided with written instructions for review at home.

PROPOFOL

Although a propofol-based conscious sedation technique has been used and is intuitively appealing, it can produce an unacceptably high incidence of upper airway obstruction. In addition, troublesome behavioral disinhibition seems to occur frequently (Young and Pile-Spellman, 1994). Initially, start with 0.1 to 0.15 mg/kg/min IV and repeat the dose 3 to 5 times to the desired effect or administer 0.5 mg/kg as a slow IV push over 3 to 5 minutes. To maintain sedation, follow by an intravenous infusion of 0.025 to 0.075 mg/kg/min. Alternatively, 10 to 20 mg intravenous incremental injections may be followed by a continuous infusion of 25 to 200 μg/kg/min. These regimens are useful and popular among anesthesiologists. Addition of midazolam reduces the requirement of propofol.

All patients should receive supplemental oxygen during conscious sedation. A variety of other sedation regimens and variations are possible (Eskridge, 1989; O'Mahony and Bosin, 1998). However, these must be based on the experience of the practitioner and the goals of anesthetic management for a particular procedure.

OPIOIDS

For conscious sedation, an ideal opioid would have a rapid onset and strong analgesia, cause minimal respiratory depression, and have a brief duration of action with minimal side effects. None of the currently available opioids fulfill these desirable characteristics. Despite the availability of opioids such as alfentanil, sufentanil, and remifentanil, morphine, meperidine, and fentanyl remain the most commonly used drugs for conscious sedation. Opioids act on specific opioid receptors located primarily in the brain stem and spinal cord. Three opioid receptors have been identified. These are mu, delta, and kappa. The mu receptor is the major site for supraspinal and spinal analgesia.

Morphine has a slow onset with peak effect at ~15 to 30 minutes. This, along with a longer duration of action, tends to limit its use, especially in short procedures. On the contrary, meperidine remains a popular opioid for conscious sedation because most clinicians and nurses are familiar with its use. Moreover, being one tenth as potent as morphine and with a shorter duration of action, it is suitable even for short procedures. However, both morphine and meperidine can cause respiratory depression and orthostatic hypotension. Nausea and vomiting can occur with the use of either of these drugs. Prolonged nausea and vomiting in an occasional patient can prevent same-day discharge.

Fentanyl is 100 times more potent than morphine. A dose of 1 to 2 μg/kg provides an adequate degree of analgesia for most interventional radiology procedures. One half to one third the initial dose may be repeated intermittently for more prolonged procedures. Fentanyl is a more suitable agent for conscious sedation because of its more rapid onset and shorter duration of action as compared with morphine and meperidine. It is less likely to cause hypotension due to the relative lack of histamine release. However, it can cause respiratory depression similar to morphine and meperidine. At times, the fentanyl-associated respiratory depression can be delayed. This is related to reabsorption of the sequestrated fentanyl from the gastrointestinal tract and washout from the lungs. Of note is that the combination of fentanyl with a benzodiazepine (such as midazolam) may result in respiratory depression and hypotension not seen with either drug alone. This is attributed to their synergistic action.

Respiratory depression produced by an opioid can be reversed by naloxone (Narcan). Full respiratory reversal can be achieved with a dose of 0.1 to 0.4 mg IV. Because of the short duration

of action of naloxone (30–45 minutes), repeat dosages may be necessary to avoid recurrence of ventilatory depression.

DEXMEDETOMIDE

The α 2 agonist dexmedetomide is a new sedative and analgesic agent that is licensed for postoperative intensive care sedation. It produces sedation, anxiolysis, and analgesia. Patients remain easily rouseable and do not suffer significant respiratory depression. Consequently, dexmedetomide may be useful for conscious sedation when close supervision by trained staff is available. A loading dose of 1.0 μg/kg over 10 minutes may be followed by an infusion of 0.2 to 0.7 μg/kg/hr to the desired effect.

DRUG COMBINATIONS

Fentanyl and midazolam are currently considered an ideal combination for conscious sedation in interventional radiology because both drugs are relatively short acting and cause minimal respiratory depression, and midazolam has a useful amnesic property (Vaselis et al, 1997). Ninety-two percent of U.S. conscious sedation practitioners use midazolam and 62% use fentanyl, either alone or in combination. On the other hand, European practitioners providing conscious sedation for interventional radiology administer midazolam and fentanyl in 58% and 33% of cases, respectively (Haslam et al, 2000).

Levels of Conscious Sedation for Different Procedures

Various levels of conscious sedation are used (Holzman et al, 1994). At the University of North Carolina Hospitals, the degree of sedation for interventional radiology procedures has been divided into the following levels:

5 Fully awake
4 Arouses easily
3 Arouses with tactile stimuli
2 Arouses with vigorous stimuli
1 Responsive to painful stimuli
0 Unresponsive

Level of conscious sedation requirement differs not only with the type of procedure but also among the U.S. and European centers (JCAHO, 2001). Vascular procedures are generally performed in the alert/awake level of sedation, whereas visceral interventions are done in a deeper level of sedation. In Europe, lesser levels of conscious sedation are used for the same procedures than in the United States (Haslam et al, 2000).

Complications

The principal concern during conscious sedation is hypoxemia or respiratory arrest or both. This complication can result from an absolute or relative overmedication and occurs when the sedative/narcotic drugs are administered at inappropriately high dosages for the size of the patient and repeated too soon. Sometimes, the patient may simply be more sensitive to the drugs, leading to a relative overmedication. This is often encountered when advanced age and concurrent medical conditions such as cardiorespiratory, renal, or hepatic diseases have not been considered in sedation planning. Therefore, it is important to reiterate that the primary role of the designated RN or anesthesiologist is to detect bradypnea and apnea. This is consistent with the ASA guidelines recommending that ventilatory function be continually monitored by observation (Practice Guidelines, 1996). When oxygen saturation level reaches 90% or less, the procedure should be stopped and respiration assisted. Below this oxygen saturation level, further desaturation occurs along the

steep portion of oxyhemoglobin dissociation curve, resulting in a greater risk of hypoxia-related complications such as cardiac or cerebral ischemia and arrhythmias.

Hypotension, vasovagal attack, and ischemic catastrophes may occur during conscious sedation. Prompt control of airway, respiration, and circulation forms the mainstay of the emergency management.

Placement of a nasopharyngeal airway can cause troublesome bleeding in anticoagulated patients and is best avoided. If the need for a nasopharyngeal airway is anticipated, it is prudent to place it before anticoagulation is initiated and observe hemostasis.

Patient-Controlled Sedation for Interventional Radiology

Propofol's sedative and hypnotic effects, fast onset, and extremely short duration have made it an ideal agent for patient-controlled sedation analgesia (PCSA) using 25 to 50 μg/kg boluses in adults. It has also been used by anesthesiologists for magnetic resonance imaging (MRI) procedures as a continuous IV infusion of 25 to 100 μg/kg/min (Kaplan, 2000). PCSA for relieving pain and anxiety during extracorporeal shock wave lithotripsy in adult patients was shown to have no cardiorespiratory depression (Maroof et al, 1993). Self-administration of a dose of 0.3 mg/kg of propofol and 0.15 μg/kg of fentanyl via a patient-controlled analgesia infusion pump (PCA pump) with a 3-minute obligatory lockout interval between consecutive doses provided sedation cum analgesia during extracorporeal shock wave lithotripsy with safety, effectiveness, and high patient satisfaction. However, respiratory depression has been reported during PCA (White and Parker, 1992; Etches, 1994). Advanced age, hypovolemia, large incremental doses, and use of a background continuous-infusion were possible contributing factors. Though a combination of propofol and fentanyl for PCSA may appear to be attractive, we recommend that until further studies are published on its safety for use during interventional radiology, it be used only by anesthesiologists in near-operating-room conditions.

GENERAL ANESTHESIA

Small children and uncooperative adult patients require general anesthesia with tracheal intubation. General anesthesia is also used for certain specific procedures such as aneurysm ablation, sclerotherapy, and some cases of chemotherapy. General anesthesia for interventional radiology is essentially similar to that administered in the operating room. During neurointerventional procedures, a theoretical argument could be made for not using nitrous oxide because of the possibility of introducing air emboli into the cerebral circulation. However, no data support this apprehension.

Chest excursions during positive pressure ventilation can interfere with road mapping. Radiologists frequently request apnea and immobility for improving the quality of the images. An effective alternative to apnea is to adjust the ventilator to a relatively rapid rate and small tidal volume. Adequate gas exchange can be maintained during brief periods without degrading the image quality by the chest excursions. If available, this may be an ideal application for high-frequency-jet ventilation.

PEARLS AND PITFALLS_____

- Fentanyl and midazolam are considered an ideal combination for conscious sedation in interventional radiology because both drugs are relatively short acting and cause minimal respiratory depression, and midazolam is also amnesic.
- Because conscious sedation requires the administration of drugs known to have the potential for respiratory depression, pulse oximetry should be used routinely for the detection of hypoxemia.
- Hypoxemia can result from an absolute or relative overmedication and occurs when the drugs are administered at inappropriately high dosages for the patient size or are repeated too soon or the patient is more sensitive to the drugs.

Further Reading

Eskridge JM. Interventional neuroradiology. Radiology 1989;172:991–1006

Etches RC. Respiratory depression associated with patient-controlled analgesia: a review of eight cases. Can J Anaesth 1994;41:125–132

Gilbertson LI. Hospital standards and requirements. Int Anesthesiol Clin 1999;37:1–18

Gravenstein JS. Monitoring with our good senses. J Clin Monit Comput 1998;14:451–453

Haslam PJ, Yap B, Mueller PR, et al. Anesthesia practice and clinical trends in interventional radiology: a European survey. Cardiovasc Intervent Radiol 2000;23:256–261

Hirsch IB. Approach to the patient with diabetes undergoing a vascular or interventional procedure. J Vasc Interv Radiol 1997;8:329–336

Holzman RS, Cullen DJ, Eichorn JH, et al. Guidelines for sedation by nonanesthesiologists during diagnostic and therapeutic procedures. J Clin Anesth 1994;6:265–276

JCAHO. Revision to Anesthesia Care Standards: Comprehensive Accreditional Manual for Ambulatory Care. Effective January 1, 2001. http://www.jcaho/standard/anesamb.html

Kaplan RF. Sedation and analgesia for children undergoing procedures outside the operating room In: Schwartz AJ, ed. Refresher Courses in Anesthesiology. Vol 28. 2000:69–79

Maroof M, Khan RM, Bhatti TH, et al. Evaluation of patient controlled sedation and analgesia for ESWL. J Stone Dis 1993;5:240–243

Mallampatti SR, Gatt SP, Gugino LD, et al. A clinical sign to predict difficult tracheal intubation: a prospective study. Can Anaesth Soc J 1985;32:429–434

O'Mahony BJ, Bosin SN. Anesthesia for closed embolisation of cerebral arteriovenous malforations. Anaesth Intensive Care 1998;16:318–323

Practice Guidelines for Sedation and Analgesia by Nonanesthesiologists (ammended October 17, 2001). www.asa.hq/practice/sedation 1017.pdf

Practice guidelines for sedation and analgesia by non-anesthesiologists: a report by the American Society of Anesthesiologists Task Force on Sedation and Analgesia by Non-Anesthesiologists. Anesthesiology 1996;84:459–471

Spies JB, Bakal CW, Burke DR, et al. Standards of Practice Committee of the Society of Cardiovascular and Interventional Radiology standards for interventional radiology. J Vasc Interv Radiol 1991;2:59–65

Stoelting RK. Pharmacology and Physiology in Anesthetic Practice. Philadelphia: Lippincott-Raven; 1999:77–145

Vaselis RA, Reinsel RA, Feshchenko VA, et al. The comparative amnestic effects of midazolam, propofol, thiopental and fentanyl at equisedative concentrations. Anesthesiology 1997;87:749–764

White PF, Parker RK. Is the risk of using "basal" infusion with patient controlled analgesia therapy justified? [Letter]. Anesthesiology 1992;76:489

Young WL, Pile-Spellman J. Anesthetic consideration for interventional neuroradiology. Anesthesiology 1994;80:427–456

CHAPTER 52 Infection and Sepsis: An Overview for the Interventional Radiologist

Edgar Turner Overton, Hilary M. Babcock, and Nigar Kirmani

Many issues in infectious diseases are of concern to the interventional radiologist. This chapter addresses abdominal and pelvic infections, infection control issues, central venous catheter infections, and bloodborne pathogen exposure, risks, and management for health care workers.

Abdominal and Pelvic Infections

Most abdominal and pelvic infections that require an interventional radiology procedure are abscesses or closed space infections. In these cases, the primary mode of treatment is drainage of the fluid collection. Drainage is necessary even if the abscess is caused by an organism that is easily treated because antibiotics penetrate poorly into unvascularized spaces such as abscesses and may not perform well in the often acidic environment of the abscess cavity. Specifics of radiological diagnosis and techniques of drainage approaches are covered elsewhere. This section focuses on likely bacteriology and the medical management of such infections.

Intra-abdominal Abscess

Intra-abdominal infection usually results from perforation of the gastrointestinal tract. It may occur as a complication of appendicitis, diverticulitis, biliary tract disease, trauma, inflammatory bowel disease, perforated ulcers, or surgery. The location of the abscess is usually related to the site of primary disease and the direction of dependent peritoneal drainage. Most patients present with fever, chills, abdominal pain, and tenderness over the involved areas. In critically ill, intensive care unit (ICU) patients, fever may be the only clue until the abscess is found on computed tomography (CT) or ultrasound. After drainage and initiation of antimicrobial therapy, most patients undergo rapid clinical improvement. The prognosis after drainage of the abscess is usually good. However, a residual or recurrent infection due to inadequate drainage, often in the setting of multiple abscesses, is associated with increased mortality (Montgomery and Wilson, 1996).

Percutaneous drainage of infected fluid collections can serve several purposes: (1) confirmation that infection is present, (2) determination of microbial etiology, (3) definitive therapy by drainage, and (4) temporizing therapy. Temporary drainage allows stabilization of a critically ill patient before definitive surgical intervention is undertaken. It may also allow definitive therapy to be limited to one surgical procedure instead of two. For example, the percutaneous drainage of a diverticular abscess allows the surgeon to perform resection with primary anastomosis instead of a two-step procedure with a temporary colostomy (McClean et al, 1994). Percutaneous drainage may be less successful with multiloculated collections, with fungal abscesses containing very viscous fluid and often with tissue invasion, and with hematomas or large amounts of necrotic tissue where adequate drainage through a catheter is less likely (McClean et al, 1994). In most cases, the drainage catheter should be left in place until the daily output drops below 10 mL/day. At this point, repeat cross-sectional imaging is performed to confirm collapse of the abscess cavity prior to drainage catheter removal. Most patients defervesce within 24 to 48 hours of abscess drainage. If the patient remains febrile, the adequacy of drainage should be reevaluated and other undrained collections excluded.

In all cases, the drainage serves both a diagnostic and a therapeutic purpose. For microbial analysis, a fluid sample should be aspirated into a syringe and either capped immediately to prevent oxygen from entering or immediately transferred into an anaerobic transport system. Although 2 to 3 mL aspirate usually provides an adequate sample, if available, a larger volume of aspirated fluid should be sent to the laboratory to ensure adequate material for all requested studies. These include

Table 52-1   Flora of the Gastrointestinal Tract

Location	Bacterial Load	Likely Organisms
Stomach, duodenum, proximal small bowel	Sparse	Viridans strep, microaerophilic strep, *Candida* spp., *Lactobacillus, Bacteroides, Fusobacterium*
Distal small bowel	Moderate	*Enterococcus, Enterobacteriaceae* (*Escherichia coli, Klebsiella, Proteus), Bacteroides fragilis*
Colon	Abundant (10^{12} organisms/gm of feces)	Anaerobes>> aerobes (1000:1) Anaerobes: *B. fragilis* (most common), Ebacterium, *Bifidobacterium* Aerobes: *Enterobacteriaceae: E. coli* (most common), Enterococcus

Table 52-2   Common Intra-abdominal Pathogens

Aerobic Gram Positive Cocci	Aerobic Gram Negative Bacilli	Anaerobes	Yeast
Staphylococcus spp. *Streptococcus Enterococcus*	*Enterobacteriaceae* (*E. coli, Klebsiella, Proteus, Serratia) Pseudomonas*	*Bacteroides fragilis Fusobacterium Peptostreptococcus*	*Candida* spp. (*albicans, krusei, glabrata, parapsilosis*)

Gram stain and aerobic and anaerobic cultures. Fluid can be transported at room temperature and should be received in the laboratory within 2 hours of sampling, to maximize the likelihood of a positive culture result (Murray, 1998). Most aerobic organisms can survive for several hours without oxygen but many anaerobes cannot survive in the presence of oxygen.

If biopsies are obtained from the abscess wall, the tissue should be placed in an anaerobic transport vial and the top replaced immediately. A 0.5 cm cube of tissue is usually adequate for culture. Tissue should be kept moist during transport by addition of a few mL of sterile saline (Schwartz, 1999; Levison and Bush, 2000). Preservatives should not be used. Culture results will often be positive, even from patients on systemic antibiotics, because there is poor penetration of most antibiotic agents into the abscess cavity. Fungal cultures may also be indicated, especially in immuno-compromised patients. The culture results allow more targeted antibiotic choices and ensure that the important infectious agents are covered.

Bacterial isolates from abdominal abscesses vary according to the part of the gastrointestinal tract that is involved but are usually polymicrobial and include anaerobes (**Table 52-1**). Until specific culture results are available, antimicrobial agents should be selected for broad coverage of expected organisms, including anaerobes. This usually requires combination drug therapy. Traditionally, this has included clindamycin for aerobic gram-positive as well as anaerobic coverage, and an aminogly-coside for aerobic gram-negatives. This regimen is still effective but its use is limited due to the side effects of the aminoglycosides, primarily ototoxicity and nephrotoxicity. Substitutes for gram-negative coverage include third generation cephalosporins (e.g., ceftriaxone), which can be combined with metronidazole for anaerobic coverage. Cephamycins (cefoxitin and cefotetan) combine gram-negative and anaerobic coverage. Combination products with β-lactam/β-lactamase inhibitors such as ampicillin/sulbactam, ticarcillin/clavulanate, and piperacillin/tazobactam offer good gram-negative and anaerobic coverage (**Table 52-2**).

Table 52-3 Empirical Antibiotic Regimen for Intra-abdominal Infections (Solokin et al, 2003)

Severity of Illness	Possible Empirical Antimicrobial Regimens	Organisms Not Covered
Mild–moderate Cephalosporin monotherapy	Cefoxitin Cefotetan	*Pseudomonas, Enterobacter, Serratia;* *Enterococcus;* ORSA; fungus
Mild–moderate β-lactam/β-lactamase monotherapy	Ampicillin/sulbactam	*Pseudomonas, Enterobacter,* *Serratia;* ORSA; fungus
Mild–moderate Quinolone based	Metronidazole + ciprofloxacin	*Enterococcus;* ORSA; fungus
Mild–moderate Cephalosporin based	Ceftriaxone + metronidazole	*Enterococcus;* ORSA; fungus
Severe	Ampicillin + Aminoglycoside + Metronidazole	ORSA; fungus
Severe Monotherapy with carbapenem or β-lactam/β-lactamase	Imipenem, Meropenem Piperacillin/tazobactam Ticarcillin/clavulanic acid	ORSA; fungus
Severe Cephalopsorin therapy	Cefotaxime + metronidazole Cefepime + metronidazole	ORSA; fungus
Severe with MRSA risk	Vancomycin + Imipenem	Fungus
Severe with MRSA risk	Vancomycin + cefepime + metronidazole	Fungus

MRSA, methicillin-resistant *Staphylococcus aureus;* ORSA, oxacillin-resistant *Staphylococcus aureus.*

The foregoing regimens do not provide satisfactory coverage for *Pseudomonas, Enterobacter*, and *Serratia. Pseudomonas* is seen in <7% of peritoneal isolates, though the incidence increases to 24% in perforated appendices (McClean, 1994). The incidence of *Pseudomonas* is also higher in hospitalized patients. If these organisms are found or are thought to be potential pathogens in a specific patient, flouroquinolones (ciprofloxacin) can be used for broader gram-negative coverage. Anaerobic coverage would still be necessary, with either clindamycin or metronidazole. Imipenem/cilastatin is a carbapenem that combines coverage for most sensitive gram-positive and gram-negative organisms, including *Pseudomonas, Serratia*, and *Enterobacter* spp., as well as anaerobes.

For empirical coverage in severely ill patients, combination therapy with imipenem/cilastatin is indicated for anaerobes and gram-negatives. In moderately ill patients, monotherapy with a cephamycin or a β-lactam/β-lactamase inhibitor is usually adequate. In the setting of a prolonged hospitalization, the frequency of *Pseudomonas* and other resistant gram-negative rods increases and antibiotic coverage for these organisms requires an aminoglycoside, flouroquinolone, or imipenem (**Table 52-3**).

Enterococcus is often seen in polymicrobial abdominal collections, but its role is often unclear. Many patients improve with drainage and broad-spectrum antibiotics that do not treat *Enterococcus*. In general, the addition of enterococcal antimicrobial therapy is indicated only if it is the primary organism isolated from a collection or if there is concurrent enterococcal bacteremia. Patients at increased risk for enterococcal infections include those with recent urinary tract instrumentation, malignancy, renal failure, diabetes mellitus, burns, major surgery, or a prolonged hospitalization. If *Enterococcus* is suspected, ampicillin can be added to the regimen. In patients allergic to penicillin, vancomycin is used.

Candida isolates are often not clinically significant, although they can be found in up to 20% of cultures from patients with gastrointestinal perforation (Schwartz, 1999). Individuals at increased risk

for candidal infections include those with diabetes mellitus, malignancy, T cell defects, malnutrition, or receiving total parenteral nutrition (TPN), and multiple abdominal surgeries. Both *Enterococcus* and *Candida* are found with increased frequency among patients who have received prolonged courses of antibiotics (McClean et al, 1994). Guidelines for treatment are similar to those with *Enterococcus*. Treatment should be reserved for cases when *Candida* is the predominant organism in the culture, there is accompanying candidemia, or fungal tissue invasion is seen on pathology. Treatment may also be indicated for patients who are immunosuppressed. Most candidal infections can be treated with fluconazole; however, some species such as *Candida krusei* and *glabrata* have higher rates of resistance to fluconazole and may require amphotericin B.

Pancreatic Infections

Pancreatic infections can be divided into two types: infected pancreatic necrosis and pancreatic abscess. Infected pancreatic necrosis develops in 40 to 60% of patients with severe, acute pancreatitis and in patients with necrosis of >50% of the pancreas (Montgomery and Wilson, 1996; Schwartz, 1999). Clinically, pancreatic infection is difficult to distinguish from severe pancreatitis without infection because the clinical presentation (fever, leukocytosis, and hemodynamic instability) can occur with or without infection. The presence of gas on CT or a percutaneous aspirate with a positive Gram' stain and culture can make the diagnosis. Usually, these infections are caused by a mixed bacterial flora including *Escherichia coli, Klebsiella, Pseudomonas,* and *Enterococcus* as well as anaerobes such as *Bacteroides. Staphylococcus* and *Streptococcus* are found in ~20% and *Candida albicans* in 5 to 10% (Montgomery and Wilson, 1996). In this setting, percutaneous drainage may be inadequate because the infected fluid is thick and the presence of particulate material occludes the drainage catheters (also see Chapters 32 and 33). Surgical debridement is usually required and 20% of patients will require more than one operation. Mortality ranges from 10 to 35% (Schwartz, 1999).

Pancreatic abscesses are localized collections of pus in or near the involved pancreas. These often occur as a late complication of pancreatitis (i.e., 3–4 weeks after the acute episode). Clinically, they can be difficult to distinguish from sterile pseudocysts. As with infected necrosis, air is seen in the fluid collection on CT or there is a positive Gram stain and culture on aspirated fluid. Percutaneous drainage may be adequate in this setting, with reported success rates ranging from 32 to 79% (Montgomery and Wilson, 1996). However, if the fluid is very thick, if the patient has a poor clinical response, or if there is significant surrounding necrosis, surgical drainage and debridement may be necessary. Mortality in pancreatic abscess can reach 20% (Schwartz, 1999).

Hepatic Abscess

Hepatic abscesses can be divided into two categories: pyogenic and amebic. Pyogenic abscesses are uncommon, with an incidence of 0.36% at autopsy. Immunocompromised patients are at increased risk (Schwartz, 1999). They occur with equal frequency in men and women and are usually secondary to an infection elsewhere. The most common source is ascending infection from the biliary tract followed by hematogenous spread due to bacteremia. *Staphylococcus aureus* can cause multiple microabscesses in this setting, usually in patients with impaired host defenses, as with chronic granulomatous disease. *Candida* may also invade the liver under similar circumstances. Hematogenous spread can also occur via the portal veins from intestinal tract infection, including appendicitis, diverticulitis, and inflammatory bowel disease. Less commonly, infection can be caused by direct extension from an intraperitoneal source or secondary to penetrating trauma. In up to 20% of cases, the primary source is unknown. Single and multiple abscesses occur with equal frequency (Schwartz, 1999).

Needle aspiration serves both diagnostic and therapeutic purposes. Cultures are positive in 90% of cases and 25% of pyogenic abscesses are polymicrobial. Fluid should be sent for both aerobic and anaerobic culture. The most commonly isolated organisms are enteric gram-negative bacteria, including *E. coli*, *Klebsiella*, *Streptococcus*, and anaerobes. *Bacteroides* spp., *Fusobacterium*, and *Actinomyces* spp. have been reported but may be missed if anaerobic cultures are not obtained.

Treatment consists of systemic antibiotics, usually for 4 to 6 weeks, as well as drainage of the abscess. (also see Chapter 16) Empirical antibiotic regimens are similar to those already outlined for intra-abdominal abscesses. These are adjusted as culture results become available. Most patients require drainage for clinical improvement, though there have been some reports of improvement without drainage. Mortality with drainage ranges from 7.5 to 20% and is higher among patients with multiple abscesses. Without drainage, mortality can be as high as 50% (Schwartz, 1999). Even after drainage, some patients may take several weeks to defervesce.

Amebic liver abscesses are caused by *Entamoeba histolytica*, are usually solitary, and usually occur in the right lobe of the liver. Diagnosis can be confirmed by serology and indirect hemagglutination testing, which is positive in 90 to 100% of cases. This infection is most common in developing countries but is seen in the United States in travelers, recent immigrants, and male homosexuals. It is transmitted by ingestion of food or water contaminated with feces containing the cystic form of the parasite, or through sexual practices involving fecal–oral contact. In the host intestine, the cysts develop into trophozoites, which invade the host tissues. Colonic disease occurs with equal frequency in men and women, but a liver abscess occurs more frequently in men (9:1). The disease is more severe in children, pregnant women, in patients on corticosteroids, with cancer, or malnutrition.

Most cases of amebic abscess can be managed medically. With metronidazole therapy alone, the cure rates in uncomplicated cases have been as high as 90% and the mortality is low, less than 1%. Possible complications include secondary infection (22%) and rupture. The latter can occur into the peritoneum, the pleural cavity, or pericardium. Indications for percutaneous drainage include very large abscesses at imminent risk for rupture, abscesses in the left lobe at increased risk for rupture into the pericardium, and failure of medical treatment, with persistent fever and pain after 5 days of metronidazole. The aspirate has a classic "anchovy paste" reddish brown consistency. Resolution of the cavity can be slow and cavity size may actually enlarge over the first few weeks, even with successful treatment. Most amebic abscesses resolve within 6 months (Li and Stanley, 1996).

Patients with Liver Transplantation

Liver transplantation patients represent a special situation that deserves additional mention. Due to the technical difficulty and duration of the surgical procedure, the presence of coagulopathy in many patients with end-stage liver disease, and the compromised nutritional status, liver transplantation has a much higher rate of postoperative infectious complications than either kidney or heart transplantion (Dummer and Ho, 2000). Intra-abdominal infections with bacterial or fungal pathogens are the most common (Paya et al, 1989). Thirty-five to 70% of transplant recipients develop an infection and half of these infections occur within 2 weeks of the surgery (Kusne et al, 1988; Paya et al, 1989). Liver abscesses and cholangitis are common problems. Liver abscesses usually present with fever and leukocytosis, with or without bacteremia. The diagnosis is made with CT or ultrasound. These infections are usually polymicrobial, with gram-negative rods, enterococci, and anaerobes being the most commonly encountered organisms. Treatment involves both antibiotic therapy and adequate drainage. Empirical administration of broad-spectrum antibiotics such as imipenem/cilastin with or without vancomycin (depending on the risk for methicillin resistant *Staphylococcus aureus* [MRSA]) is the initial treatment while awaiting culture results.

Other intra-abdominal abscesses also occur in liver transplant recipients. The clinical presentation is similar to that of the liver abscess. In addition to the potential microbial etiologies already noted, coagulase-negative staphylococci and *S. aureus* are commonly found. Therefore, the empirical antibiotic regimen should include vancomycin while results are pending (Dummer and Ho, 2000). Fungal pathogens are more common after liver transplantation and usually occur within the first 2 months after transplantation. *Candida* spp. are the most frequent pathogen, although *Aspergillus* spp. are also reported. Patients are less likely to present with fever. In one retrospective series, candidal etiologies were more common among patients with impaired renal function, a prolonged duration of operation, repeat transplantation, and colonization with *Candida* spp. at the time of surgery (Collins et al, 1994). Due to the concern for a wide range of potential pathogens and the underlying condition of these patients, it is important to send cultures for aerobes, anaerobes, and fungi in fluid collections drained from liver transplant patients.

Splenic Abscess

Splenic abscesses are uncommon and usually occur in patients with sickle hemoglobinopathies, trauma victims, bacteremic patients, or intravenous drug abusers. Prior to the antibiotic era, these infections were uniformly fatal. With antibiotics, patient survival has improved markedly. The symptoms are the triad of fever, abdominal pain, and leukocytosis. Ultrasound or CT usually provides the diagnosis. At time of diagnosis, 25% of abscesses are solitary (Gadacz et al, 1974; Levison and Bush, 2000). The presence of multiple small abscesses suggests hematogenous spread. The key to survival is the combination of drainage and antimicrobial therapy. Solitary abscess cavities that are not located in the splenic hilum are generally amenable to percutaneous drainage under ultrasound or CT guidance. Several retrospective studies have shown that in the proper context, percutaneous drainage is as effective as surgical intervention and prevents splenectomy (Ng et al, 2002; Thanos et al, 2002).

Agents that may cause splenic abscesses are numerous. When occurring as a complication of bacterial endocarditis, multiple small abscesses are often seen, and the most common causative agents are *S. aureus* or *Streptococcus*. In other cases, gram-negative rods, notably *Salmonella*, have been responsible. In one series, 36% of cases were polymicrobial with the frequent presence of anaerobes (Phillips et al, 1997). Additionally, fungal infections have become more common as the population with risk factors for disseminated candidiasis has increased (e.g., patients receiving cancer chemotherapy or high-dose steroids or having undergone multiple abdominal surgeries) (Levison and Bush, 2000). Treatment consists of empirical broad-spectrum antibiotic coverage for gram-negative, gram-positive, and anaerobic organisms at the time of diagnosis until drainage and culture results become available. In patients who are bacteremic, therapy is directed against the isolated organism.

Biliary Infections

Acute cholecystitis is related to obstruction of the cystic duct with subsequent distension of the gallbladder causing obstruction of the blood supply and lymph drainage, which leads to tissue necrosis with proliferation of bacteria and clinically manifested infection. Complications of acute cholecystitis include empyema, gangrene, emphysematous cholecystitis, pericholecystic or intraperitoneal abscess, peritonitis, cholangitis, liver abscess, and bacteremia. Biliary pathogens consist of intestinal flora, which includes enterococci and enteric gram-negative bacilli such as *Klebsiella, Enterobacter*, and *Proteus*. Anaerobes are also found frequently, especially in patients who have undergone multiple biliary tract procedures. *Pseudomonas aeruginosa* is commonly isolated from patients who have biliary stents. Treatment consists of broad-spectrum antibiotics for specific coverage of these gram-negative bacteria. This consists of flouroquinolones, aminoglycosides, or cefepime, in combination metronidazole for anaerobic coverage. Piperacillin/tazobactam or imipenem are single agents that also provide adequate coverage for both anaerobic and gram-negative organisms. Surgical intervention is required for gangrenous cholecysitis, perforation, and pericholecystic abscess. In clinically unstable patients, cholecystostomy and stone removal may be a temporizing measure prior to definitive intervention (also see Chapters 30 and 31).

Percutaneous transhepatic cholangiography is used for the evaluation of the biliary tree in cases where ERCP cannot be performed and allows for the removal of obstructing stones, drainage of infected bile, dilatation of strictures, and placement of stents (Kavanaugh et al, 1997). In patients with obstructive jaundice, prophylactic antibiotics should be given at the time of the procedure to prevent biliary sepsis. Cephalosporins have been used and are generally effective because gram-negative bacilli are the most common pathogens. The cephalosporins have no activity against enterococci, which have been documented to cause biliary sepsis in cases where a cephalosporin was used. Thus it is prudent to use ampicillin and an aminoglycoside to cover gram-negative rods (GNRs) and enterococci in patients undergoing cholangiography. A flouroquinolone can be substituted for the aminoglycoside if there is concern for renal toxicity. Care should be taken to decompress the biliary tree prior to contrast injection to prevent biliary sepsis (Wu et al, 1997). In all procedures involving the biliary tree, aspirates should be sent for both aerobic and anaerobic culture.

Perinephric Abscesses

Perinephric abscess is an uncommon complication of urinary tract infection. Patients with diabetes mellitus and urinary tract calculi are at increased risk. Abscesses can result from urinary tract obstruction or from bacteremia. Most patients have fever and flank pain and have often been ill for 1 to 2 weeks. As many as 30% of patients have a normal urinalysis and 40% have sterile urine cultures (Sobel and Kaye, 2000). In most cases, pyelonephritis is due to enteric gram-negative bacilli. Less commonly, gram-positive cocci (especially *S. aureus*) are found as a result of hematogenous spread, which is more likely to cause intrarenal abscesses. Anaerobes are usually not involved. In previously healthy outpatients without history of instrumentation, *E. coli* is the most common organism. Empirical treatment consists of coverage with ampicillin or cefazolin. Patients with a history of frequent or prolonged hospitalizations, multiple urinary tract procedures, or immunosuppression, are at risk for more resistant organisms such as *Pseudomonas* or *Klebsiella*. These patients may require broader coverage with a flouroquinolone or cefepime. In patients who have not been on therapy prior to drainage, dual therapy with a flouroquinolone and aminoglycoside can be used to speed up clearance of bacteria.

The diagnosis of a perinephric abscess is established by CT or ultrasound. Needle aspiration confirms the diagnosis, at which time a drainage catheter can be placed. Cultures of the fluid can help to guide antibiotic coverage. In most cases, percutaneous decompression and drainage are adequate. Surgical intervention is reserved for cases in which percutaneous drainage fails. Intrarenal abscesses do not always require drainage. Lesions <5 cm will often resolve with antibiotic therapy alone, whereas larger abscesses may require drainage. Patients with emphysematous pyelonephritis may need nephrectomy.

Pelvic Abscesses

Pelvic abscesses occur most often as a late complication of surgery. Many can be treated successfully with antibiotics alone. Because *Bacteroides fragilis* is often isolated from these collections, antibiotic regimens should include clindamycin or metronidazole for anaerobic coverage (Mead, 2000). If conservative management fails, percutaneous or surgical drainage should be undertaken. Fluid should be sent for both aerobic and anaerobic culture. Tubo-ovarian abscesses usually respond to medical management with broad-spectrum antibiotics. Drainage may be necessary if the clinical response is poor and if the abscess is large (>10 cm).

Infection-Control Precautions for Antibiotic-Resistant Organisms

Interventional procedures may need to be performed on patients who have been colonized or infected with antibiotic-resistant organisms, such as methicillin-resistant *S. aureus* (MRSA), or vancomycin-resistant *Enterococcus* (VRE). For procedures on these patients, isolation precautions must be followed and most facilities have infection-control policies to manage such cases. In general, patients on contact precautions should be transported directly into the procedure area and not held in hallways or holding areas. If the patient must go to a holding area, contact precautions should be observed, including the use of gowns, gloves, and dedicated equipment such as stethoscopes. Meticulous hand hygiene must be maintained and gowns and gloves disposed of between patient contacts.

During the procedure, the number of personnel should be limited to those needed, and the presence of students and observers should be minimized. After the procedure, any equipment that came in contact with the patient or the personnel taking care of the patient should be disinfected. Reusable equipment such as monitors, cautery devices, blood pressure cuffs, telephones, and instrument stands that cannot be soaked in disinfectant should be wiped down with disinfectant and allowed to air dry, per the recommendations of the disinfecting agent manufacturer. Preparation for the next case should not begin until the patient has left the room and the room has been cleaned and all equipment disinfected. Reuse of syringes between patients and the use of multidose medicine vials between patients have been associated with transmission of hepatitis B and C and should be avoided (CDC, 2003;52).

Central Venous Catheter–Associated Infections

The use of central venous catheters (CVCs) has increased dramatically over the last decade. In the United States, an estimated 5 million CVCs are placed annually (Oppenheim, 2000). As their use increases, infectious complications have also increased. There are three major infectious complications: exit site infections, tunnel infections, and catheter-related bloodstream infections.

Exit Site Infection

This is defined as a localized cellulitis within 2 cm of the skin exit site. Microbiological diagnosis includes a positive culture of any exudate at the exit site. These are usually minor infections that can often be managed with oral antibiotics. Parenteral antibiotics may be required for more resistant infections and in immunocompromised patients. Catheter removal is usually not required.

Tunnel Infections

These are more difficult to treat. They should be suspected if there is pain and an erythema track along the subcutaneous tunnel of the catheter. Parenteral antibiotics and catheter removal are usually necessary.

Catheter-Related Bacteremia

This is the most serious infectious complication of central venous catheter (CVC) use. Guidelines have been published outlining strategies for the prevention of these serious hospital-acquired infections

(CDC, 2002;51). The use of these catheters should be reserved for patients with a proven need and the catheter should be removed as soon as clinically feasible (Henderson, 2000). Manipulation of the catheter should be minimized and careful hand disinfection performed before and after use. Catheter insertion location is important in terms of the incidence of infection. The highest risk of infection is associated with a femoral site, followed by the internal jugular. The lowest risk for infection is associated with subclavian placement.

The risk of infection can be minimized by using strict sterile precautions at the time of CVC insertion, that is skin disinfection with chlorhexidine or iodinated prep solutions and standardized use of full-barrier precautions such as gowns, masks, caps, gloves, and large sterile drapes. Routine replacement of catheters has not been shown to decrease infection rates. Antibiotic (rifampin, minocycline) or antiseptic (chlorhexidine silver-sulfadiazine) treated catheters have been associated with lower rates of infection. However, adverse reactions to chlorhexidine have been observed in Japan and the effect of these catheters on antibiotic resistance has not been fully elucidated. Their widespread use cannot yet be strongly recommended, although they may be useful in high-risk (e.g., immunocompromised) patients, or in other high-risk settings or when other interventions already outlined have not lowered the rates of infection (Mermel et al, 2001).

Defining a catheter-related bacteremia and distinguishing it from contamination or from systemic bacteremia unrelated to the CVC can be difficult. Most definitions call for cultures to be positive with the same organism from the catheter (either blood drawn through the catheter or a catheter-tip culture) and from a peripheral site. Clinical signs and symptoms of infection should be present and no other source of bacteremia should be evident.

Infection rates for peripheral intravenous catheters are low (0.2–0.5%). For CVCs, reported rates range from 3.8 to 12% (Corona et al, 1990). The organisms most commonly associated with CVC infections are coagulase-negative *Staphylococcus* and *S. aureus*. Occasionally, gram-negative rods such as *Klebsiella, Enterobacter, Pseudomonas*, or *Serratia* are found. These organisms may be associated with contaminated infusate. Candidal CVC infections are most often associated with TPN.

Defining optimal management of CVC-related bacteremia can be difficult. Most clinicians agree that, optimally, all infected catheters would be removed. However, because many patients have limited options for intravenous access, preservation of the line is a frequent goal. Infections with coagulase-negative *Staphylococcus* are the most amenable to line preservation. In patients with fever and mild to moderate clinical illness, the catheter can be retained until microbiological data are available. In patients with more severe illness, with clinical signs and symptoms suggestive of CVC infection, or with complications of infection such as embolic phenomena, the catheter should be removed promptly. Candidal CVC infections also require prompt catheter removal (Mermel et al, 2001). Increased mortality has been related to the duration of time that the catheter remains in place after positive cultures for yeast (Corona et al, 1990).

In cases where the source of the patient's bacteremia is unclear but may be from the CVC, catheter tip cultures can be helpful. The skin around the exit site should be carefully cleansed with alcohol prior to removal. Once the catheter is removed aseptically, the distal 5 cm tip should be clipped with sterile scissors and placed into a sterile tube or cup. This container should be taken directly to the laboratory. Drying of the specimen prior to processing should be prevented because it could result in false-negative cultures (Murray, 1998). If the CVC has been changed over a wire and the tip cultures are positive, the new catheter should also be removed and another catheter placed at a new site (Reed et al, 1995).

In most cases, systemic antibiotics are given, although duration of therapy can be debated. If a new access is desired, there should be at least a 2- to 3-day device-free interval between removal and replacement. If possible, the new CVC should be placed only after negative blood cultures have been obtained following removal of the original CVC.

Infected Hemodialysis Access Catheters

Infections of hemodialysis catheters can present a special challenge. The frequent access of a long-term device can result in high rates of colonization and infection. Diagnosing these infections requires blood cultures from the catheter and from a peripheral source, if possible. The most common cause of catheter-associated infections in this setting is *S. aureus.* Penicillinase-resistant penicillins are the drugs of choice for these infections. Infections with methicillin-resistant *S. aureus* can be treated with vancomycin. Management of these catheters is similar to that already outlined. Efforts to retain the catheter may include long-term parenteral antibiotics (Mermel et al, 2001).

Occupational Exposures

Health care workers (HCWs) are at risk for occupational exposures to the blood and body fluids of patients infected with bloodborne pathogens. The three pathogens of most concern are human immunodeficiency virus (HIV), hepatitis B, and hepatitis C. Strategies to prevent body substance exposures can be broken down into three categories: behaviors, work practice modifications, and engineering advances. Protective behaviors include use of universal precautions such as gloves, gowns, and face shields during every procedure; using double gloves for surgical procedures, including CVC insertion; and avoiding recapping of sharps. Work practice modifications include announcement of sharps passage during procedures involving assistants, and when possible, using staples instead of sutures and no-touch transfers of sharps using a tray or basin. Engineering advances include newer safety devices such as blunt suture needles, safety catheters with needle guards, and needle-less tubing.

Preexposure prophylaxis is the ideal way to prevent infections with these pathogens. Unfortunately, there are no effective preexposure prophylaxis mechanisms for either HIV or hepatitis C virus (HCV). Hepatitis B vaccination is the principal means by which HCWs can protect themselves from infection with hepatitis B virus (HBV). The vaccine has been proven to be both safe and effective and it is recommended for all HCWs (CDC, 2001;50). After completion of the three injection series, >90% of vaccinees will have an adequate antibody response (HBsAb >10 mIU/mL). This level should be determined 1 to 2 months after completion of the vaccine series. HCWs who fail to respond adequately should be tested for chronic HBV by checking their HBsAg. If this antigen is positive, the person should be referred to a specialist for further evaluation of chronic HBV. If the antigen is negative, the person should undergo a second series of HBV vaccination. Revaccination of these persons results in immunity in 25 to 50%. Those failing to have an adequate antibody response are classified as a nonresponder. Lack of response is more common among the obese, smokers, age over 50 years, and immunocompromised individuals. It is of note that responders will have a waning antibody titer that will decrease below 10 mIU/mL in 6 to 10 years. However, there is no indication for booster doses of vaccine because immunocompetent adults maintain effective immunity (Beltrami et al, 2000). Furthermore, there is no need for repeat testing of antibody titers in HCWs who have responded to vaccination.

Exposure is defined by the Centers for Disease Control and Prevention (CDC) in a publication *Public Health Service Guidelines for the Management of Health-Care Worker Exposures to HIV and Recommendations for Postexposure Prophylaxis* as: "eye, mouth, other mucous membrane, non-intact skin or parenteral (i.e., needle-stick injury) contact with blood or other potentially infectious material such as semen, vaginal secretions, cerebrospinal fluid (CSF), synovial fluid, pleural fluid, pericardial fluid, peritoneal fluid, amniotic fluid, or saliva" (CDC, 1998;47). Every exposure incident should be reported immediately to the appropriate employee health or infection control personnel. Immediate local measures include washing with soap and water or, in the case of eye or mouth contact, irrigation with normal saline. The source patient should be tested for HIV antibody, hepatitis B surface and e-antigens (markers of ongoing viral replication), and hepatitis C antibody. The exposed HCW should also have the hepatitis B surface antibody titer checked to confirm protective levels from previous vaccination, or, if unvaccinated, to ascertain baseline status.

Table 52-4 Infection Risk (%) by Exposure[a]

Type of Injury	Virus		
	Hepatitis B	Hepatitis C	HIV
Percutaneous injury	—	0–7	0.25
HBsAg+, HBeAg+	22–40	—	—
HBsAg+, HBeAg−	1–6	—	—
Anti-HBsAb	0	—	—
Hepatitis C RNA+	—	0–7	—
Hepatitis C RNA−	—	~0	—
Mucous membrane	—	0	0.9
Cutaneous	~0	~0	~0

[a]*Ippolito G, Puro V, De Carli G, Italian Study Group on Occupational Risk of HIV Infection. The risk of occupational human immunodeficiency virus in health care workers. Arch Intern Med 1993;153.*

Human Immunodeficiency Virus

The risk of transmission of HIV is the lowest of these three pathogens (**Table 52-4**). In cases of percutaneous exposure to known HIV-positive source blood, the risk of seroconversion is 0.3%. In a CDC case control study, predictors of HIV transmission after a needle-stick injury included sustaining a deep injury, sustaining an injury from a terminal patient, visible blood on the device, and the needle having been in the source patient's blood vessel (CDC, 1998;47). In cases of mucous membrane exposure, the risk drops to 0.09%. When seroconversion occurs, it is usually at a mean of 46 days after the exposure and 95% of exposed HCWs who will seroconvert have done so by 6 months. Delayed seroconversion, as late as 12 months after the exposure, has been reported in cases of simultaneous exposure to HIV and HCV.

Postexposure prophylaxis with antiretroviral medications can be given in cases of high-risk exposures or after exposures to known HIV-positive patients. The risk for transmission of HIV in HCWs exposed to HIV-positive blood who took AZT (zidovudine) postexposure was decreased by 81% (CDC, 1998;47). Postexposure prophylaxis now usually consists of combination therapy with two or three antiretroviral agents selected by an infectious disease or infection control specialist. Medications should be started as soon as possible after the exposure, within minutes to hours. The addition of a third drug should be considered in cases where there is concern for previous exposure to the standard drugs in the source patient. If the source is found to be HIV-negative, the medications can be stopped immediately. If the source is known to be or found to be HIV-positive, prophylaxis is usually continued for 4 weeks. Follow-up testing of the HCW is performed at 6 weeks, 3 months, and 6 months. Occasionally, testing at a year may be indicated (CDC, RR-7, 1998). It should be noted, that the medicines used for prophylaxis often cause side effects making completion of therapy difficult. These include nausea, malaise, fatigue, headache, diarrhea, and other gastrointestinal symptoms are common. The individual should be provided therapy to alleviate these symptoms and to help complete the course of postexposure prophylaxis.

Hepatitis B

Hepatitis B transmission to unvaccinated HCWs occurs at a higher rate than that of HIV. Rates of hepatitis B are higher in HCWs than in the general population, though this difference is decreasing with more widespread use of the vaccine. All HCWs should be vaccinated against hepatitis B. If not previously vaccinated, the worker should be offered vaccination at the time of the exposure. The risk to an unvaccinated HCW of acquiring hepatitis B from a percutaneous exposure to the blood of a patient who has circulating hepatitis B surface antigen is stratified according to the e-antigen

Table 52-5 Postexposure Prophylaxis for Exposure to Hepatitis B Virus[a]

Vaccination and Antibody Response Status of Exposed Individual[e]	Source Patient HBsAg Positive	Source Patient HBsAg Negative	Source Patient Unknown Status
Unvaccinated	HBIG[b] × 1 Initiate HBV vaccine series	Initiate HBV vaccine series	Initiate HBV vaccine series
Previously vaccinated Known responder[c]	No treatment	No treatment	No treatment
Previously vaccinated Known non-responder[d]	HBIG[b] × 1 Initiate revaccination series	No treatment	If risk high, treat as if HBeAg positive
Previously vaccinated Response unknown	Test exposed person for HBsAb —If adequate, no treatment —If inadequate, HBIG[b] × 1 and vaccine booster	No treatment	Test exposed person for HBsAb —If adequate, no treatment —If inadequate, administer vaccine booster and recheck titer in 1–2 months

[a]Taken from CDC guidelines for occupational exposures (CDC, RR-11, 2001).

[b]Hepatitis B immune globulin; dose is 0.06 mL/kg intramuscularly.

[c]A responder is a person with adequate levels of serum antibody to HBsAg (i.e., HBsAb ≥10 mIU/mL).

[d]A nonresponder is a person with inadequate levels of serum antibody to HBsAg (i.e., HBsAb ≤10 mIU/mL).

[e]Persons previously infected with HBV are immune to reinfection and do not require postexposure prophylaxis.

status of the source patient. HBeAg is present in patients who have a high level of viremia and suggests a greater probability of transmission. If the source patient is e-antigen negative, the risk of transmission is 1 to 6%. If the source patient is e-antigen positive, the risk increases to 22 to 40% (see **Table 52-4**).

If the source patient's hepatitis B status is unknown, a hepatitis B surface antigen level should be obtained at the time of the exposure incident. The unvaccinated HCW should be offered vaccination at this time (see **Table 52-5**) (CDC RR-11, 2001). If the source patient's HBsAg is negative, no further action is needed. If positive, then treatment depends on the HCW's vaccination status. If the HCW's antibody titer is not known, it should be checked at this time. If it is adequate, no further intervention is necessary. If the HCW has not been vaccinated against hepatitis B, has not completed the vaccination series, or has an inadequate antibody titer, postexposure prophylaxis can be given with hepatitis B immunoglobulin (HBIg) and a vaccination series initiated. If the HCW has been vaccinated and has had an adequate antibody titer (HBsAb >10 mIU/mL), no further treatment is necessary. Follow-up testing can be performed at 6 months (CDC, Hepatitis B virus, 1991;40).

Hepatitis C

Hepatitis C virus can also be transmitted by exposure to blood. It is probably not well transmitted by other routes because its incidence in HCW is similar to that of the general population (~1–2%). The average incidence of HCV seroconversion after a percutaneous exposure is 1 to 6%, in series prior to the hepatitis C-RNA testing. In cases where the source patient is known to have circulating hepatitis C-RNA, the risk of transmission is estimated to be 10% (see **Table 52-4**). There is no available vaccine or accepted postexposure prophylaxis regimen for hepatitis C. The source patient should be checked for hepatitis C antibody and for viral RNA at the time of the exposure. If the source patient is positive, the HCW should have HCV antibody testing at baseline and in 4 to 6 months. Recent reports of good results with treatment of acute HCV infection have prompted a more aggressive approach in some areas. HCV-RNA testing can be performed between 2 and 6 weeks after the exposure. If the HCW has repeated positive tests for HCV-RNA, early preemptive therapy with interferon may be considered (CDC, RR-19, 1998). These individuals should be referred to an infectious diseases or hepatology specialist for appropriate management.

Further Reading

Beltrami EM, Williams IT, Shapiro CN. Risk and management of blood-borne infections in health care workers. Clin Microbiol Rev 2000;13:385–407

Centers for Disease Control and Prevention (CDC). Guidelines for the prevention of intravascular catheter-related infections. MMWR Morb Mortal Wkly Rep 2002;51(RR10):1–42. http://www.cdc.gov/mmwr/preview/mmwrhtml/rr5110a1.htm

Centers for Disease Control and Prevention (CDC). Hepatitis B virus: appendix a: postexposure prophylaxis for hepatitis B. MMWR Morb Mortal Wkly Rep 1991;40:21–25

Centers for Disease Control and Prevention (CDC). Public Health Service Guidelines for the management of health-care worker exposures to HIV and recommendations for postexposure prohylaxis. MMWR Morb Mortal Wkly Rep 1998;47:1–34

Centers for Disease Control and Prevention (CDC). Recommendations for preventing transmission of human immunodeficiency virus and hepatitis B virus to patients during exposure-prone invasive procedures. MMWR Morb Mortal Wkly Rep 1991;40(RR-8):1–9. http://www.cdc.gov/mmwr/preview/mmwrhtml/00014845.htm

Centers for Disease Control and Prevention (CDC). Recommendations for prevention and control of hepatitis C virus infection and HCV-related chronic disease. MMWR Morb Mortal Wkly Rep 1998;47:1–39

Centers for Disease Control and Prevention (CDC). Transmission of hepatitis B and C viruses in outpatient settings: New York, Oklahoma, and Nebraska, 2000–2002. MMWR Morb Mortal Wkly Rep 2003;52:901–906

Centers for Disease Control and Prevention (CDC). Updated U.S. Public Health Service guidelines for the management of occupational exposures to HBV, HCV, and HIV and recommendations for postexposure prophylaxis. MMWR Morb Mortal Wkly Rep 2001;50:1–42

Collins LA, Samore MH, Roberts MS. Risk factors for invasive fungal infections complicating orthotopic liver transplantation. J Infect Dis 1994;170:644–652

Corona M, Peters SG, Narr BJ, et al. Infections related to central venous catheters. Mayo Clin Proc 1990;65:979–986

Dummer JS, Ho M. Infections in solid organ transplant recipients. In: Mandell GL, Bennett JE, Dolin R, eds. Mandell, Douglas, and Bennett's Principles and Practices of Infectious Diseases. 5th ed. Philadelphia: Churchill Livingstone; 2000:3148–3158

Gadacz T, Way LW, Dunphy JE. Changing clinical spectrum of splenic abscess. Am J Surg 1974;128: 182–187

Henderson DK. Infections due to percutaneous devices. In: Mandell GL, Bennett JE, Dolin R, eds. Mandell, Douglas, and Bennett's Principles and Practices of Infectious Diseases. 5th ed. Philadelphia: Churchill Livingstone; 2000:3005–3015

Ippolito G, Puro V, De Carli G, Italian Study Group on Occupational Risk of HIV Infection. The risk of occupational human immunodeficiency virus in health care workers. Arch Intern Med 1993;153:1451–1458

Kavanagh PV, van Sonnenberg E, Wittich GR, et al. Interventional radiology of the biliary tract. Endoscopy 1997;29:570–576

Kusne S, Dummer JS, Singh N. Infections after liver transplantation: an analysis of 101 consecutive cases. Medicine (Baltimore) 1988;67:132–143

Levison ME, Bush LM. Peritonitis and other intra-abdominal infections. In: Mandell GL, Bennett JE, Dolin R, eds. Mandell, Douglas, and Bennett's Principles and Practices of Infectious Diseases. 5th ed. Philadelphia: Churchill Livingstone; 2000:821–856

Li E, Stanley SL Jr. Protozoa: amebiasis. Gastroenterol Clin North Am 1996;25:471–492

McClean KL, Sheehan GJ, Harding GK. Intraabdominal Infection: a review. Clin Infect Dis 1994;19: 100–116

Mead PB. Infections of the female pelvis. In: Mandell GL, Bennett JE, Dolin R, eds. Mandell, Douglas, and Bennett's Principles and Practices of Infectious Diseases. 5th ed. Philadelphia: Churchill Livingstone; 2000:1240–1241

Mermel LA, Farr BM, Raad II. Guidelines for the management of intravascular catheter-related infections. Infect Control Hosp Epidemiol 2001;22:222–242

Montgomery R, Wilson S. Intra-abdominal abscesses: image-guided diagnosis and therapy. Clin Infect Dis 1996;23:28–36

Murray PR. Pocket Guide to Clinical Microbiology. 2nd ed. Washington, DC: ASM Press; 1998

Ng KK, Lee TY, Wan YL, et al. Splenic abscess: diagnosis and management. Hepatogastroenterology 2002;49:567–571

Oppenheim B. Optimal management of central venous catheter-related infections: what is the evidence? J Infect 2000;40:26–30

Paya CV, Hermans PE, Washington JA, et al. Incidence, distribution, and outcome of episodes of infection in 100 liver transplantations. Mayo Clin Proc 1989;64:555–564

Phillips GS, Radosevich MD, Lipsett PA. Splenic abscess. Arch Surg 1997;132:1331–1336

Reed CR, Sessler CN, Glauser FL, et al. Central venous catheter infections: concepts and controversies. Intensive Care Med 1995;21:177–183

Schwartz S. Principles of Surgery. 7th ed. New York: McGraw-Hill; 1999:1537–1542; 1479–1480; 1399–1401

Sobel JD, Kaye D. Urinary tract infections. In: Mandell GL, Bennett JE, Dolin R, eds. Mandell, Douglas, and Bennett's Principles and Practices of Infectious Diseases. 5th ed. Philadelphia: Churchill Livingstone; 2000:793–794

Solokin JS, Mazuski JE, Baron EJ, et al. Guidelines for the selection of anti-infective agents for complicated intra-abdominal infections. Clin Infect Dis 2003;37:997–1005

Thanos L, Dailiana T, Papaioannou G. Percutaneous CT-guided drainage of splenic abscess. AJR Am J Roentgenol 2002;179:629–632

Wu SM, Marchant LK, Haskal ZJ. Percutaneous interventions in the biliary tree. Semin Roentgenol 1997;32:228–245

CHAPTER 53 Vertebroplasty for Painful Hemangioma

Anne Cotten

Clinical Presentation

A 41-year-old man presented with a 2-year history of lumbar pain. He did not complain of any radiculopathy. Physical examination was remarkable for reproduction of the pain when percussion was performed at L3. Laboratory tests were normal.

Radiological Studies

Radiographs and computed tomography (CT) revealed a well-circumscribed osteolytic lesion involving the left side of the L3 vertebral body and the adjacent pedicle (**Fig. 53-1**). The lesion showed a characteristic coarse trabecular pattern. The CT did not demonstrate any associated degenerative disease of the lumbar spine.

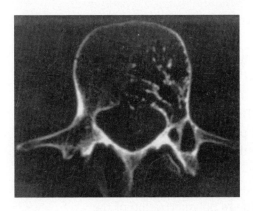

Figure 53-1 Computed tomographic scan through the L 3 vertebra demonstrates the characteristic appearance of a vertebral hemangioma with involvement of the left pedicle.

Diagnosis

Painful vertebral hemangioma

Treatment

Vertebroplasty of L3 was performed under fluoroscopic guidance using a 10 gauge needle. A left transpedicular route was used (**Fig. 53-2**) and 5 mL of methyl methacrylate was injected into the vertebral body hemangioma. Using the same route, an additional injection of 1.5 mL of cement was used to fill the left pedicle (**Fig. 53-3**). A CT scan performed in the hour following the cement injection demonstrated satisfactory filling of the hemangioma (**Fig. 53-4**). No leakage of methyl methacrylate was demonstrated. There was complete relief of pain within 12 hours of the cement injection and the patient remains free of back pain 1 year after vertebroplasty.

Discussion

Vertebral hemangiomas are common benign lesions of the spine that are often asymptomatic and discovered incidentally during radiological evaluation. Rarely, they may be painful. There must be a close correlation between the clinical findings and radiological features to ensure that the patient's

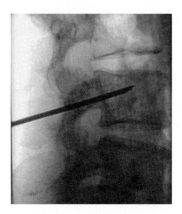

Figure 53-2 Lateral radiograph shows the left transpedicular route of the 10 gauge needle.

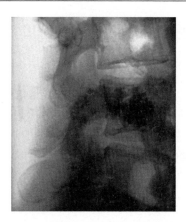

Figure 53-3 Lateral radiograph obtained after the injection of methyl methacrylate cement into the vertebral body and left pedicle.

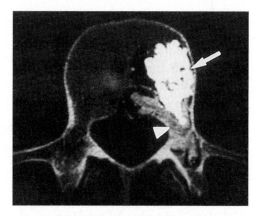

Figure 53-4 Computed tomographic scan performed after vertebroplasty demonstrates satisfactory filling of the hemangioma. The second injection of cement (arrowhead) appears less opaque than the cement injected initially (arrow).

pain is due to the vertebral hemangioma. In exceptionally rare cases, vertebral hemangiomas are aggressive, resulting in spinal cord or nerve root compression.

Vertebroplasty is an effective radiological procedure in which methyl methacrylate cement is percutaneously injected into a vertebral body lesion. This procedure is usually performed under fluoroscopic guidance, although some authors have emphasized the use of CT for needle positioning or assessment of methyl methacrylate injection (Cotten et al, 1998). The choice of needle route depends upon the experience of the radiologist, and a transpedicular or posterolateral route can be used for both the thoracic and the lumbar spine. In the patient described, the transpedicular route was chosen because the lesion also involved the left pedicle.

Once the needle is in the desired location, methyl methacrylate polymer (20 mL powder, 5–7 mL solvent) is mixed. The viscosity of this mixture increases progressively due to polymerization of the methyl methacrylate. When the cement has a consistency of paste, it is injected through the needle into the lesion. The injection is stopped when the cement fills the lesion or if leakage of cement is detected, especially foraminal, epidural, or into the venous system. A CT scan is performed within the hour following cement injection. This allows assessment of vertebral body filling and detection of methyl methacrylate leakage.

Marked or complete pain relief has been demonstrated in more than 90% of patients with vertebral hemangioma treated in this fashion (Deramond et al, 1998). Pain relief occurs within hours or days after the procedure (mean, 24 hours), sometimes after an initial, transient worsening of the pain. Why the injection of methyl methacrylate affords pain relief is not well understood. Destruction of sensitive nerve endings in surrounding tissue probably occurs in response to mechanical, vascular, chemical, and thermal forces, but stabilization of micro fractures and reduction of mechanical forces may also alleviate pain. Methyl methacrylate also allows direct embolization of the hemangiomatous vertebral body.

Vertebroplasty is contraindicated in the presence of coagulation disorders because large-bore needles are used for injection. If emergency decompressive surgery cannot be performed, neither should vertebroplasty be performed because it carries the potential risk of epidural or foraminal leakage of methyl methacrylate.

Indications of vertebroplasty include painful or aggressive hemangioma, osteolytic metastasis, myeloma, and painful osteoporotic vertebral body compression fractures (Cotten et al, 1996; Ide et al, 1996; Weill et al, 1996; Cortet et al, 1999). Whatever the disease, the decision to perform vertebroplasty should be made by a multidisciplinary team because the choice between vertebroplasty, surgery, radiation therapy, medical treatment, or a combination thereof depends upon several factors, which include the level of spinal involvement and the state of general health and life expectancy of the patient.

PEARLS AND PITFALLS

- Rarely, vertebral hemangioma may be painful. Prior to treatment, correlation of the clinical findings and radiological features is essential to ensure that the patient's pain is indeed due to the vertebral lesion.
- In vertebroplasty, methyl methacrylate is percutaneously injected into vertebral body lesions caused by painful or aggressive hemangioma, osteolytic metastasis, myeloma, and painful osteoporotic compression fractures.
- Vertebroplasty is associated with complete or significant pain relief in more than 90% of patients with painful vertebral hemangioma.

Further Reading

Cortet B, Cotten A, Boutry N, et al. Percutaneous vertebroplasty in the treatment of osteoporotic vertebral compression fractures: an open prospective study. J Rheumatol 1999;26:2222–2228

Cotten A, Boutry N, Cortet B, et al. Percutaneous vertebroplasty: state of the art. Radiographics 1998;18:311–320

Cotten A, Deramond H, Cortet B, et al. Preoperative percutaneous injection of methyl methacrylate and N-butyl cyanoacrylate in vertebral hemangiomas. AJNR Am J Neuroradiol 1996;17:137–142

Deramond H, Depriester C, Galibert P, et al. Percutaneous vertebroplasty with polymethylmethacrylate. Radiol Clin North Am 1998;36:533–589

Ide C, Gangi A, Rimmelin A, et al. Vertebral haemangiomas with spinal cord compression: the place of preoperative percutaneous vertebroplasty with methyl methacrylate. Neuroradiology 1996;38:585–589

Weill A, Chiras J, Simon JM, et al. Spinal metastases: indications for and results of percutaneous injection of acrylic surgical cement. Radiology 1996;199:241–247

CHAPTER 54 Treatment of Osteoid Osteoma

Dominik Weishaupt, William B. Morrison, and Mark E. Schweitzer

Clinical Presentation

A 35-year-old man was evaluated for right hip pain of 6 months' duration. The pain had increased in severity during the past weeks, being worse at night, and was relieved by nonsteroidal anti-inflammatory medication. Physical examination was normal.

Radiological Studies

A plain radiograph of the right hip demonstrated a well-demarcated, round, osteosclerotic lesion in the intertrochanteric region of the right femur (**Fig. 54-1**). The hip was otherwise normal. Computed tomography (CT) and magnetic resonance imaging (MRI) were obtained for further characterization of the lesion (**Figs. 54-2** and **54-3**). CT revealed a typical nidus surrounded by a sclerotic rim. The lesion was biopsied percutaneously under CT guidance using a coaxial needle drill biopsy.

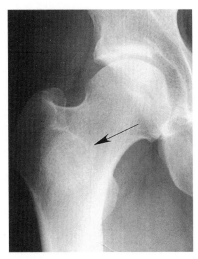

Figure 54-1 Plain radiograph of the right hip demonstrates a round, sclerotic lesion in the intertrochanteric region of the femur (arrow).

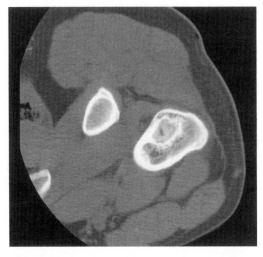

Figure 54-2 Computed tomography with the patient in the prone position demonstrates a typical nidus surrounded by osteosclerosis.

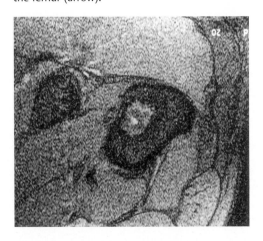

Figure 54-3 Axial gradient-echo magnetic resonance image of the right hip following intravenous contrast administration (with the patient in the prone position) shows an enhancing medullary osteoid osteoma. The nidus demonstrates intense enhancement in the center and less enhancement at the periphery.

322

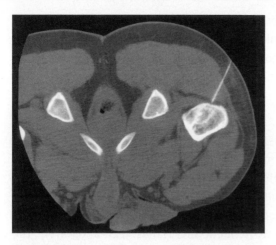

Figure 54-4 Computed tomographic image obtained after placement of a 22 gauge van Sonnenberg needle.

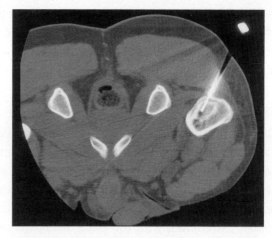

Figure 54-5 Computed tomographic image shows the 12 gauge Ackerman biopsy needle in the center of the nidus.

Diagnosis

Osteoid osteoma of the right femur

Treatment Options

Successful treatment of osteoid osteoma requires complete resection or destruction of the nidus. Several techniques have been reported for percutaneous treatment under CT guidance: a combination of percutaneous coaxial drill biopsy with intralesional ethanol injection; percutaneous total resection of the osteoid osteoma (bone trephination); and lesion destruction with laser interstitial thermal therapy, cryotherapy, or radio-frequeny (RF) ablation.

Treatment

Percutaneous coaxial drill biopsy with intralesional ethanol injection was selected as treatment. The procedure was performed with CT guidance (High Speed, General Electric Medical Systems, Milwaukee, WI) and under general anesthesia. The patient was placed in a prone position and the skin was prepped and sterile draped. Two millimeter thickness sections were obtained at a table feed of 2 mm for localization of the nidus. The needle path was determined by positioning a simple grid (made with injection needles) on the skin. The angle and depth of the trajectory were determined electronically at the console of the scanner on the scan slice passing through the center of the nidus.

The skin, subcutaneous tissues, and periosteum were anesthetized with 1% lidocaine and a small skin incision was made. A 25 cm long, 22 gauge van Sonnenberg needle (Cook, Incorp., Bloomington, IN) was advanced to the periosteal surface overlying the center of the nidus (**Fig. 54-4**). After satisfactory positioning, the inner stylet was removed, and a 15 cm long, 12 gauge hollow Ackerman biopsy needle was coaxially advanced to the bone surface over the outer cannula of the van Sonnenberg needle. After confirmation of satisfactory positioning of the needles by CT, the van Sonnenberg needle was removed, and the intact cortex overlying the nidus was drilled with the standard cutting trocar (**Fig. 54-5**). Once the nidus was reached, the drilling procedure was continued until the cutter had passed the whole nidus. Subsequently, the cutting trocar was removed leaving the Ackerman needle in place. The biopsy core containing the nidus was sent for histological examination. Subsequently, 1 mL of 96% ethanol was injected into the nidus. Because the nidus was large, a second, more proximal (than the first) drilling biopsy was performed followed by another injection of 1 mL of 96% ethanol. After removal of all instruments the skin was closed with sterile tape.

Discussion

Osteoid osteoma is a self-limited benign osteogenic tumor that consists of a well-demarcated osteoblastic vascular mass called a nidus, which is surrounded by a zone of reactive bone sclerosis. Teenagers and young adults are most frequently affected and there is a male predominance. The lesions are most frequently located in the long bones of the lower extremities, with the femoral neck being the single most frequent site. Osteoid osteomas occur less frequently in the long bones of the upper extremities, with the elbow being the most frequent site. Hands, feet, and, rarely, the axial skeleton may also be involved. Flat bones and the craniofacial bones are almost never affected. The clinical symptoms are quite characteristic. Most patients complain of pain of increasing severity that is relieved by aspirin or other nonsteroidal anti-inflammatory agents. The pain is usually worse at night and may be referred to the closest joint. On physical examination, painful swelling of the adjacent tissue may be present, if the tumor is superficially located.

Osteoid osteomas may be located in the cortex, medullary canal, or periosteum. Cortical osteoid osteomas are most frequent. On plain radiographs, most tumors demonstrate a centrally lucent area, called the nidus, located within a fusiform area of sclerotic bone. The nidus may have a variable degree of calcification. Because the plain radiographic findings may be subtle, scintigraphy, CT, and MRI are useful in identifying the nidus and characterizing the lesion. Soft tissue involvement is a rare finding that may be mistaken as being criteria of malignancy.

The classic treatment of osteoid osteoma includes en bloc surgical resection of the lesion. However, the nidus may be difficult to localize during surgery and excision of a significant portion of bone may be necessary to assure complete removal of the lesion. This may result in a prolonged period of inactivity, especially if the lesion is located in a weight-bearing bone. Therefore, the less invasive CT-guided percutaneous techniques provide an alternative method of treatment.

The use of CT in combination with percutaneous techniques allows for precise resection or destruction of the nidus through a small skin incision, without disproportionate resection of bone. Under CT guidance, the entire nidus may be resected using trephine needles. Alternatively, as in the case presented, the lesion may be treated by a combination of coaxial drill biopsy with subsequent ethanol ablation. Percutaneous CT-guided destruction of the nidus by laser interstitial thermal therapy, cryotherapy, or radio-frequeny (RF) ablation are additional therapeutic options. In general, all percutaneous CT-guided techniques for the treatment of osteoid osteomas are considered to be safe, and complications as well as recurrences are rare. However, to date, there is no consensus as to which of the percutaneous techniques is the preferred method for treatment.

PEARLS AND PITFALLS

- Osteoid osteomas are common benign osteogenic tumors occurring in teenagers and young adults. They show a predilection for the shaft of lower-extremity long bones.
- Conventional radiographs and CT establish the diagnosis, which is strongly suggested by the clinical picture.
- Treatments options include surgical excision, CT-guided percutaneous resection, or destruction of the nidus.

Further Reading

Adam G, Neuerburg J, Vorwerk D, et al. Percutaneous treatment of osteoid osteomas: combination of drill biopsy and subsequent ethanol injection. Semin Musculoskelet Radiol 1997;1:281–284

Gangi A, Dietemann JL, Gasser B, et al. Percutaneous laser photocoagulation of osteoid osteomas. Semin Musculoskelet Radiol 1997;1:273–279

Parlier-Cuau C, Champsaur P, Nizard R, et al. Percutaneous removal of osteoid osteoma. Radiol Clin North Am 1998;36:559–566

Rosenthal DI, Hornicek FJ, Torriani M, et al. Osteoid osteoma: percutaneous treatment with radiofrequency energy. Radiology 2003;229:171–175

White LM, Schweitzer ME, Deely DM. Coaxial percutaneous needle biopsy of osteolytic lesions with intact cortical bone. AJR Am J Roentgenol 1996;166:143–144

Woertler K, Vestring T, Boettner F, et al. Osteoid osteoma: CT-guided percutaneous radiofrequency ablation and follow-up in 47 patients. J Vasc Interv Radiol 2001;12:717–722

CHAPTER 55 Postoperative Pelvic Lymphocele

Khaled Toumeh and Corey J. Jost

Clinical Presentation

A 76-year-old diabetic woman was evaluated for intermittent hematuria. A transitional cell carcinoma of the bladder with perivesical tissue invasion was diagnosed (T3N0M0) and she underwent radial cystectomy with ileal conduit, hysterectomy, and pelvic lymphadenectomy. The immediate post-operative course was uncomplicated. One month later, she returned with lower-extremity swelling, shortness of breath, and a moderate probability ventilation perfusion (VQ) lung scan. She was treated for pulmonary embolus with intravenous anticoagulation and was subsequently started on coumadin. Four months after the surgery, she developed intractable lower-extremity edema. She remained afebrile and had not experienced night sweats or malaise. There was no leucocytosis on the complete blood count (CBC).

Radiological Studies

A computed tomographic (CT) scan of the pelvis revealed an 11 × 7 cm, homogeneous, fluid density mass in the left side of the pelvis (**Fig. 55-1**). No solid component or postcontrast enhancement was seen.

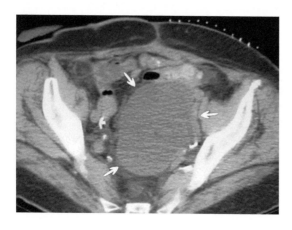

Figure 55-1 Computed tomography of the pelvis shows a large, left-sided fluid collection (arrows).

Differential Diagnosis

This included an abscess, urinoma, seroma, and chronic hematoma. An abscess was unlikely because the patient did not have fever or leucocytosis. A lymphocele was most likely because of the late manifestation.

Diagnosis

Postoperative lymphocele with secondary lower-extremity lymphedema

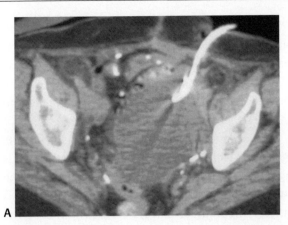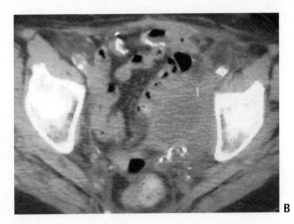

Figure 55-2 (**A**) Computed tomography obtained for evaluation of recurrent symptoms shows reaccumulation of the lymphocele. A drainage catheter has been placed. (**B**) Examination prior to sclerotherapy shows decrease in the size of the lymphocele.

Treatment

CT-guided drainage was performed. A micropuncture set was used to obtain access and a 6F pigtail type drainage catheter was inserted. The aspirated fluid was clear and cytology showed only a few white blood cells. There were no organisms seen on Gram stain. The catheter was left to drainage via gravity. Initially, there was a high-volume output (200 mL/day), which subsequently decreased to 30 mL/day, and the catheter was removed. Three weeks after catheter removal, the patient redeveloped lower-extremity swelling. A repeat CT scan showed a recurrent lymphocele. A drainage catheter was reinserted using CT guidance (**Fig. 55-2**). In addition, the lymphocele was sclerosed with absolute alcohol. On a follow-up evaluation 6 months after treatment, there was mild lower-extremity edema (left > right). A pelvic ultrasound examination (not shown) showed no recurrence of the lymphocele.

Discussion

A lymphocele is an abnormal collection of lymphatic fluid without a true epithelial lining, which typically develops in response to an injury to the lymphatic vessels. Such injury is most commonly iatrogenic but may result from other forms of trauma. A lymphocele may also develop secondary to a tumor. Postoperative lymphoceles are an uncommon complication of renal transplantation, and vascular, retroperitoneal, and pelvic surgery. The incidence is higher after lymphadenectomy and renal transplantation. It is estimated that up to 25% of radical pelvic dissections may be complicated by lymphocele formation.

Most lymphoceles are due to an injury to a larger lymphatic vessel and develop within 3 months of major surgery or trauma. The majority are asymptomatic. Symptoms, when present, are typically due to a mass effect and include pain, venous obstruction, deep venous thrombosis, lymphedema, and hydronephrosis. Secondary infection can also occur.

In the past, lymphoceles were treated by surgical marsupialization using open or laparoscopic techniques. Surgical treatment is effective in over 90% of cases. Over the last 2 decades, there has been an increasing interest in less invasive options and percutaneous treatment. Several techniques have been advocated for the percutaneous treatment and include image-guided simple aspiration, aspiration and catheter drainage, drainage, and sclerotherapy. Among these, sclerotherapy has been the most effective.

Contraindications to sclerotherapy include active infection, cancer, and possible exposure of the sclerosing agent to a vascular graft in the proximity of the lesion being treated.

Technique and Outcome

The most commonly used sclerosing agents are absolute alcohol, 10% povidone iodine, doxycycline, and bleomycin. These agents induce an inflammatory reaction in the cavity wall that leads to its collapse and obliteration. Cost and operator preference are the major factors in the selection of the sclerosing agent. Povidone iodine and absolute alcohol are inexpensive and widely available. Doxycycline and bleomycin are expensive but may have to be used in cases that are resistant to the former.

In preparation for the procedure, the patient is given a single dose of intravenous cefazolin. Image-guided catheter insertion is performed using a strict sterile technique, and the lymphocele is drained. The fluid is evaluated to confirm the diagnosis by laboratory studies and to exclude the presence of an infection or malignancy by Gram stain and cytology, respectively. Following this, a cystogram is performed using 60% iodinated contrast medium to calculate the volume of the lymphocele and to exclude contrast leak. Subsequently, the cavity is evacuated completely and absolute alcohol is instilled. The volume of alcohol instilled should equal ~30 to 50% of the original volume. After instilling the alcohol, the catheter is clamped for 10 to 15 minutes and the patient is asked to rotate into left and right lateral decubitus positions to expose the entire cavity to the sclerosing agent. After aspiration of the alcohol, the catheter is placed to gravity drainage. The daily output is charted and the catheter is removed when the daily output decreases to <10 mL.

Two injections per treatment session have been advocated and the repetition of treatment on a weekly basis, if needed. For sclerotherapy with povidone iodine, the same technique is used. However, with bleomycin, the dose is limited to 20 units per session. If the cyst is very large, an initial attempt at drainage may reduce the size of the cavity and thus decrease the required volume of the sclerosing agent.

Complications of the procedure are uncommon. Zuckerman et al (1997) reported 9% infection rate without antibiotic prophylaxis; however, these cases responded to antibiotic treatment. Other complications include catheter dislodgment.

The reported success rate is between 80 and 94% and the average catheter dwell time is 1 to 3 weeks. Most patients can be treated on an outpatient basis.

PEARLS AND PITFALLS_____

- Percutaneous sclerotherapy is a relatively safe and effective form of treatment for postoperative lymphoceles.
- Absolute alcohol and povidone iodine are the most commonly used agents.
- Thirty to 50% of the aspirated volume is instilled and left in place for 10 to 15 minutes.
- The catheter is removed after fluid output decreases to below 10 mL/day.

Further Reading

Akhan O, Cehirge S, Ozman M, et al. Percutaneous transcatheter sclerotherapy of post operative lymphoceles. Cardiovasc Intervent Radiol 1992;15:224–227

Caliendo MV, Lee DE, Queiroz DL. Sclerotherapy with use of doxycycline after percutaneous drainage of post operative lymphoceles. J Vasc Interv Radiol 2001;12:73–77

Doehn C, Fornara P, Fricke L, et al. Laparoscopic fenestration of post transplant lymphoceles. Surg Endosc 2002;16:690–695

Kerlan RK, LaBerge JM, Gordon RL, et al. Bleomycin sclerosis of pelvic lymphoceles. J Vasc Interv Radiol 1997;8:885–887

Khorram O, Stern JL. Bleomycin sclerotherapy of an intractable inguinal lymphocyst. Gynecol Oncol 1993;50:244–246

Kim JK, Jeong YY, Kim YY, et al. Post operative pelvic lymphocele: treatment with simple percutaneous catheter drainage. Radiology 1999;212:390–394

McDowell GC II, Babaian RJ, Johnson DE. Management of symptomatic lymphocele via percutaneous drainage and sclerotherapy with tetracycline. Urology 1991;37:237–239

Montalvo BM, Yrizarry JM, Casillas VJ, et al. Percutaneous sclerotherapy of lymphoceles related to renal transplantation. J Vasc Interv Radiol 1996;7:117–123

Sawhney R, D'Agostino HB, Zink S, et al. Treatment of post operative lymphoceles with percutaneous drainage and alcohol sclerotherapy. J Vasc Interv Radiol 1996;7:241–245

Seelig MH, Klinger PJ, Oldenburg WA. Treatment of post operative cervical chylous lymphocele by percutaneous sclerosing with povidone-iodine. J Vasc Surg 1998;27:1148–1151

Teiche PE, Pauer W, Schmid N. Use of talcum in sclerotherapy of pelvic lymphoceles. Tech Urol 1999;5:52–53

Zuckerman DA, Yeager TD. Percutaneous ethanol sclerotherapy of post operative lymphoceles. AJR Am J Roentgenol 1997;169:433–437

INDEX

Page numbers followed by f or t indicate figures and tables, respectively.